European Observatory on Health Systems and Policies Series

The European Observatory on Health Systems and Policies is a unique project that builds on the commitment of all its partners to improving health systems:

- World Health Organization Regional Office for Europe
- Government of Belgium
- Government of Finland
- Government of Ireland
- Government of the Netherlands
- Government of Norway
- Government of Slovenia
- Government of Spain
- Government of Sweden
- Veneto Region of Italy
- European Commission
- European Investment Bank
- World Bank
- UNCAM
- London School of Economics and Political Science
- London School of Hygiene & Tropical Medicine

The series

The volumes in this series focus on key issues for health policy-making in Europe. Each study explores the conceptual background, outcomes and lessons learned about the development of more equitable, more efficient and more effective health systems in Europe. With this focus, the series seeks to contribute to the evolution of a more evidence-based approach to policy formulation in the health sector.

These studies will be important to all those involved in formulating or evaluating national health policies and, in particular, will be of use to health policy-makers and advisers, who are under increasing pressure to rationalize the structure and funding of their health system. Academics and students in the field of health policy will also find this series valuable in seeking to understand better the complex choices that confront the health systems of Europe.

The Observatory supports and promotes evidence-based health policy-making through comprehensive and rigorous analysis of the dynamics of health care systems in Europe.

Series Editors

Josep Figueras is the Director of the European Observatory on Health Systems and Policies, and Head of the European Centre for Health Policy, World Health Organization Regional Office for Europe.

Martin McKee is Head of Research Policy and Head of the London Hub of the European Observatory on Health Systems and Policies. He is Professor of European Public Health at the London School of Hygiene & Tropical Medicine as well as a co-director of the School's European Centre on Health of Societies in Transition.

Elias Mossialos is the Co-director of the European Observatory on Health Systems and Policies. He is Brian Abel-Smith Professor in Health Policy, Department of Social Policy, London School of Economics and Political Science and Director of LSE Health.

Richard B. Saltman is Associate Head of Research Policy and Head of the Atlanta Hub of the European Observatory on Health Systems and Policies. He is Professor of Health Policy and Management at the Rollins School of Public Health, Emory University in Atlanta, Georgia.

Reinhard Busse is Associate Head of Research Policy and Head of the Berlin Hub of the European Observatory on Health Systems and Policies. He is Professor of Health Care Management at the Berlin University of Technology.

European Observatory on Health Systems and Policies Series

Series Editors: Josep Figueras, Martin McKee, Elias Mossialos, Richard B. Saltman and Reinhard Busse

Published titles

Regulating entrepreneurial behaviour in European health care systems
Richard B. Saltman, Reinhard Busse and Elias Mossialos (eds)

Hospitals in a changing Europe
Martin McKee and Judith Healy (eds)

Health care in central Asia
Martin McKee, Judith Healy and Jane Falkingham (eds)

Funding health care: options for Europe
Elias Mossialos, Anna Dixon, Josep Figueras and Joe Kutzin (eds)

Health policy and European Union enlargement
Martin McKee, Laura MacLehose and Ellen Nolte (eds)

Regulating pharmaceuticals in Europe: striving for efficiency, equity and quality
Elias Mossialos, Monique Mrazek and Tom Walley (eds)

Social health insurance systems in western Europe
Richard B. Saltman, Reinhard Busse and Josep Figueras (eds)

Purchasing to improve health systems performance
Joseph Figueras, Ray Robinson and Elke Jakubowski (eds)

Human resources for health in Europe
Carl-Ardy Dubois, Martin McKee and Ellen Nolte (eds)

Primary care in the driver's seat
Richard B. Saltman, Ana Rico and Wienke Boerma (eds)

Mental health policy and practice across Europe: the future direction of mental health care
Martin Knapp, David McDaid, Elias Mossialos and Graham Thornicroft (eds)

Decentralization in health care
Richard B. Saltman, Vaida Bankauskaite and Karsten Vrangbæk (eds)

Health systems and the challenge of communicable diseases: experiences from Europe and Latin America
Richard Coker, Rifat Atun and Martin McKee (eds)

Caring for people with chronic conditions: a health system perspective
Ellen Nolte and Martin McKee (eds)

Nordic health care systems: recent reforms and current policy challenges
Jon Magnussen, Karsten Vrangbæk and Richard B. Saltman (eds)

Diagnosis-related groups in Europe: moving towards transparency, efficiency and quality in hospitals
Reinhard Busse, Alexander Geissler, Wilm Quentin and Miriam Wiley (eds)

Migration and health in the European Union

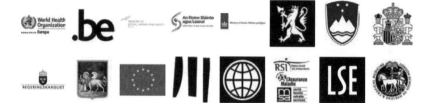

The European Observatory on Health Systems and Policies is a partnership between the World Health Organization Regional Office for Europe, the Governments of Belgium, Finland, Ireland, the Netherlands, Norway, Slovenia, Spain, Sweden and the Veneto Region of Italy, the European Commission, the European Investment Bank, the World Bank, UNCAM (French National Union of Health Insurance Funds), the London School of Economics and Political Science and the London School of Hygiene & Tropical Medicine.

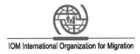 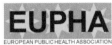 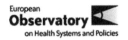

Migration and health in the European Union

Editors

Bernd Rechel, Philipa Mladovsky, Walter Devillé, Barbara Rijks, Roumyana Petrova-Benedict, Martin McKee

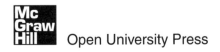 Open University Press

Open University Press
McGraw-Hill Education
McGraw-Hill House
Shoppenhangers Road
Maidenhead
Berkshire
England
SL6 2QL

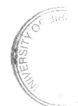

email: enquiries@openup.co.uk
world wide web: www.openup.co.uk

and Two Penn Plaza, New York, NY 10121-2289, USA

First published 2011

A catalogue record of this book is available from the British Library

ISBN-13: 978-0-33-524567-3 (pb)
eISBN: 978-0-33-524568-0

Library of Congress Cataloging-in-Publication Data
CIP data applied for

Typeset by RefineCatch Limited, Bungay, Suffolk
Printed in Great Britain by Ball and Bain Ltd, Glasgow

Fictitious names of companies, products, people, characters and/or data that may be used herein (in case studies or in examples) are not intended to represent any real individual, company, product or event.

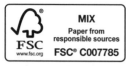

The McGraw-Hill Companies

26372509

Contents

List of tables and figures   xi
About the authors   xiii
Acknowledgements   xvii
Abbreviations   xix

Section I   **Introduction**

one   **Migration and health in the European Union:**
                  an introduction   3
                  Bernd Rechel, Philipa Mladovsky, Walter Devillé, Barbara Rijks,
                  Roumyana Petrova-Benedict and Martin McKee

Section II   **Context**

two   **Trends in Europe's international migration**   17
                  John Salt

three   **Asylum, residency and citizenship policies**
                  and models of migrant incorporation   37
                  Anthony M. Messina

Section III   **Access to health services**

four   **The right to health of migrants in Europe**   55
                  Paola Pace

five   **Migrants' access to health services**   67
               Marie Nørredam and Allan Krasnik

Section IV   Monitoring migrant health

six   **Monitoring the health of migrants**   81
               Bernd Rechel, Philipa Mladovsky and Walter Devillé

Section V   Selected areas of migrant health

seven   **Non-communicable diseases**   101
               Anton Kunst, Karien Stronks and Charles Agyemang

eight   **Communicable diseases**   121
               Tanja Wörmann and Alexander Krämer

nine   **Maternal and child health – from conception
               to first birthday**   139
               Anna Reeske and Oliver Razum

ten   **Occupational health**   155
               *Andrés A. Agudelo-Suárez, Elena Ronda-Pérez and
               Fernando G. Benavides*

eleven   **Mental health of refugees and asylum-seekers**   169
               Jutta Lindert and Guglielmo Schinina

Section VI   Policy response

twelve   **Migrant health policies in Europe**   185
               Philipa Mladovsky

thirteen   **Differences in language, religious beliefs and
               culture: the need for culturally responsive
               health services**   203
               Sophie Durieux-Paillard

fourteen   **Good practice in emergency care: views
               from practitioners**   213
               *Stefan Priebe, Marija Bogic, Róza Ádány, Neele V. Bjerre,
               Marie Dauvrin, Walter Devillé, Sónia Dias, Andrea
               Gaddini, Tim Greacen, Ulrike Kluge, Elisabeth Ioannidis,
               Natasja K. Jensen, Rosa Puigpinós i Riera, Joaquim
               J.F. Soares, Mindaugas Stankunas, Christa Straßmayr,
               Kristian Wahlbeck, Marta Welbel and Rosemarie McCabe*

fifteen   **Good practice in health service provision
               for migrants**   227
               David Ingleby

Section VII   **Conclusions**

sixteen   **The future of migrant health in Europe**   **245**
                    Bernd Rechel, Philipa Mladovsky, Walter Devillé,
                    Barbara Rijks, Roumyana Petrova-Benedict and
                    Martin McKee

                    Index   251

List of tables and figures

Tables

2.1 Three largest groups of foreign citizens residing in
selected European countries by citizenship and as a percentage
of all non-nationals, 2008   23
2.2 Inflows of foreign labour into selected European
countries, 1995–2008 (thousands)   26
2.3 Asylum applications in selected European countries,
1995–2008 (thousands)   29
3.1 EU member state decisions on asylum applications (2009)   40
3.2 Quality of migrant access to long-term residence
across the EU (2007)   42
3.3 Components of citizenship policies across the EU (2008)   44
3.4 Acquisition of citizenship across the EU (2007–08)   45
6.1 Information on national or ethnic origin, religion
and language and their equivalents collected in
official statistics in Council of Europe countries   82
6.2 Examples of health and migration indicators
collected through surveys in selected European countries   89
6.3 Selected European surveys collecting information on
health and migration   93
7.1 Available information on NCDs (other than cancer,
heart disease and DM) among migrants, and estimated
differences with locally born residents in the Netherlands   109

7.2 Rank order of conditions posing the greatest burden of
disease among non-western migrants in the Netherlands, 2005,
compared to the rank order for the locally born population 114
8.1 Target groups of TB screening in selected European countries 130
8.2 Type of TB screening methods targeting migrants in
selected European countries 132
10.1 Distribution of the Spanish and foreign working population
by occupation and sex (as %) 158
10.2 List of studies on occupational injuries among migrants
in the European Union 160
11.1 Selected pre-migration, migration and post-migration
factors potentially associated with psychopathology 174
12.1 Coverage regulations for asylum-seekers, selected EU countries 190
14.1 Selected A&E departments in each country 215
14.2 Questions and case vignettes used in the interviews 217

Figures

1.1 Policy measures tackling the determinants of health for migrants 8
2.1 Foreign citizens as a percentage of the total population in EU
member states, Norway and Switzerland 2008 21
2.2 Net migration (per thousand) in Europe, EU, Russian Federation
and in other regions of Europe, 1985–2009 24
2.3 Natural increase, net migration and total population increase
(per thousand) in the "new" and "old" EU member states,
1985–2009 25
2.4 Total number of apprehended aliens for selected European
countries, 2000 and 2007 32
2.5 Total number of apprehended aliens for selected European
countries, 2006–2007 33
7.1 Self-reported NCD prevalence in Amsterdam in populations born
in the Netherlands, Morocco and Turkey, 1999–2000, men
and women combined 107
7.2 Cancer incidence in migrant groups and the respective countries
of origin compared to the locally born Dutch population
(set at 100), 1996–2002, men and women combined 112
8.1 Map of global prevalence of chronic HBV infections, 2006 124
9.1 Factors influencing perinatal outcomes among migrants 140
10.1 Foreign labour force stocks in Europe (% of total labour force),
1998–2007 156

About the authors

Róza Ádány is Medical Specialist in Preventative Medicine and Public Health at the Faculty of Public Health, Medical and Health Science Centre, University of Debrecen, Hungary.

Andrés A. Agudelo-Suárez is Lecturer at the Faculty of Dentistry at the University of Antioquia, Medellín, Colombia, and Researcher at the Centre for Research in Occupational Health (CISAL) in Barcelona and at the Public Health Department of the University of Alicante, Spain.

Charles Agyemang is Assistant Professor at the Department of Public Health, Academic Medical Centre, University of Amsterdam, the Netherlands.

Fernando G. Benavides is Professor at the Pompeu Fabra University and Director of the Centre for Research in Occupational Health (CISAL) in Barcelona, Spain.

Neele Bjerre is Research Assistant at the Unit for Social and Community Psychiatry, Barts and the London School of Medicine and Dentistry, Queen Mary, University of London, United Kingdom.

Marija Bogic is Researcher at the Unit for Social and Community Psychiatry, Barts and the London School of Medicine and Dentistry, Queen Mary, University of London, United Kingdom.

Marie Dauvrin is Research Fellow of the Institute of Health and Society, Catholic University of Louvain, Belgium.

Walter Devillé is Senior Researcher at NIVEL (Netherlands Institute for Health Services Research) and Endowed Professor for Pharos at the University of Amsterdam, Amsterdam Institute of Social Sciences Research, the Netherlands.

Sónia Dias is Assistant Professor in Public Health at the Institute of Hygiene and Tropical Medicine, Universidade Nova de Lisboa, Portugal.

Sophie Durieux-Paillard is in charge of the migrants health programme of university hospitals in Geneva, Switzerland.

Andrea Gaddini is psychiatrist at the Public Health Agency for the Lazio Region, Italy.

Tim Greacen is Director of the Maison Blanche Research Laboratory at the Etablissement public de santé Maison Blanche, France.

David Ingleby is Professor of Intercultural Psychology at Utrecht University, the Netherlands, and a member of the European Research Centre on Migration and Ethnic Relations (ERCOMER).

Elisabeth Ioannidis is Senior Researcher in the Department of Sociology, National School of Public Health, Athens, Greece.

Natasja K. Jensen is Researcher at the Danish Research Centre for Migration, Ethnicity and Health (MESU), Unit of Health Services Research, Department of Public Health, University of Copenhagen, Denmark.

Ulrike Kluge is Research Fellow at the Department for Psychiatry and Psychotherapy, Charité - University Medicine Berlin, Germany.

Alexander Krämer is Head of the Department of Public Health Medicine in the School of Public Health at the University of Bielefeld, Germany.

Allan Krasnik is Professor at the Unit of Health Services Research, Department of Public Health, University of Copenhagen and Director of the Danish Research Centre for Migration, Ethnicity and Health, Denmark.

Anton E Kunst is Associate Professor at the Department of Public Health, Academic Medical Centre, University of Amsterdam, the Netherlands.

Jutta Lindert is Professor of Public Health at the Protestant University of Applied Sciences Ludwigsburg, Germany.

Rosemarie McCabe is Senior Lecturer at Barts and the London School of Medicine and Dentistry, Queen Mary, University of London, United Kingdom.

Martin McKee is Professor of European Public Health at the London School of Hygiene & Tropical Medicine and Director of Research Policy at the European Observatory on Health Systems and Policies.

Anthony M. Messina is the John R. Reitemeyer Professor in the Department of Political Science at Trinity College, United States.

Philipa Mladovsky is Research Fellow at the European Observatory on Health Systems and Policies and at LSE Health, United Kingdom.

Marie Nørredam is Associate Professor at the Unit of Health Services Research, Department of Public Health, University of Copenhagen and Research Director of the Danish Research Centre for Migration, Ethnicity and Health, Denmark.

Paola Pace is Migration Law Specialist at the International Organization for Migration.

Roumyana Petrova-Benedict is Senior Regional Migration Health Manager for Europe and Central Asia at the International Organization for Migration.

Rosa Puigpinós i Riera is Medical Researcher at the Agency of Public Health of Barcelona, Spain.

Stefan Priebe is Professor of Social and Community Psychiatry, Barts and the London School of Medicine and Dentistry, Queen Mary, University of London, United Kingdom.

Oliver Razum is Head of the Department of Epidemiology & International Public Health at Bielefeld University, Germany.

Bernd Rechel is Researcher at the European Observatory on Health Systems and Policies and Honorary Senior Lecturer at the London School of Hygiene & Tropical Medicine, United Kingdom.

Anna Reeske is Researcher at the Institute for Prevention Research and Social Medicine at the University of Bremen. Until 2009 she was Researcher at the Department of Epidemiology & International Public Health at the University of Bielefeld, Germany.

Barbara Rijks is Migration Health Programme Coordinator at the Migration Health Division of the International Organization for Migration.

Elena Ronda-Pérez is Senior Lecturer at the Public Health Department of the University of Alicante and Researcher at the Centre for Research in Occupational Health (CISAL) in Barcelona, Spain.

John Salt is Emeritus Professor of Geography at University College London, United Kingdom.

Guglielmo Schinina is Coordinator for Mental Health, Psychosocial and Cultural Medical Integration at the International Organization for Migration.

Joaquim J.F. Soares is Associated Professor of Psychology at the Department of Public Health Sciences, Section of Social Medicine, Karolinska Institutet, Stockholm, Sweden.

Mindaugas Stankunas is Lecturer in the Department of Health Management, Lithuanian University of Health Sciences, Kaunas, Lithuania.

Christa Straßmayr is Research Sociologist at the Ludwig Boltzmann Institute for Social Psychiatry, Vienna, Austria.

Karien Stronks is Professor at the Department of Public Health, Academic Medical Centre, University of Amsterdam, the Netherlands.

Kristian Wahlbeck is Researcher at the National Institute for Health and Welfare (THL), Department for Mental Health and Substance Abuse Services, Helsinki, Finland.

Marta Welbel is Research Sociologist at the Institute of Psychiatry and Neurology, Warsaw, Poland.

Tanja Wörmann is Research Associate and Lecturer at the Department of Public Health Medicine in the School of Public Health at the University of Bielefeld, Germany.

Acknowledgements

This book is the result of a collaboration between the European Observatory on Health Systems and Policies, the EUPHA Section on Migrant and Ethnic Minority Health, and the International Organization for Migration. We are especially grateful to all the authors for their valuable contributions.

We are also very grateful to the reviewers of this volume, Carin Björngren-Cuadra, Sandro Cattacin, Mark Johnson, Ursula Karl-Trummer, Sijmen A. Reijneveld, Harald Siem and María Luisa Vázquez, for their very helpful comments and suggestions on the whole manuscript, and to David Ingleby, Elena Ronda Pérez, Oliver Razum and Tanja Wörmann for their comments on individual chapters.

Finally, this book would not have appeared without the hard work of the production team led by Jonathan North, with the able assistance of Alison Chapman, Aki Hedigan and Caroline White.

Bernd Rechel
Philipa Mladovsky
Walter Devillé
Barbara Rijks
Roumyana Petrova-Benedict
Martin Mckee

Abbreviations

A&E	accident and emergency
AIDS	acquired immune-deficiency syndrome
AMAC	Assisting Migrants and Communities
BCG	Bacillus Calmette-Guérin immunization
BME	black and minority ethnic
CALD	culturally and linguistically diverse
CEAS	Common European Asylum System
CHD	coronary heart disease
CI	confidence interval
CLAS	culturally and linguistically appropriate services
COPD	chronic obstructive pulmonary disease
CXR	chest X-ray
DALY	disability-adjusted life year
d.f.	degrees of freedom
DM	diabetes mellitus
DSM	Diagnostic and Statistical Manual
ECHI	European Health Interview Survey
ECHP	European Community Household Panel
ECRI	European Commission against Racism and Intolerance
EEA	European Economic Area
EMN	European Migration Network
EPSCO	Employment, Social Policy, Health and Consumer Affairs Council
EU	European Union
EU8	the eight central and eastern European countries that joined the EU in 2004

EU10	the 10 countries that joined the EU in 2004
EU12	the 12 countries that joined the EU in 2004 and 2007
EU15	the 15 countries that were members of the EU before 2004
EU-SILC	European Union Statistics on Income and Living Conditions
FGM	female genital mutilation
GDP	gross domestic product
GP	general practitioner
HAV	hepatitis A virus
HBsAg	hepatitis B surface antigen
HBV	hepatitis B virus
HCV	hepatitis C virus
HDI	Human Development Index
HDV	hepatitis delta virus
HELIUS	Healthy Life in an Urban Setting
HEV	hepatitis E virus
HIV	human immunodeficiency virus
HPV	human papilloma virus
HUMA	Health for Undocumented Migrants and Asylum seekers
ICMPD	International Centre for Migration Policy Development
ILO	International Labour Organization
IOM	International Organization for Migration
MEHO	Migration and Ethnic Health Observatory
MMR	measles, mumps and rubella
MONICA	MONItoring of trends and determinants in CArdiovascular disease
NCD	non-communicable disease
NGO	non-governmental organization
NHS	National Health Service
NIVEL	Netherlands Institute for Health Services Research
OR	odds ratio
OECD	Organisation for Economic Co-operation and Development
POLS	Permanent Research Life Situation
PTSD	post-traumatic stress disorder
RR	risk ratio
SHARE	Survey of Health, Ageing and Retirement in Europe
SLAN	Survey of Lifestyles, Attitudes, and Nutrition
STI	sexually transmitted infection
TB	tuberculosis
TCN	third-country national
TST	tuberculin skin test
UN	United Nations
UNHCR	United Nations High Commissioner for Refugees
WHO	World Health Organization

Section I

Introduction

chapter **one**

Migration and health in the European Union: an introduction

Bernd Rechel, Philipa Mladovsky,
Walter Devillé, Barbara Rijks,
Roumyana Petrova-Benedict and
Martin McKee

Introduction

This book explores key features of health and migration in the European Union (EU). The increasing diversity of populations in Europe creates new challenges for health systems, which have to adapt in order to remain responsive. These challenges are increasingly recognized with regard to migrants, who comprise a growing share of European populations. Eurostat data on the size of the population in the EU without EU citizenship provide indications of the scale of migration to Europe: in 2009, 4.0% of the EU's total population were citizens of countries outside the EU (Vasileva 2010). However, citizenship is an imprecise measure of migrant status, since it does not include naturalized migrants who have assumed the citizenship of their host country (Castles and Davidson 2000; Nielsen et al. 2009). In addition, there is an unknown number of irregular or undocumented migrants, believed to account for 0.39–0.77% of the population in the 27 EU member states in 2008 (Vogel 2009), although other estimates suggest that this proportion could be as high as 4% (Karl-Trummer et al. 2009). Taken together, this means that the size of the migrant population in the EU is considerably higher than the Eurostat data indicate.

Another complicating factor is that the very definition of migrants differs from country to country (IOM 2010). While the UN Recommendations on Statistics of International Migration define a long-term migrant as a "person who moves to a country other than that of his or her usual residence for a period of at least a year" (United Nations Department of Economic and Social

Affairs 1998: 18), not all countries follow this definition. This makes it difficult to compare data from different countries. It should also be noted that there is a need to look beyond the generation that has moved from one country to another. Although the term "second-generation migrant" is a contradiction in terms (Kobayashi 2008), the challenges for the health of the descendants of migrants are sometimes greater than for those who migrated (Ingleby 2009; Gushulak 2010; WHO Regional Office for Europe 2010).

While a number of publications on migrant health in Europe have appeared in recent years (Fernandes and Miguel 2009; Peiro and Benedict 2009; Björngren-Cuadra and Cattacin 2010), comprehensive information on different aspects of health and migration, and how these can best be addressed by health systems, is still not easy to find. This volume attempts to fill this gap in the literature. We hope that the book will be of value to researchers, policy-makers and practitioners.

Information on migration and health

While migrants are often comparatively healthy, a phenomenon known as the "healthy migrant effect", they often face particular health challenges and are vulnerable to a number of threats to their physical and mental health. However, all too often, the specific health needs of migrants are poorly understood, communication between health care providers and migrant clients remains poor, and health systems are not prepared to respond adequately. The situation is compounded by the problems migrants face in realizing their human rights; accessing health and other basic services; and being relegated to low paid and often dangerous jobs, with the most acute challenges being faced by undocumented migrants, trafficked persons and asylum-seekers.

One major reason for this lack of understanding is the scarcity of data. Apart from the above-mentioned lack of clarity about who constitutes a migrant – and how many migrants there are in any given country (Aung et al. 2010) – high-quality data on health determinants, health status and health service utilization by migrants are not available in most EU countries (Rafnsson and Bhopal 2008; Ingleby 2009; Padilla and Miguel 2009). For example, registry data on health care utilization that allow for identification of migrants at a national or sub-national level are only available in 11 of the 27 EU member states (Nielsen et al. 2009).

Where data on migrant health are available, they often point in contradictory directions, due to the diversity of migrants in terms of age, gender, country of origin and destination, socioeconomic status and type of migration. In general, many health discrepancies disappear after controlling for socioeconomic status (WHO Regional Office for Europe 2010), though poor socioeconomic status may itself be a result of migrant status and ethnicity. This is related to processes of social exclusion and illustrates that migration is an important social determinant of health (Davies et al. 2009; Ingleby 2009; Davies et al. 2010). Research into migration and health is further complicated by the complexity of the relationship between migration and health; the health of migrants is shaped by many factors throughout the migration process, including ethnic identity and genetic characteristics (Ingleby et al. 2005), and health needs change with time of residence in the host country. It has therefore been described as "foolish to attempt any generalisations about the general level of health of all migrants" (Ingleby 2009: 11).

To the limited extent that generalizations are possible and information is available across countries and migrant groups, migrants seem to be more vulnerable to communicable diseases, as well as to occupational diseases and poor mental health, which is in part due to patterns of disease in their countries of origin, poor living conditions, precarious employment and the trauma that can be associated with various causes of migration (Gushulak et al. 2010). In terms of non-communicable disease, migrants to Europe seem initially to have a lower risk of cancer but higher risk of diabetes and some other diseases, while the risk of cardiovascular disease varies among different groups (see Chapter 7 on "Non-communicable disease"). Migrants are also at higher risk of maternal and child health problems, with differences in perinatal outcomes persisting between migrants and non-migrants, and evidence that both the utilization and quality of antenatal care is lower among migrant women (see Chapter 9 on "Maternal and child health").

Where available, utilization rates provide information on how migrants access services. A systematic review of migrants' utilization of somatic health services in Europe found that they tend to make less use of mammography and cervical cancer screening, have more contacts with general practitioners, the same or higher utilization of specialist care, and higher, equal or lower levels of utilization of emergency care (Uiters et al. 2009; Nørredam et al. 2010), although without detailed information on health needs, these findings are difficult to interpret. In general, rather than suffering from exotic diseases, most migrants seek help for "common-or-garden" (Ingleby 2009) complaints that are also common among the non-migrant population.

A much clearer picture emerges with regard to either asylum-seekers (Watson 2009) or undocumented migrants (Karl-Trummer, Novak-Zezula et al. 2010). In 2003, the Council of the European Union outlined minimum standards for the reception of asylum-seekers which include emergency care, essential treatment of illness, and necessary medical or other assistance for applicants with special needs (Council of the EU 2003). However, in 2004, ten of 25 EU countries provided only emergency care to asylum-seekers (Nørredam et al. 2006).

With regard to undocumented migrants, there is a tendency in many EU member states to restrict entitlements to health services "to discourage the entry of new migrants" (Björngren-Cuadra and Cattacin 2010). In 2010, nine of 27 EU countries restricted access to health services in such a way to make emergency care inaccessible to undocumented migrants and only five countries (Netherlands, France, Italy, Portugal and Spain) offered undocumented migrants access to health services beyond emergency care, such as including primary care. In only four EU member states (Netherlands, France, Portugal and Spain) were undocumented migrants entitled to access the same range of services as nationals of that country as long as they met certain pre-conditions, such as proof of identity or residence (Björngren-Cuadra and Cattacin 2010; Karl-Trummer, Björngren-Cuadra et al. 2010).

Apart from legal restrictions on entitlements to health care, which are most pronounced for undocumented migrants and asylum-seekers, migrants may be particularly affected by user fees (Nielsen et al. 2009), as well as by impeded access to health insurance. Other barriers include language, unfamiliarity with rights, entitlements and the overall health system, underdeveloped health literacy, administrative obstacles, social exclusion, and direct and indirect discrimination.

The political response so far

There is a growing body of knowledge on ways in which to foster health systems' responsiveness to the needs of migrants, including many examples of good practices (Fernandes and Miguel 2009; MIGHEALTHNET 2010). Ideally, the needs of migrants should be incorporated into all elements of health systems, including regulation, organization, financing and planning, to ensure non-discrimination and equal entitlement to health services. Specific steps that can help health systems to meet the needs of migrants typically involve measures to overcome linguistic, cultural and administrative barriers, such as interpretation and translation services; culturally informed models of care; culturally tailored public health programmes; the use of cultural support staff (such as health mediators); training of staff in diversity; diversification of the workforce; and the involvement of migrants in all aspects of health care delivery (Fernandes and Miguel 2009; WHO 2010). However, more needs to be done to evaluate the effectiveness of "best practices" that are rarely, if ever, subject to rigorous assessment (Ingleby 2009). Furthermore, good practices "do not fix the system" and, for long-term sustainability, structural changes are required that embed good practices in health policy and practice (Fernandes and Miguel 2009; Ingleby 2009).

Yet, health systems in Europe are only slowly waking up to the need to become more responsive to migrant populations by establishing appropriate and accessible health services. In contrast to traditional countries of immigration, such as Australia, Canada and the United States, few European countries have adopted explicit migrant health policies (Ingleby 2006).

At last, however, the issue of migrant health is receiving increasing attention in Europe. Of major importance in this respect were the EU presidencies of Portugal in 2007 and Spain in 2010. The Portuguese EU presidency held a conference on "Health and Migration in the European Union – Better Health for All in an Inclusive Society" in Lisbon in 2007, with the conference conclusions adopted by the Employment, Social Policy, Health and Consumer Affairs Council (EPSCO) in December 2007. Under the Spanish EU presidency, migration and health were considered within the overarching theme of health inequalities. This led to the adoption, by the European Council, of "Council conclusions on Equity and Health in All Policies: Solidarity in Health" (Peiro and Benedict 2009; Peiro and Benedict 2010).

Other international and European organizations have also contributed to the greater recognition of the migrant health agenda. In November 2007, a conference of ministers of health of the Council of Europe adopted the "Bratislava Declaration on health, human rights and migration" (Council of Europe 2007). In 2009, the project on "Assisting Migrants and Communities" (AMAC), led by the International Organization for Migration (IOM) and co-financed by the EU and Portugal, ran an EU-level consultation on "Migration Health – Better Health for All" in Lisbon (Peiro and Benedict 2009). In May 2008, the World Health Assembly adopted the resolution on the "Health of Migrants" (World Health Assembly 2008). The World Health Organization (WHO), the IOM and the Spanish Ministry of Health and Social Policy co-convened a "Global Consultation on Migrant Health" in Madrid in 2010 (WHO 2010). Yet, despite these positive developments, there is the danger that many policies and programmes will be short-lived, as funding by the EU and member states for migrant health initiatives declined between 2007 and 2010 (Peiro and Benedict 2010).

There are wide differences in the extent to which European countries have considered and implemented national migrant health policies. So far, only eleven (including one country from outside the EU) seem to have adopted specific national policies aimed at improving migrant health (see Chapter 12 on "Migrant health policies in Europe"). One obvious reason for the variation across countries is the size of the migrant population, which is still very small in countries in central and eastern Europe. Another issue is the overall political climate. On the other hand, Italy, Portugal and Spain have only experienced large-scale immigration relatively recently but have already adopted national migrant health policies (Vazquez et al. 2010). While some countries with a relatively extended history of immigration, such as the United Kingdom and the Netherlands, have established national migrant health policies, others, such as France, have not.

The political attention paid to the health of migrants is also related to prevailing attitudes towards migrants and immigration (Ingleby 2009). While there has been an increasing harmonization of immigration policies in EU member states, the dominant emphasis has been on restriction and control (Bendel 2007). The overall political climate in a country is an important factor that can help or hinder health systems in becoming more responsive to the needs of migrants (Ingleby 2006). A number of European countries, including Germany, have historically been reluctant to even consider themselves as countries of immigration. Furthermore, there has been a political backlash against immigration in a number of European countries, with a particularly hostile reception for asylum-seekers and a rise in anti-Muslim rhetoric. In 2010 alone, far-right anti-immigrant parties made electoral gains in Austria, Italy, the Netherlands, Hungary and Sweden, whereas France made headlines by establishing a ministry of national identity and deporting Roma originating from central and eastern Europe. Germany's Chancellor Angela Merkel declared that multiculturalism had "utterly failed" (Chrisafis 2010), and Switzerland voted in a referendum to ease the expulsion of foreigners convicted of crimes. This political environment, in which mainstream parties find themselves in the grip of populism, is made even more challenging as the economic crisis and cutbacks in public expenditure result in growing unemployment, not least among migrant workers. In this general political and economic context it will be crucial to counteract discrimination and not to retreat from efforts to establish and implement national migrant health policies.

The range of areas that need to be addressed by such policies is illustrated in Figure 1.1, adapted from the well-known "rainbow" on determinants of

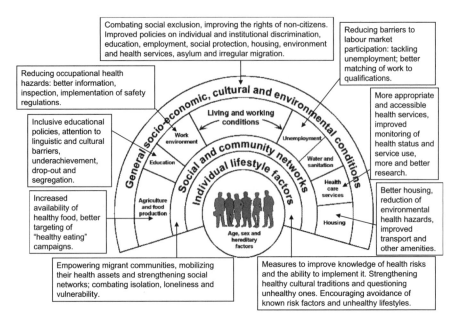

Figure 1.1 Policy measures tackling the determinants of health for migrants

Source: Adapted from WHO Regional Office for Europe (2010)

health (Dahlgren and Whitehead 1991). It becomes clear that policies need to go beyond improving health services to encompass actions addressing the social exclusion of migrants and their employment, education and housing conditions.

Outline of the book

This book is structured in seven sections. Following the introductory section, Section 2 explores the overall context of migration and health in the EU; Section 3 addresses the rights of migrants to health and looks at problems in accessing health services; Section 4 explores challenges and opportunities in monitoring migrant health; Section 5 is devoted to the health issues faced by migrants in Europe; Section 6 discusses the policy response so far, the need for culturally responsive health services and examples of best practice; and the final section is devoted to the conclusions that can be drawn from the material presented in this volume.

Following this introduction, Chapter 2 reviews the scale and nature of migration flows to post-war Europe. The chapter discusses the availability and quality of available data, the stocks and flows of foreign populations, the scale and nature of labour migration, and the challenges related to asylum-seekers and undocumented migration.

Chapter 3 is concerned with asylum, residency and citizenship policies and models of incorporating migrants into Europe. It argues that national provision of health services for migrants cannot be divorced from broader immigration policies. The chapter finds large variations across Europe in all four policy areas examined.

The next section of the book investigates human rights and access to health care for migrants in Europe. Chapter 4 describes international, European and national provisions on the right to health and how far these are being implemented in practice. It includes a discussion of United Nations, Council of Europe and EU provisions, mechanisms for their enforcement, and evidence on implementation.

Chapter 5 addresses migrants' access to health care. It reviews the current knowledge about health care utilization by migrants in Europe and finds that they tend to have a lower uptake of preventive services (such as for cancer screening and reproductive health care) but higher use of general practitioners; there is inconclusive evidence on emergency care, hospital care and specialist care. The chapter argues that differences in access are due to the formal and informal barriers migrants face in accessing health care, such as legal restrictions, language barriers, sociocultural factors, and migrants' lack of information about their rights and the health system of the host country.

The next section of the book aims to unravel the often diverging health needs of migrants. Chapter 6 is concerned with the questions of what data are available and how much use they are. It finds that there is a lack of high-quality information on the health of migrants, as routine data on migrant health are available in only a few EU countries and the understanding of exactly who constitutes a migrant differs widely from country to country. The chapter explores some of the political and methodological complexities involved, and considers what would be needed to improve the availability of data on health and migration in Europe.

Chapter 7 discusses the issue of non-communicable diseases. While findings vary among different migrant groups, the chapter reports that migrants tend to have a lower risk of cancer, are experiencing steep increases in diabetes and have a higher occurrence of stroke. As integration progresses, with migrants adopting the same lifestyles and facing the same environmental risks as locally born people, the epidemiological profiles of migrants tend to converge towards those of the host country. However, convergence appears to be a slow process.

Chapter 8 presents the available evidence on communicable diseases among migrants in Europe and discusses the practice in several European countries of screening migrants at entry. Migrants coming from high-prevalence countries tend to have higher than average rates of tuberculosis, hepatitis B and HIV/AIDS compared to majority populations in Europe. Of the 27 EU member states, 13 have specific screening programmes for tuberculosis among migrants, with screening most commonly directed at asylum-seekers and refugees.

Chapter 9 discusses maternal and child health. It focuses on the antenatal period and the first year of life, with particular consideration of unfavourable birth outcomes that are at least partly avoidable, such as stillbirths, neonatal and infant mortality, low birth weight, preterm birth and malformations. The authors find persisting differences in perinatal outcomes between migrants and non-migrants in Europe. There tend to be higher rates of stillbirth and infant mortality among migrants, with refugees, asylum-seekers and undocumented migrants being particularly vulnerable. There is also evidence that both the utilization and quality of antenatal care is lower among migrant women.

Chapter 10 reviews available research on employment and working conditions and their effects on the health of migrants. The majority of studies conducted in Europe in 1990–2010 found that rates of occupational injury were higher among migrants. However, due to a possible systematic bias in reporting, true differences might be even greater than these studies suggest. Unskilled and undocumented labour migrants working in sectors such as construction, mining and agriculture are particularly at risk.

Chapter 11 explores what is known about the mental health of refugees and asylum-seekers. It examines their psychopathology, ranging from psychological distress to mental disorders (e.g. depressive disorders and depression, and post-traumatic stress disorders), and draws lessons on how mental health care providers can meet the needs of refugees and asylum-seekers. In almost every study that has been done, refugees and asylum-seekers who reported exposure to political violence prior to migration were more likely to meet diagnostic criteria for the presence of psychopathology.

The next section of the book is concerned with policy responses and best practices. Chapter 12 reviews the migrant health policies that have been adopted so far in Europe at national and regional levels. It finds that only eleven European countries (one of which is outside the EU) have so far adopted specific policies on migrant health. There is considerable variation in terms of which population groups are targeted by these policies, the health issues addressed, whether providers or patients are the focus of interventions, and whether policies are actually being implemented. In England, Ireland and the Netherlands, for example, migrant policies are integrated into broader policies that also encompass ethnic minorities, while in Austria, Germany, Italy, Portugal, Spain, Sweden and Switzerland, the focus is more specifically on migrants.

Chapter 13 argues that there is a need for culturally responsive health care, in order to overcome differences in language, religion and culture. It examines how language barriers can be addressed through interpretation services, what it means to interact with patients of different cultural backgrounds, and how to address religious concerns. The chapter cautions against common preconceptions and argues in favour of a more open-minded approach that puts mutual understanding at the heart of the dialogue between health workers and patients.

Chapter 14 presents findings on best practice in accident and emergency departments. It is based on in-depth interviews with practitioners in areas with relatively high levels of migrants in 16 European countries. The chapter identifies a number of crucial factors for providing migrants with high-quality services, including the provision of good quality and easily accessible professional interpreting services, the promotion of cultural awareness among health workers, informing migrants about treatment expectations and the health system, ensuring legal and financial access to health services, and investing time and organizational resources.

Chapter 15 reviews good practice in health service provision for migrants generally. It first reviews how concern about adapting health services to the needs of migrants has arisen and then examines how service delivery can be modified. Among the mechanisms the chapter identifies are ensuring entitlements of migrants to health care, providing information on health and the health system, improving the geographical and administrative accessibility of health services and addressing language and cultural barriers. The chapter also identifies ways of making change sustainable and argues for more research on the effectiveness of interventions in the area of migrant health.

The final section of the book brings together the key findings and conclusions. Chapter 16 pays particular attention to the policy implications of the findings presented in this book and what can be done at the European, national and regional levels to improve migrant health in Europe.

References

Aung, N., Rechel, B. and Odermatt, P. (2010) Access to and utilisation of GP services among Burmese migrants in London: a cross-sectional descriptive study. *BMC Health Services Research*, 10: 285.

Bendel, P. (2007) Everything under control? The European Union's policies and politics of immigration. In: Faist, T. and Ette, A. (eds) *The Europeanization of National Policies and Politics of Immigration*. Basingstoke: Palgrave Macmillan: 32–48.

Björngren-Cuadra, C. and Cattacin, S. (2010) *Policies on Health Care for Undocumented Migrants in the EU27: Towards a Comparative Framework. Summary Report*. Malmö: Health Care in NowHereland, Malmö University.

Castles, S. and Davidson, A. (2000) *Citizenship and Migration: Globalization and the Politics of Belonging*. Basingstoke: Palgrave.

Chrisafis, A. (2010) 'It's still a ghetto here. Apartheid exists here. But that suits the politicians.' *The Guardian*, 17 November (http://www.guardian.co.uk/world/2010/nov/16/france-racism-immigration-sarkozy, accessed 6 June 2011).

Council of Europe (2007) *Bratislava Declaration on Health, Human Rights and Migration, 23 November 2007, 8th Conference of European Health Ministers*. Bratislava: Council of Europe.

Council of the EU (2003) Council Directive 2003/9/EC of 27 January 2003 laying down minimum standards for the reception of asylum seekers. *Official Journal of the European Union*, L 31/18.

Dahlgren, G. and Whitehead, M. (1991) *Policies and Strategies to Promote Social Equity in Health*. Stockholm: Institute for Futures Studies.

Davies, A.A., Basten, A. and Frattini, C. (2009) *Migration: A Social Determinant of the Health of Migrants*. Background paper developed within the framework of the IOM project "Assisting Migrants and Communities (AMAC): Analysis of social determinants of health and health inequalities". Geneva: International Organization for Migration.

Davies, A.A., Basten, A. and Frattini, C. (2010) Migration: a social determinant of migrants' health. *Eurohealth*, 16(1): 10–12.

Fernandes, A. and Miguel, J.P. (eds) (2009) *Health and Migration in the European Union: Better Health for All in an Inclusive Society*. Lisbon: Instituto Nacional de Saude Doutor Ricardo Jorge.

Gushulak, B. (2010) Monitoring migrants' health. In: *Health of Migrants – The Way Forward*. Report of a global consultation, Madrid, Spain, 3–5 March 2010. Geneva: World Health Organization: 28–42.

Gushulak, B., Pace, P. and Weekers, J. (2010) Migration and health of migrants. In: Koller, T. (ed.) *Poverty and Social Exclusion in the WHO European Region: Health systems respond*. Copenhagen: WHO Regional Office for Europe: 257–81.

Ingleby, D. (2006) Getting multicultural health care off the ground: Britain and the Netherlands compared. *International Journal of Migration, Health and Social Care*, 2(3/4): 4–14.

Ingleby, D. (2009) *European Research on Migration and Health*. Background paper developed within the framework of the IOM project "Assisting Migrants and Communities (AMAC): Analysis of social determinants of health and health inequalities". Geneva: International Organization for Migration.

Ingleby, D., Chimienti, M., Hatziprokopiou, P., Ormond, M. and De Freitas, C. (2005) The role of health in integration. In: Fonseca, M.L. and Malheiros, J. *Social Integration and Mobility: Education, Housing and Health*. Lisbon: Centro de Estudos Geográficos: 101–37.

IOM (2010) *World Migration Report 2010. The future of migration: Building capacities for change*. Geneva: International Organization for Migration.

Karl-Trummer, U., Björngren-Cuadra, C. and Novak-Zezula, S. (2010) *Two Landscapes of NowHereland*. Fact Sheet Policies (http://files.nowhereland.info/760.pdf, accessed 25 May 2011).

Karl-Trummer, U., Metzler, B. and Novak-Zezula, S. (2009) *Health Care for Undocumented Migrants in the EU: Concepts and Cases*. Geneva: International Organization for Migration.

Karl-Trummer, U., Novak-Zezula, S. and Metzler, B. (2010) Access to health care for undocumented migrants in the EU: a first landscape of NowHereland. *Eurohealth*, 16(1): 13–16.

Kobayashi, A. (2008) A research and policy agenda for second generation Canadians. *Canadian Diversity*, 6(23): 3–6.

MIGHEALTHNET (2010) *Information network on good practice in health care for migrants and minorities in Europe* (http://www.mighealth.net/index.php/Main_Page, accessed 25 May 2011).

Nielsen, S., Krasnik, A. and Rosano, A. (2009) Registry data for cross-country comparisons of migrants' healthcare utilization in the EU: a survey study of availability and content. *BMC Health Services Research*, 9: 210.

Nørredam, M., Mygind, A. and Krasnik, A. (2006) Access to health care for asylum seekers in the European Union – a comparative study of country policies. *European Journal of Public Health*, 16(3): 286–90.

Nørredam, M., Nielsen, S. and Krasnik, A. (2010) Migrants' utilization of somatic healthcare services in Europe – a systematic review. *European Journal of Public Health*, 20(5): 555–63.

Padilla, B. and Miguel, J.P. (2009) Health and migration in the EU: building a shared vision for action. In: Fernandes, A. and Miguel, J.P. (eds) *Health and Migration in the European Union: Better Health for All in an Inclusive Society*. Lisbon: Instituto Nacional de Saude Doutor Ricardo Jorge: 15–22.

Peiro, M.-J. and Benedict, R. (2009) *Migration Health: Better Health for All in Europe*. Brussels: International Organization for Migration.

Peiro, M.-J. and Benedict, R. (2010) Migrant health policy: The Portugese and Spanish EU Presidencies. *Eurohealth*, 16(1): 1–4.

Rafnsson, S.B. and Bhopal, R.S. (2008) Migrant and ethnic health research: report on the European Public Health Association Conference 2007. *European Journal of Public Health*, 122(5): 532–4.

Uiters, E., Devillé, W., Foets, M., Spreeuwenberg, P. and Groenewegen, P. (2009) Differences between immigrant and non-immigrant groups in the use of primary medical care: a systematic review. *BMC Health Services Research*, 9: 76.

United Nations Department of Economic and Social Affairs (1998) *Recommendations on Statistics of International Migration, Revision 1*. New York: Statistics Division, UN DESA (Statistical Papers, Series M, No. 58, Rev.1).

Vasileva, K. (2010) Foreigners living in the EU are diverse and largely younger than the nationals of the EU Member States. *Statistics in Focus*, 45. Luxembourg: Eurostat, European Commission.

Vazquez, M-L., Terraza-Nunez, R., Vargas, I., Rodriquez, D. and Lizana, T. (2010) Health policies for migrant populations in three European countries: England; Italy and Spain. *Health Policy* [Epub ahead of print].

Vogel, D. (2009) *Size and development of irregular migration to the EU*. Clandestino Research Project. Athens: Hellenic Foundation for European and Foreign Policy (http://research.icmpd.org/fileadmin/Research-Website/Startseite/Clandestino/clandestino_policy_brief_comparative_size-of-irregular-migration.pdf, accessed 25 May 2011).

Watson, R. (2009) Migrants in Europe are losing out on care they are entitled to. *BMJ*, 339: b3895.

World Health Assembly (2008) *Health of Migrants, Resolution 61.17*. Geneva: World Health Organization.

WHO (2010) *Health of Migrants – The Way Forward*. Report of a global consultation, Madrid, Spain, 3–5 March 2010. Geneva: World Health Organization.

WHO Regional Office for Europe (2010) *How Health Systems can Address Health Inequities Linked to Migration and Ethnicity*. Copenhagen: WHO Regional Office for Europe.

Section II

Context

chapter two

Trends in Europe's international migration

John Salt

Introduction

In 1989, governments across Europe were confronted with a new and largely uncharted situation. The Iron Curtain, which had created two separate migration spaces in Europe, fell, raising the possibility of mass migration from the east, towards the "lotus lands" of western Europe. Meanwhile, growing flows from the countries of the south were creating a new "migration frontier" along the northern shores of the Mediterranean. Italy, Greece, Spain and Portugal, traditionally countries of emigration, became countries of net immigration. A new asylum regime came into being, as the problems stemming from the break-up of Yugoslavia led to widespread use of temporary protection. In central and eastern Europe, ethnically-based migrations were common, frequently continuations of those that had begun in the aftermath of the Second World War but which ceased with the raising of the Iron Curtain. Other ethnic movements were of co-nationals "returning" to a "motherland", such as populations displaced in communist times, especially in the former USSR. New economic flows developed, between east and west and within central and eastern Europe. Some were permanent, many were short-term and a new lexicon grew up to describe them – labour tourism, pendular migration, circular migration, petty trading and transit migration.

The 1990s were characterized by the increasing integration of central and eastern Europe into the European migration sphere. In political terms attention turned more and more to the management of migration. By the mid-1990s Europe had largely adapted to changed migration flows, although there was great uncertainty about how to handle the fall-out from the Yugoslavian crisis. Elements of the picture were still blurred, especially in eastern Europe and the former USSR, where data systems remained inadequate. Furthermore, the growing importance of irregular migration, human smuggling and migrant trafficking were already causing concern. As the formerly separate western and eastern European migration systems increasingly fused into one, some eastern European countries also became countries of immigration.

New migrations appeared, some reflecting the emergence of new areas of origin. There were an estimated 63,000 Chinese migrants in Germany in 2001, twice the figure of 1993 and 10 times more than in 1988 (Giese 2003). In Italy, 68,000 residence permits were granted to Chinese citizens in 2001, more than 5 times more than in 1993 (Ceccagno 2003). Albanians were also on the move, remittances from whom represent an important source of income for the country; by 2000, 133,000 Albanians had permits to stay in Italy (Mai and Schwander-Sievers 2003).

There was also evidence of new types of flows. Peraldi (2004) described radical change in Algerian migratory routes over the previous ten years. The traditional labour migration into France was replaced by forms of circulation in which many Algerians became suitcase traders throughout the Mediterranean region. Often serving tourist markets, their moves took place within family networks which allowed them to seize trading opportunities in whichever city they presented themselves. Romanians were observed to circulate within informal transnational networks which they would use to exploit whatever "work niches" opened to undocumented workers (Potot 2008). Some "ethnic" migrations metamorphosed into circulatory ones. Michalon (2004) demonstrates that the migration of ethnic Germans from Transylvania (Romania) to Germany in the early 1990s became a circulatory movement, with periods of work in Germany interspersed with living back in Romania. The new migratory flows that have emerged in the 1990s and 2000s have given rise to a variety of policy responses across Europe (see Chapter 3 on "Asylum, residency and citizenship policies and models of migrant incorporation").

The data problem

The lack of available data and the enormous variation from country to country mean that it is not easy to detect European patterns or trends. Europe is highly geographically differentiated in both its physical and human geography and its migrations, not only from east to west and north to south, but also between adjacent countries. The image of Europe is, therefore, one of diversity. This diversity relates not only to existing flows and trends but also to the methods of registering and measuring them.

Although the provision of statistical data has improved immeasurably in recent years, the situation remains far from ideal. In western Europe, the existing data still pose a wide range of problems for users, arising largely from incompatibility of sources, as well as conceptual and definitional problems (Poulain et al. 2006). In central and eastern Europe and parts of the former USSR, data availability has improved but is still patchy.

A fundamental problem is the complexity of migration. For the most part, the concepts of migration used as the basis for collecting statistics do not reflect many of the realities of today's movements, characterized as they are by new forms and dynamics. Particularly difficult to capture are short-term movements and status changes, as well as, most obviously, undocumented migrations. Changes in the stocks of foreign nationals (i.e. those holding a different citizenship than that of the host country) do not only reflect the balance of flows, but also rates of naturalization which have greater or lesser effects, depending on the policies of destination countries. All this means that the identification of common patterns and trends is difficult, if not impossible (see Chapter 6 on "Monitoring the health of migrants").

Stocks of foreign population

What constitutes a foreign population is not immediately apparent. Some countries use the notion of "people of immigrant background", normally referring to the birthplace or nationality of a parent or grandparent. Those of foreign origin who have subsequently naturalized to become citizens of host countries may also have been included. In this chapter "foreign" relates to passport held and the terms "foreign national" and "foreign citizen" are used interchangeably. In cases where people have been born in countries outside that in which they are now living, the term "foreign born" is used. This group may include people of various nationalities. In most countries, statistics on the foreign population are available only by nationality or place of birth (see Chapter 6 on "Monitoring the health of migrants").

It is impossible to produce a complete picture of trends in stocks of foreign population in Europe since 1989, due to data inadequacies in some countries. Hence, estimations of migrant stocks and changes over time must be treated with caution. First, the data reflect what the national collecting organizations are able to make available. For some countries, statistics from the same source are available annually, but for others they are not. In the case of France, for example, the only source on the stock of foreign population is the periodic census. There are no data for the Russian Federation since 1997, while the first figures for Ukraine appeared in 2004. Second, sources of data may change. Recent statistics for Spain are from municipal registers, while those for earlier years are from residence permits, the numbers of which are lower. Third, statistics may be revised. This is particularly pertinent for Germany where a lower figure for 2004 compared with earlier years was the result of administrative procedures, involving cross-checking different registers to produce a revised figure. Data for the United Kingdom have also been revised periodically, resulting in different figures for some years than had previously been reported. More recent data are more comprehensive, although in the most recent Eurostat data for 2008 those for several countries have been estimated and are not the result of direct counts.

Total numbers

International compilations of statistics, like those of Eurostat, are based on the contributions of individual states. As far as possible, they adhere to a common template, but this is not always possible. The statistics used here are those recorded by the surveys and administrative systems of individual countries and do not include undocumented migrants. Although aggregate numbers are imprecise, there is evidence of a steady rise in Europe's foreign population. In the late 1980s, the total was probably in the region of 15 million, rising to around 19 million by the mid-1990s and to 25.5 million in 2004 (Salt 2006). The vast majority of this foreign population was living in western Europe. The annual rate of increase of the foreign population has fluctuated. During much of the 1980s and 1990s, it was around 1.5%, but rose to about 8% between 1989 and 1993. Since 2000, the annual increase has been about 3.7% per year. Most of this increase was in western Europe, particularly the four Mediterranean countries of Greece, Italy, Portugal and Spain, whose share of the western European total more than doubled to about 25%, an absolute increase of over 3 million. However, the statistics are misleading. Much of this rise can be attributed to regularization programmes, which had the effect of converting unrecorded migrants into recorded ones. Furthermore, the more than doubling of the Spanish stock of foreign population was related to the change in the statistical source for Spain referred to above, rather than a sudden increase in immigration (Salt 2006).

By 2008, an estimated 30.8 million foreign citizens lived in the 27 member states of the European Union (EU), equivalent to approximately 6% of the total population (Vasileva 2009). However, it is important to note that the ratio between the domestic and foreign populations is influenced by the rate of naturalization, which affects both components in the calculation. In the United Kingdom, for example, less than half of those born in the Indian sub-continent have citizenship of that region, whereas 83% of those born in countries of the European Economic Area (EEA) have retained their original citizenship.

Origins and destinations[1]

In 2008, over a third of foreign nationals living on the territory of the 27 EU member states had EU citizenship, about a fifth were from other European countries, and the remainder were from outside Europe, including about 15% from Africa, 12% from Asia and 10% from the Americas. Since the formation of the European Economic Community in 1957, around a third of foreigners in the 15 states that were members of the EU before 2004 (EU15) have been EU citizens, which means that the pattern for them has been relatively constant.

About three-quarters of the EU's foreign nationals live in five countries: Germany, Spain, United Kingdom, France and Italy (Vasileva 2009). The foreign share of total populations varies considerably (Figure 2.1). Proportions are generally higher in western European countries, with Luxembourg, at 43%, holding a traditional top spot and with Switzerland, Spain and Austria also exceeding 10%. High proportions in Latvia and Estonia are due to the large share of Russian-speaking minorities in these countries, many members of which hold Russian citizenship or are stateless. In contrast, proportions in Romania, Poland, Bulgaria and Slovakia are less than 1%.

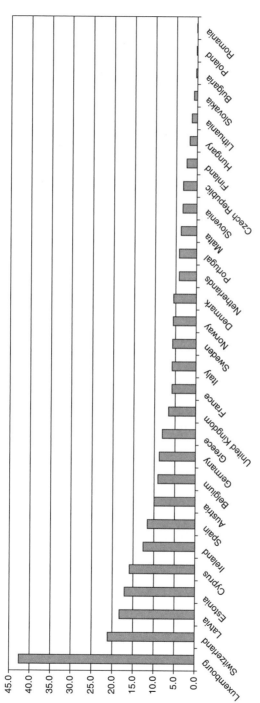

Figure 2.1 Foreign citizens as a percentage of the total population in EU member states, Norway and Switzerland, 2008

Source: Vasileva, A. (2009)

The composition of the foreign population in western Europe is a reflection of successive waves of post-war migration, associated first with labour shortage and more recently (especially since the mid-1970s) with family reunion, as well as the flight of refugees from war-torn areas both within and outside Europe. The dominant foreign groups within each country reflect the sources from which labour has been recruited since the Second World War, historical links and bilateral relations with former colonies, and ease of access (in terms of geography or policy) for refugees and asylum-seekers from different places. Despite their recent status as immigration countries, the largest groups of foreign nationals continue to be from the countries of southern Europe from where workers were recruited (Italy, Portugal, Spain and Greece), plus Turkey and the former Yugoslavia, and more recently northern Africa. The major newcomer to the scene is Romania, whose citizens are the biggest non-national group in Spain, Italy and Hungary. In addition to immigration from Romania, changes since 2001 include increases in the number of citizens of Poland living in other EU countries and in those from China.

The availability of historical data on the nationalities of the foreign population in central and eastern Europe varies from country to country. During most years since 1989, the largest groups of foreign nationals seem to have come from other central and eastern European states, although the picture is clearly not static and is further complicated by changes in numbers resulting from changes in citizenship. In recent years, eastern European states have received increasing numbers of nationals from Ukraine and the Russian Federation.

Table 2.1 summarizes the situation across the EU according to the most recent data. In 2008, in the EU27 as a whole, Turks were the largest group (2.4 million), constituting 7.9% of all non-nationals, followed by Moroccans (1.7 million, 5.6%) and Romanians (1.7 million, 5.4%). There continue to be major variations between destination countries in the nationalities of those who choose to live in them. In some cases, such as Turks, Algerians and Ecuadorians, more than 70% of those living in the EU have settled in one particular member state.

Flows of foreign population

The data problems discussed earlier apply even more to migration flows. Data for European countries are now more comprehensive than they have ever been, but significant gaps remain. Statistics on emigration are particularly problematic; many countries do not collect them, and those that do tend to underestimate emigration (Salt et al. 1994; Poulain et al. 2006). Even in countries with well developed data collection systems, more often than not, there are substantial differences between the estimates of origin and destination countries. Furthermore, many of the movements seen in much of central and eastern Europe during the last 20 years defy most collection systems. Because statistics for all countries are not available for every year it is impossible to produce an accurate set of annual inflows of foreign population for the whole of Europe. Some countries have no usable data at all, while others have only a partial record.

Table 2.1 Three largest groups of foreign citizens residing in selected European countries by citizenship and as a percentage of all non-nationals, 2008

	Citizens of	Numbers	%	Citizens of	Numbers	%	Citizens of	numbers	%
EU 27	**Turkey**	**2,419,000**	**7.9**	**Morocco**	**1,727,000**	**5.6**	**Romania**	**1,677,000**	**5.4**
Austria	Serbia/Montenegro	132,600	15.9	Germany	119,800	14.3	Turkey	109,200	13.1
Belgium	Italy	169,000	17.4	France	130,600	13.4	Netherlands	123,500	12.7
Bulgaria	Russian Federation	9000	36.7	Ukraine	2200	8.8	Greece	1600	6.6
Czech Republic	Ukraine	103,400	29.7	Slovakia	67,900	19.5	Viet Nam	42,300	12.2
Denmark	Turkey	28,800	9.7	Iraq	18,300	6.1	Germany	18,000	6
Finland	Russian Federation	26,200	19.8	Estonia	20,000	15.1	Sweden	8300	6.3
France*	Portugal	492,000	13.6	Algeria	477,500	13.2	Morocco	461,500	12.7
Germany	Turkey	1,830,100	25.2	Italy	570,200	7.9	Poland	413,000	5.7
Greece	Albania	577,500	63.7	Ukraine	22,300	2.5	Georgia	17,200	1.9
Hungary	Romania	65,900	37.3	Ukraine	17,300	9.8	Germany	14,400	8.2
Italy	Romania	625,300	18.2	Albania	402,000	11.7	Morocco	365,900	10.7
Latvia	Rec. non-citizens[1]	371,700	89.5	Russian Federation	28,500	6.9	Lithuania	3400	0.8
Lithuania	Russian Federation	12,800	29.7	Belarus	4700	10.9	Stateless	4200	9.7
Luxembourg	Portugal	76,600	37.2	France	26,600	12.9	Italy	19,100	9.3
Malta	Ukraine	4100	26.5	India	900	6	Serbia	800	5.1
Netherlands	Turkey	93,700	13.6	Morocco	74,900	10.9	Germany	62,400	9.1
Norway	Sweden	29,900	11.2	Poland	26,800	10.1	Denmark	20,500	7.7
Poland	Germany	11,800	20.5	Ukraine	6100	10.6	Russian Federation	3700	6.4
Portugal	Brazil	70,100	15.7	Cape Verde	64,700	14.5	Ukraine	39,600	8.9
Romania	Rep. of Moldova	5500	21	Turkey	2200	8.4	China	1900	7.3
Slovakia	Czech Rep.	6000	14.6	Poland	4000	9.8	Ukraine	3700	9.2
Slovenia	Bosnia and Herzegovina	32,500	47.3	Serbia	13,800	20.1	FYR Macedonia	7400	10.9
Spain	Romania	734,800	14	Morocco	649,800	12.3	Ecuador	423,500	8
Sweden	Finland	80,400	15.3	Iraq	40,000	7.6	Denmark	38,400	7.3
Switzerland	Italy	291,200	18.2	Germany	203,200	12.7	Portugal	183,000	11.4
United Kingdom	Poland	392,800	9.9	Ireland	347,900	8.8	India	296,500	7.5

NOTES: *2005 data; [1]a recognized non-citizen is a person who is neither a citizen of the reporting country nor of any other country, but who has established links to that country which include some but not all rights and obligations of full citizenship.

Source: Vasileva, A. (2009)

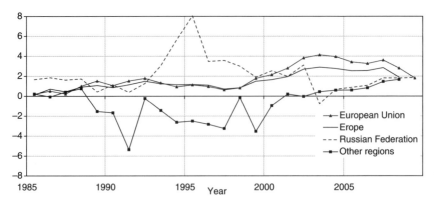

Figure 2.2 Net migration (per thousand) in Europe, EU, Russian Federation and in other regions of Europe, 1985–2009

NOTE: Data for Europe include the Asian parts of the Russian Federation and exclude Turkey; data for "other regions" include the Balkans.

Source: Sobotka (2009)

Net migration in Europe between 1985 and 2009 is summarized in Figure 2.2. This has been compiled from various sources by Sobotka (2009). For Europe as a whole and for the EU net gain generally increased, mainly after 1999, although after that growth fell back as recession took hold. Gains in the Russian Federation fluctuated in the 1990s, as ethnic Russians moved back from other parts of the former USSR. Other parts of Europe, including the Balkans, Ukraine and the Republic of Moldova, experienced substantial net emigration. Recent projections of population by national origin for a number of European countries suggest that by 2050 populations of foreign origin will rise to 15–35% of the total (Coleman 2009).

Sobotka (2009) points out the contrasting trends between the EU15 and the EU12 countries (the 12 countries that joined the EU in 2004 and 2007) in total population increase, net migration and natural increase (Figure 2.3). Most of the EU15 countries showed above-average population gains, with net migration the more important component of change every year since 1990. In contrast, after 1990 population increase in the EU12 fell and natural increase became negative. Poor emigration data for some countries prevent meaningful overall estimates of net migration in recent years, but even some EU12 countries have recorded considerable immigration in recent years: for example, net migration to the Czech Republic (including Czech citizens) rose from 18 600 in 2004 to 71 800 in 2008 (Maresova 2009).

The trends described here are complex and represent considerable variations from country to country and at different time periods. In the circumstances, explanations will also be complex, related to general economic conditions in the countries of central and eastern Europe, the effects of Balkan wars, national policy initiatives, regularization programmes, levels of asylum-seeking and the efforts of smugglers and traffickers, as well as other factors. Even so, it should be noted that the trends described above underestimate total flows, since for the

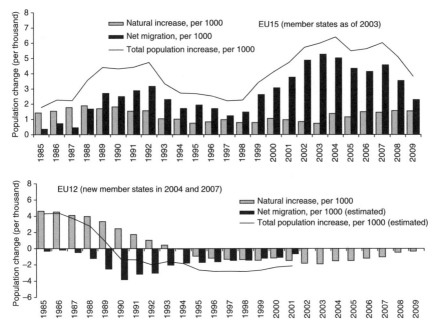

Figure 2.3 Natural increase, net migration and total population increase (per thousand) in the "new" and "old" EU member states, 1985–2009

Source: Sobotka (2009)

most part they exclude asylum-seekers, some categories of temporary migrants, and undocumented migrants.

Flows of labour

There are major difficulties in estimating inflows of foreign labour to individual countries and Europe as a whole. There is a multiplicity of (usually) administrative sources which are frequently partial in coverage. For example, work permits are a common source, but they exclude nationals of the EEA in other EEA member states, for which other sources have to be used. Only non-Nordic citizens are included in the figures in Nordic states. There are also severe problems in relation to the recording of seasonal, frontier and other short-term workers; they are included in the data for some countries, but not for others.

Recorded inflows of foreign labour have been modest in most countries in recent years, the biggest recipient being Germany (Table 2.2). In the majority of the countries of western Europe for which data are available, the numbers recorded per year are less than 20,000, with an emphasis on the recruitment of skilled workers. Even so, across western Europe, patterns of foreign labour recruitment and use echo those of the 1960s. In the United Kingdom Worker Registration Scheme for EU8 (the eight central and eastern European countries that joined the EU in 2004) workers, almost all registrations since 2004 have

Table 2.2 Inflows of foreign labour into selected European countries, 1995–2008 (thousands)

(a) Western Europe

	1995	1996	1997	1998	1999	2000	2001	2002	2003	2004	2005	2006	2007	2008
Austria[1]	15.4	16.3	15.2	15.4	18.3	25.4	27.0	24.6	24.1	24.5	23.2	22.6	29.6	–
Belgium	2.7	2.2	2.5	7.3	8.7	7.5	7.0	6.7	4.6	4.3	6.3	12.5	23.0	25.0
Denmark[2]	2.2	2.8	3.1	3.3	3.1	3.6	5.1	4.8	2.3	4.3	7.4	13.6	19.3	10.3
Finland	–	–	–	–	–	10.4	14.1	13.3	13.8	15.2	18.7	22.0	24.0	–
France	10.6	9.6	9.9	9.7	12.1	13.9	18.8	17.8	17.0	17.0	19.3	21.0	27.0	23.8
Germany[3]	470.0	439.7	285.4	275.5	304.9	333.8	373.8	374.0	372.2	380.3	–	–	–	–
Ireland	15.7	–	4.5	5.7	6.3	18.0	36.4	40.3	47.6	34.1	27.1	24.9	23.6	13.6
Italy	–	–	–	21.6	21.4	58.0	92.4	139.1	87.1	71.6	75.3	69.0	150.1	167.8
Luxembourg[4]	16.5	18.3	18.6	22.0	24.2	27.3	–	22.4	22.6	22.9	24.8	28.0	31.0	–
Netherlands[5]	–	9.2	11.1	15.2	20.8	27.7	30.2	34.6	38.0	44.1	46.1	74.1	50.0	15.6
Norway	–	–	–	–	14.0	14.8	17.8	23.5	25.2	33.0	28.3	40.5	54.8	52.6
Portugal	2.2	1.5	1.3	2.6	4.2	7.8	136.0	55.3	16.4	19.3	13.1	13.8	–	–
Spain	36.6	36.6	25.9	48.1	49.7	172.6	154.9	101.6	74.6	158.9	648.5	108.8	102.5	–
Sweden	–	–	–	2.4	2.4	3.3	3.3	–	10.2	8.5	13.3	18.1	–	–
Switzerland[6]	32.9	29.8	25.4	26.8	31.5	34.0	41.9	40.1	35.4	40.0	40.3	46.4	74.3	76.7
Turkey	–	–	–	–	–	24.2	22.4	22.6	21.7	27.5	22.1	–	–	–
United Kingdom[7]	51.0	50.0	59.0	68.0	61.2	86.5	76.2	99.0	80.0	89.4	86.2	96.7	88.0	–

(b) *Central and eastern Europe*

	1995	1996	1997	1998	1999	2000	2001	2002	2003	2004	2005	2006	2007	2008
Bulgaria[8]	0.3	0.1	0.1	0.1	0.1	0.3	0.3	0.3	0.4	1.0	0.6	1.1	1.1	1.6
Hungary	–	–	19.7	22.6	29.6	40.2	47.3	49.8	57.4	79.2	72.6	71.1	55.2	–
Czech Republic[9]	–	71.0	61.0	49.9	40.3	40.1	40.1	44.6	47.7	34.4	55.2	–	–	–
Lithuania	0.4	0.5	0.8	1.0	1.2	0.7	0.6	0.5	0.6	0.9	1.6	3.0	3.0	7.1
Poland[10]	–	–	–	–	–	7.0	5.9	5.8	5.8	7.0	6	6.6	7.7	12.4
Romania[11]	0.7	0.7	1.0	1.3	1.5	–	–	–	–	–	2.7	5.5	–	–
Slovakia[12]	3.0	3.3	3.2	2.5	2.0	1.8	2.0	–	–	–	–	–	–	–

Sources: Council of Europe, National Statistical Offices, OECD SOPEMI correspondents

NOTES:

[1.] Data for all years covers initial work permits for both direct inflow from abroad and for first participation in the Austrian labour market of foreigners already in the country.

[2.] Residence permits issued for employment. Nordic citizens are not included.

[3.] Break in series 1998–1999.

[4.] Data cover both arrivals of foreign workers and residents admitted for the first time to the labour market.

[5.] Number of temporary work permits (WAV). 2002 data refer to January–September. *Source:* CWI.

[6.] Seasonal and frontier workers are not taken included.

[7.] Data from the Labour Force Survey.

[8.] Number of new work permits.

[9.] Work permits issued for foreigners.

[10.] Number of first work permits.

[11.] New work permits issued to foreign citizens.

[12.] Work permits granted. Czech nationals do not need work permits in Slovakia.

been for low-skilled work. Germany's bilateral agreement with Poland brought in more than 250,000 seasonal workers a year, mostly in agriculture (Dietz and Kaczmarczyk 2008). In Ireland, the most rapid increases in issued work permits in the late 1990s were for agriculture, hotels and catering (Hughes 2004). The Netherlands tells a similar story, with increasing numbers of temporary work permits, especially for agriculture, horticulture and a range of low-skilled service jobs, such as drivers and hotel and catering workers (Snel et al. 2004). In Austria, agriculture and forestry and parts of the tourist sector have been increasing their foreign labour intake (Biffl 2004). Only with the recession starting in 2008, and the availability of workers from Bulgaria and Romania after 2007, do numbers of recorded recruits from beyond the EU appear to have gone down. However, any reduction may be because employers have preferred to use irregular workers in order to reduce labour costs.

In the years following the collapse of communism, the central and eastern European countries developed their own migration patterns, characterized by a wide range of circulatory and informal flows, sometimes referred to by the epithet "pendular". By 2000, labour migration within and to the central and eastern European countries was highly differentiated according to the duration, skills and origins of migrants (Wallace 1999; Kraler and Iglicka 2002). Migrants were more likely than indigenous workers to be in the private sector and working in small firms, generally in more insecure jobs.

The current situation in the central and eastern European region shows some similarities with western Europe during its guestworker phase of the 1960s and early 1970s. Then, migrants from the Mediterranean moved into northwest Europe to work in the more unpleasant and low-paid jobs in agriculture, construction, manufacturing and low-paid services. In the EU8 states today, (Czech Republic, Estonia, Hungary, Latvia, Lithuania, Poland, Slovakia and Slovenia), foreign workers from further east are working (often illegally) in the agriculture and construction industries and in the low-skilled and low-paid service sector. Often, they are replacing the nationals of these countries who have moved to work in western Europe.

Asylum-seeking in Europe

Much of the discussion about the scale of migration into and within Europe separates asylum-seekers from what are considered "normal" (predominantly labour and family reunion) migration flows. There are sound reasons for this. Not only are the motivations of the two sets of moves different, but the data are also collected and presented differently. However, the distinction between the two has become increasingly blurred, as indicated by the high rates of refusal of asylum claims by host governments.

Trends in the number of applications

Since the mid-1990s, the number of applications for asylum has fluctuated (Table 2.3). In western Europe, the figure for 2008 was similar to that for 1995, but well down on the peak of 1999. Trends across countries have varied.

Table 2.3 Asylum applications in selected European countries, 1995–2008 (thousands)

(a) Western Europe

	1995	1996	1997	1998	1999	2000	2001	2002	2003	2004	2005	2006	2007	2008
Austria	5.9	7.0	6.7	13.8	20.1	18.3	30.1	39.4	32.3	24.6	22.5	13.3	11.9	12.8
Belgium	11.4	12.4	11.8	22.0	35.8	42.7	24.6	18.8	16.9	15.4	16.0	11.6	11.1	17.1
Denmark	5.1	5.9	5.1	9.4	12.3	12.2	12.5	6.1	4.6	3.2	2.3	1.9	1.9	2.4
Finland	0.9	0.7	1.0	1.3	3.1	3.2	1.7	3.4	3.1	3.9	3.6	2.3	1.4	4.0
France	20.4	17.4	21.4	22.4	30.9	38.8	47.3	59.0	60.0	58.6	49.7	30.7	29.4	42.0
Germany	127.9	116.4	104.4	98.6	95.1	78.6	88.3	71.1	50.6	35.6	29.0	21.0	19.2	6.0
Greece	1.3	1.6	4.4	3.0	1.5	3.1	5.5	5.7	8.2	4.5	9.1	12.3	25.1	33.3
Iceland	0.0	–	0.0	0.0	0.0	0.0	0.1	0.1	0.1	0.1	0.1	0.0	0.0	0.0
Ireland	0.4	1.2	3.9	4.6	7.7	11.1	10.3	11.6	7.9	4.8	4.3	4.3	4.0	6.8
Italy	1.7	0.7	1.9	11.1	33.4	15.6	9.6	16.0	13.5	9.7	9.5	10.3	14.1	30.3
Liechtenstein	–	–	–	0.2	0.5	0.0	0.1	0.1	0.1	0.1	0.0	0.0	0.0	0.0
Luxembourg	0.4	0.3	0.4	1.7	2.9	0.6	0.7	1.0	1.6	1.6	0.8	0.5	0.4	0.8
Netherlands	29.3	22.2	34.4	45.2	42.7	43.9	32.6	18.7	13.4	9.8	12.4	14.5	7.1	13.4
Norway	1.5	1.8	2.3	8.4	10.2	10.8	14.8	17.5	16.0	8.0	5.4	5.3	6.5	20.5
Portugal	0.5	0.3	0.3	0.4	0.3	0.2	0.2	0.3	0.1	0.1	0.1	0.1	0.2	0.2
Spain	5.7	4.7	5.0	6.7	8.4	7.9	9.5	6.3	5.8	5.4	5.3	5.3	7.7	4.5
Sweden	9.1	5.8	9.7	12.8	11.2	16.3	23.5	33.0	31.4	23.2	17.5	24.3	36.4	40.5
Switzerland	17.0	18.0	24.0	41.3	46.1	17.6	20.6	26.1	21.1	14.3	10.1	10.5	10.4	16.6
United Kingdom	55.0	37.0	41.5	58.5	91.2	98.9	91.6	103.1	60.1	40.6	30.8	28.3	28.3	30.5
Totals (western Europe)	**293.5**	**253.4**	**278.2**	**361.4**	**453.4**	**419.8**	**423.6**	**437.3**	**346.8**	**263.5**	**228.5**	**196.5**	**215.1**	**281.7**

Continued overleaf

Table 2.3 *Continued*

(b) Central and eastern Europe

	1995	1996	1997	1998	1999	2000	2001	2002	2003	2004	2005	2006	2007	2008
Bulgaria	0.5	0.3	0.4	0.8	1.3	1.8	2.4	2.9	1.6	1.1	0.8	0.6	1.0	0.7
Czech Republic	1.4	2.2	2.1	4.1	7.3	8.8	18.1	8.5	11.4	5.5	4.2	3.0	1.9	2.7
Estonia	–	–	–	0.0	0.0	–	0.0	0.0	0.0	0.0	0.0	0.0	0.0	0.0
Hungary	0.1	0.2	0.2	7.1	11.5	7.8	9.6	6.4	2.4	1.6	1.6	2.1	3.4	3.1
Latvia	–	–	–	0.1	0.0	–	0.0	0.0	0.0	0.0	0.0	0.0	0.0	0.0
Lithuania	–	–	0.3	0.2	0.1	0.2	0.3	0.3	0.2	0.2	0.1	0.2	0.1	0.2
Poland	0.8	3.2	3.5	3.4	3.0	4.6	4.5	5.2	6.9	8.1	6.9	4.2	7.2	7.7
Romania	–	0.6	1.4	1.2	1.7	1.4	2.4	1.2	1.1	0.7	0.6	0.4	0.7	1.2
Slovakia	0.4	0.4	0.7	0.5	1.3	1.6	8.2	9.7	10.3	11.4	3.6	2.9	2.6	1.0
Slovenia	–	0.0	0.1	0.5	0.9	9.2	1.5	0.7	1.1	1.3	1.8	0.5	0.0	0.2
Totals (central and eastern Europe)	**3.2**	**6.9**	**8.7**	**17.9**	**27.1**	**35.4**	**47.0**	**34.9**	**35.0**	**29.7**	**19.6**	**13.9**	**16.9**	**16.8**

Source: Governments, UNHCR. Compiled by UNHCR (Population Data Unit). http://www.unhcr.org/pages/49c3646c4d6.html

Germany and, to a lesser extent the Netherlands, have experienced a general reduction, while Sweden and France have moved in the opposite direction. The most common characteristic was for numbers to rise around the year 2000, followed by falls up to 2008. Data on asylum-seeking in central and eastern Europe are still very partial. For the most part, the numbers recorded are low, but the region displays similar trends to its western neighbours.

Most of the literature on asylum has focused on policy, legislation and procedures (see Chapter 3 on "Asylum, residency and citizenship policies and models of migrant incorporation"). Several interconnected factors appear to be very important for explaining the patterns of destination for asylum-seekers: existing communities of compatriots, colonial bonds, knowledge of the language, smugglers and traffickers, and national asylum policies. Chain migration effects seem important, especially in terms of friendship and kinship networks. One major study in the 1990s, mainly carried out in the Netherlands, Belgium and the United Kingdom, but with reference to the north American literature as well, found that most asylum-seekers are not well informed with regard to possible destination countries; indeed, the influence of rumour is strong (Böcker and Havinga 1998). A more recent study in the United Kingdom found that facilitators/smugglers were primarily responsible for the choice of destination (Gilbert and Koser 2004). Asylum policy and reception vary between countries and this information is used by facilitators, as well as by individual asylum-seekers. Since the mid-2000s, most European countries have tightened their asylum procedures through a combination of policy instruments, including speedier processing of applications and reviews of benefit levels (OECD 2008, 2010). It should be noted that various forms of temporary protection were offered by European governments in the 1990s, mainly to citizens of the former Yugoslavia. Such schemes are beyond the United Nations High Commissioner for Refugees (UNHCR) Convention system and other formal humanitarian statuses and assume that once conflict ends those persons given protection will return home. Such returns help explain increased rates of emigration from Germany in the years following conflict in the former Yugoslavia.

Trends in the number of asylum decisions

Statistics on asylum decisions are difficult to interpret because of the time lag between an application being made and a decision being reached. A further complication is the appeals procedure which may mean several "decisions" on a single case. For Europe as a whole, the proportions of decisions granting asylum (based on the 1951 United Nations Convention Relating to the Status of Refugees) or humanitarian status have remained low; neither exceeded 20% of total decisions made in any year and in some years their proportions fell to under 10%.

There are substantial variations in the proportions from different countries granted protection. In 2008, almost three-quarters of decisions made by EU27 member states on behalf of Somalis and Eritreans were positive, compared to almost half for Iraqis, and only one in eight for Turks (Juchno 2009).

Irregular migration

Most migrants are fully authorized and one estimate suggests that only approximately 10–15% of migrants worldwide are in an irregular situation, most of them having entered legally but overstaying their authorized stay (IOM 2010). Estimating the numbers of irregular migrants in Europe is fraught with obvious difficulties. The International Centre for Migration Policy Development (ICMPD) carried out an annual survey and analysis of border management and apprehension data within the framework of the Clandestino project, while the European Migration Network (EMN) has begun to publish data on apprehensions and removals.

Many statistics on flows of irregular migrants come from border apprehension statistics, poorly accounting for the variety of routes into irregularity. Border apprehension data provide only a poor approximation of flows and stocks of irregular migrants, as they exclude by definition those who entered legally, as well as those who successfully make it to the destination country in an irregular way. Data also vary according to the nature of the border and the effort put in by the authorities to control flows. Statistics may also fluctuate markedly from year to year as a result of general amnesties. Thus, between 2001 and 2002, the number of apprehensions by Greece fell from 220,000 to 44,000.

It does appear that the overall trend in the level of apprehensions across European countries has been downward (Figures 2.4 and 2.5). Of nine countries for which EMN data are available for 2000 and 2007, only Poland, France and Hungary showed increases.

In 2010, Greece accounted for 90% of all detections of irregular border crossing along the EU's external borders, with 75,000 detections between January and October 2010. Most detections took place at the land and sea borders with Turkey and most detected irregular migrants came from Afghanistan (Frontex 2010).

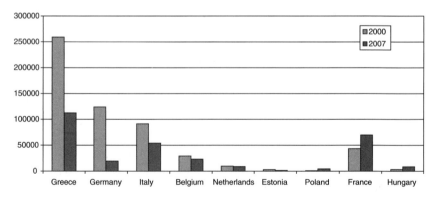

Figure 2.4 Total number of apprehended aliens for selected European countries, 2000 and 2007

Source: European Migration Network, (http://emn.sarenet.es/Downloads/prepareShowFiles. do;jsessionid=8055094C0294CB136F9A8065E23F2F69?directoryID=119, accessed 25 May 2011)

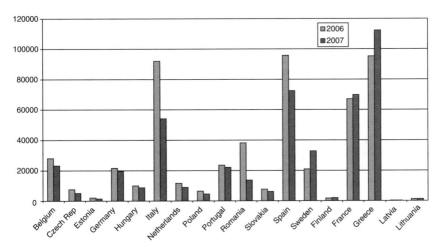

Figure 2.5   Total number of apprehended aliens for selected European countries, 2006–2007

Source: European Migration Network, (http://emn.sarenet.es/Downloads/prepareShowFiles. do;jsessionid=8055094C0294CB136F9A8065E23F2F69?directoryID=119, accessed 25 May 2011)

Other sources of information on undocumented migrants include population censuses, files from government administrative bodies, surveys, and regularization programmes (IOM 2010). Numerous amnesty programmes, mainly in Mediterranean countries, have shown the numbers of migrants living irregularly to be considerable. Attempts have also been made in some countries to estimate the size of irregular populations indirectly, but these are indicative at best (Van der Leun et al. 1998; Baldassarini 2001; Piguet and Losa 2002; Pinkerton et al. 2004; Woodbridge 2005; Gordon et al. 2009).

Human smuggling (where the agent procures, for direct or indirect benefit, illegal entry of an individual into another state) and migrant trafficking (where an agent exploits the individual, often with coercion) are major elements in the discourse on irregular migration. Unfortunately, there is a fundamental lack of hard evidence relating to both of these. Methodologies for studying both traffickers/smugglers and their clientele are barely developed, the theoretical basis for analysis is weak and, most importantly, substantial empirical surveys are few and far between (Koser 2011). The annual survey of central and eastern European countries carried out by the ICMPD provides information on apprehensions of human smugglers and traffickers. In 2008, the total number of apprehensions of smugglers was 5942 (up from 5290 in 2007), while 647 traffickers were apprehended (up from 619 in 2007) (ICMPD 2010). There were wide variations between countries in the numbers they apprehended. Greece (2211) and Turkey (1305) accounted for the largest numbers of smugglers apprehended in 2008, followed by Slovenia (622) and Croatia (448). Turkey (253) and Greece (162) apprehended the largest numbers of traffickers. These numbers are indicative only; no one knows how many smugglers and traffickers are involved in the business. It is likely that those apprehended at borders are relatively low-level operatives, with most of the higher level smuggling and trafficking organization done in origin countries.

Conclusions

Today, the burning issues are no longer those of the early 1990s or 2000s. Recorded migration is now relatively stable, the main exceptions being the incorporation of large numbers of amnestied former irregular migrants in some countries and of economic migrants in the aftermath of EU enlargement in others. Both western and eastern European countries are growing more concerned with the challenges of their ageing demographics and the role that international migration could play. There is also a realization that the demographic profile of immigrants is an important element in future population developments in Europe (Haug et al. 2002; Coleman 2009). The response to some skill shortages is increasing openness to those from abroad and there is ample evidence of global competition for highly qualified people (OECD 2008, 2010). Unrecorded and irregular migrations continue to pose challenges, but there is no hard evidence that their scale is increasing. Indeed, some data suggest the numbers might be declining, although this may reflect the diversion of irregular flows into new and less policed routes.

What seems to be emerging is a more integrated European economic and social space, characterized by both new and older forms of mobility. However, distinctive spatial migration fields in western, central and eastern Europe and the former USSR are still clearly identifiable. In the continent as a whole, there is now widespread circulation of people in informal and short-term movements. In both western and eastern Europe there are also some remarkable parallels with the guestworker phase in the decades after the Second World War (Dobson et al. 2009). These include the occupations migrants take up and the transition of temporary movements by single migrants into a settled family migration.

Note

1   Much of the information in this section, particularly in relation to 2008, is taken from Vasileva (2009).

References

Baldassarini, A. (2001) *Non Regular Foreign Input of Labour in the New National Accounts Estimates*. OECD Meeting of National Accounts Experts, Paris (STD/NA(2001)30).

Biffl, G. (2004) *International Migration and Austria*. The report of the Austrian SOPEMI correspondent to the OECD. Paris: OECD.

Böcker, A. and Havinga, T. (1998) *Asylum Migration to the European Union: Patterns of Origin and Destination*. Luxembourg: European Commission.

Ceccagno, A. (2003) New Chinese migrants in Italy. *International Migration*, 41(3): 187–213.

Coleman, D. (2009) Migration and its consequences in 21st century Europe. In: Coleman, D. and Ediev, D. (eds) *Vienna Yearbook of Population Research 2009: Impact of migration on demographic change and composition in Europe*. Vienna: Institute of Demography: 1–18.

Dietz, B. and Kaczmarczyk, P. (2008) On the demand side of international labour mobility: the structure of the German labour market as a causal factor of Polish seasonal migration. In: Bonifazi, C., Okolski, M., Schoorl, J. and Simon, P. (eds) *International Migration in Europe: New Trends and New Methods of Analysis*. Amsterdam: IMISCOE Research, Amsterdam University Press: 37–64.

Dobson, J., Latham, A. and Salt, J. (2009) *On the move? Labour migration in times of recession. What can we learn from the past?* London: Policy Network Paper.

Frontex (2010) *Current migratory situation in Greece (update 29 November 2010)*. Warsaw: Frontex (http://www.frontex.europa.eu/rabit_2010/background_information/, accessed 14 May 2011).

Giese, K. (2003) New Chinese migration to Germany: historical consistencies and new patterns of diversification within a globalised migration regime. *International Migration*, 41(3): 155–85.

Gilbert, A. and Koser, K. (2004) *Information dissemination to potential asylum seekers in countries of origin and/or transit*. London: Home Office (Research findings 220).

Gordon, I., Scanlon, K., Travers, T. and Whitehead, C. (2009) *Economic Impact on the London and UK Economy of an Earned Regularisation of Irregular Migrants to the UK*. London: GLA Economics.

Haug, W., Compton, P. and Courbage, Y. (eds) (2002) *The Demographic Characteristics of Immigrant Populations*. Strasbourg: Council of Europe.

Hughes, G. (2004) *International Migration*. The report of the Irish SOPEMI correspondent to the OECD. Dublin: Economic and Social Research Institute.

ICMPD (2010) *Year Book on Illegal Migration, Human Smuggling and Trafficking in Central and Eastern Europe*. Vienna: International Centre for Migration Policy Development.

IOM (2010) *World Migration Report 2010*. Geneva: International Organization for Migration.

Juchno, P. (2009) Asylum decisions in 2008. In: *Population and Social Conditions, Statistics in Focus 92/2009*. Luxembourg: Eurostat, European Commission.

Juhasz, J. (2000) Migrant trafficking and human smuggling in Hungary. In: Laczko, F. and Thompson, D. *Migrant Trafficking and Human Smuggling in Europe*. Geneva: International Organization for Migration: 167–232.

Klinchenko, T. (2000) Migrant trafficking and human smuggling in Ukraine. In: Laczko, F. and Thompson, D. *Migrant Trafficking and Human Smuggling in Europe*. Geneva: International Organization for Migration: 329–416.

Koser, K. (2011) Why take the risk? Explaining migrant smuggling. In: Modood, T. and Salt, J. (eds) *Migration and Ethnicity*. Basingstoke: Palgrave Macmillan.

Kraler, A. and Iglicka, K. (2002) Labour migration in Central European Countries. In: Laczko, F., Stacher, I. and Klekowski von Koppenfels, A. (eds) *New Challenges for Migration Policy in Central and Eastern Europe*. The Hague: TMC Asser Press: 27–56.

Mai, N. and Schwander-Sievers, S. (2003) Albanian migration and new transnationalisms. *Journal of Ethnic and Migration Studies*, 29(6): 939–48.

Maresova, J. (2009). *Report of the Hungarian SOPEMI correspondent to the OECD*. Paris: OECD.

Michalon, B. (2004) Playing on ethnicity to be there and here: the three paradoxes of 'ethnic migrations'. In: *International Migration in Europe: New trends and new methods of analysis*. Papers from the 2nd Conference of the EAPS Working Group on International Migration in Europe, Rome, Italy, 25–27 November 2004.

OECD (2008) *International Migration Outlook*. Paris: Organisation for Economic Co-operation and Development.

OECD (2010) *International Migration Outlook*. Paris: Organisation for Economic Co-operation and Development.

Peraldi, M. (2004) Algerian routes: a new perspective on migrant and social mobilities. In: *International Migration in Europe: New trends and new methods of analysis*. Papers from the 2nd Conference of the EAPS Working Group on International Migration in Europe, Rome, Italy, 25–27 November 2004.

Piguet, E. and Losa, S. (2002) *Travailleurs de l'ombre? Demande de main-d'œuvre du domaine de l'asile et ampleur de l'emploi d'étrangers non déclarés en Suisse*. Zurich: Seisomo.

Pinkerton, C., McLaughlan, G. and Salt, J. (2004) *Sizing the illegally resident population in the UK*. London: Home Office (Home Office Online Report 58/04) (http://css.escwa.org.lb/SD/1017/Illegal-resident_UK.pdf, accessed 8 June 2011).

Potot, S. (2008) The Romanian circulatory migration: a case study. In: Bonifazi, C., Okolski, M., Schoorl, J. and Simon, P. (eds) *International Migration in Europe: New Trends and New Methods of Analysis*. Amsterdam: IMISCOE Research, Amsterdam University Press: 87–103.

Poulain, M., Perrin, N. and Singleton, A. (eds) (2006) *THESIM: Towards Harmonised European Statistics on International Migration*. Louvain: Presses Universitaire de Louvain.

Salt, J. (2006) *Current Trends in International Migration in Europe*. Strasbourg: Council of Europe.

Salt, J., Singleton A. and Hogarth, J. (1994) *Europe's International Migrants: Data Sources, Patterns and Trends*. London: HMSO.

Snel, E., de Boom, J. and Engbersen, G. (2004) *International Migration and the Netherlands*. The report of the Dutch SOPEMI correspondent to the OECD. Paris: OECD.

Sobotka, T. (2009) Data and Trends: Migration continent Europe. In: Coleman, D. and Ediev, D. (eds) *Vienna Yearbook of Population Research 2009: Impact of migration on demographic change and composition in Europe*. Vienna: Institute of Demography: 217–33.

Van der Leun, J.P., Engbersen, G. and van der Heijden, P. (1998) *Illegaliteit en criminaliteit. Schattingen, aanhoudingen en uitzettingen [Illegality and crime. Estimates, detentions and deportations.]* Rotterdam: Erasmus University.

Vasileva, K. (2009) Citizens of European countries account for the majority of the foreign population in EU-27 in 2008. In: *Population and Social Conditions, Statistics in Focus 92/2009*. Luxembourg: Eurostat, European Commission.

Wallace, C. (1999) Economic hardship, migration and survival strategies in East-Central Europe. *Sociological Series*, 35. Vienna: Institute of Advanced Studies.

Woodbridge, J. (2005) *Sizing the Unauthorised (Illegal) Population of the United Kingdom in 2001*. London: Home Office.

chapter three

Asylum, residency and citizenship policies and models of migrant incorporation

Anthony M. Messina

Introduction

This chapter examines the immigration and migrant incorporation (a more neutral concept than "integration") policies of European Union (EU) member states. Its main focus is third-country nationals (TCNs), i.e. citizens of countries outside the EU. Excluded from its purview are EU migrants who, in addition to enjoying the rights of residence and free movement throughout the Union as recognized under the Maastricht Treaty (EU 1992), can readily access health services in any member state and be reimbursed thanks to the coordination of national social security systems across the EU.

Three critical features can be distinguished that are common to the experience of TCNs migrating to the EU. First, both regular and irregular migrants face serious obstacles to acquiring or exercising basic social rights, including access to health care (Cholewinski 2005). Second, against a backdrop of general disadvantage, there are substantial disparities in accessing health care among different groups of migrants (such as asylum-seekers, family dependants, workers and undocumented migrants), disparities that are grounded in their different legal and social status (Huber et al. 2008). Finally, the degree to which migrants can access health care often varies significantly (Nørredam et al. 2005). Although TCNs everywhere face challenges in accessing health services and are among the least well cared-for populations within the EU (Chauvin et al. 2007), differences among categories of migrants within individual countries and across countries persist, despite a growing Europeanization of immigration policies (Rosenow 2009).

What accounts for these differences? One possible explanation – that health care provision and incorporation regimes for TCNs are more or less generous depending on the size of the TCN population – can be summarily dismissed, since high incorporation scores have been earned by some EU countries (such as Italy, Spain and Ireland) with medium to high numbers of TCNs as a percentage of the total population, while countries with low incorporation scores (such as Malta, Poland and Slovakia) have a much smaller share of TCNs as a percentage of the total population (Münz 2006; Niessen et al. 2007). Rather, this chapter argues that national differences in the ability of migrants to access health care reflect the patchwork of national immigration and migrant incorporation regimes currently prevailing in Europe. Differences in national policies on asylum, residency, citizenship and broader aspects of migrant incorporation contribute to much, if not most, of the variation evident in the ability of migrants to access health care across the EU (Sicakkan 2008a). In essence, health services for migrants in each country cannot be divorced from the broader immigration policy regimes in which they are embedded. The central purpose of this chapter is to delineate some of the key differences among the 27 EU member states on asylum, residency and citizenship policies and their respective models of migrant incorporation.

Asylum

The Treaty of Amsterdam (1997) established the EU's legal competence in the areas of freedom, security and justice (EU 1997). Extending this foundation, the 1999 Tampere and 2004 Hague Programmes set out to create a Common European Asylum System (CEAS) whose core objective is to implement a policy regime which mandates common standards based on fair and efficient asylum procedures. The first phase of constructing the CEAS came to fruition with the adoption of the legal instruments created by the Temporary Protection Mechanism Directive (2001), the Dublin Regulation (2003), the Reception Conditions Directive (2003), the Qualification Directive (2004), and the Asylum Procedures Directive (2005). Reflecting the CEAS's aspirations, the Qualification Directive establishes minimum standards for the qualification and status of TCNs and stateless persons, either as refugees or persons who otherwise need international protection. The Asylum Procedures Directive, in turn, seeks to ensure that all national asylum procedures in the first instance satisfy the same minimum standards throughout the EU. With some exceptions, the Asylum Procedures Directive mandates that asylum-seekers be allowed the opportunity of a personal interview concerning their application. It also establishes basic principles and guarantees for scrutinizing their claims, including *inter alia* the provision of comprehensive information at the start of the process about the procedures that will take place, access to legal assistance and interpretation services, and the obligation on EU member states to meet the needs of unaccompanied minors.

Since Tampere, the EU's legal jurisdiction over asylum and immigration policy has steadily expanded. Indeed, most of the policy-making authority for asylum and immigration under the EU's Justice and Home Affairs pillar was changed from unanimous to majority voting within the European Council beginning in 2005, increasing the decision-making power of the Council in this policy area. Furthermore, in 2002, the European Commission was granted the prerogative to propose new legislation. In 2008, the French Presidency of the European Council proposed a new "European Pact on Immigration" which established the goal of achieving a Common Asylum Policy by 2012, an aspiration reinforced in the Stockholm Programme adopted in 2009 (Council of the EU 2009).

As a result of these and other initiatives, the goal of forging a common European asylum policy has undeniably moved closer in recent years. Indeed, the degree of asylum policy coordination achieved thus far at the EU level has created interdependency among member states. Nevertheless, despite common rules and the fact that asylum has increasingly been subsumed within the EU's jurisdiction, national practices continue to vary, especially with regard to the conditions for receiving migrants, the processing of asylum claims and migrant return policies (European Council on Refugees and Exiles 2010). Moreover, even after having been granted asylum, refugees tend to be treated differently across member states, so that some EU countries are perceived by asylum-seekers as far more attractive destinations than others.

Across the EU as a whole, just over one quarter of all persons seeking asylum in 2009 were recognized as genuine in the first instance. Of the 78,800 persons who were ultimately granted protection status, 39,000 were granted refugee status, 29,900 subsidiary protection and 9600 authorization to stay for humanitarian reasons. Yet, primarily as a consequence of divergent national practices, the chances of being granted protection vary significantly from one member state to the next. The extent of this variation is illustrated by Table 3.1. The chances of obtaining asylum in the first instance were virtually nil in Greece in 2009. In contrast, persons seeking asylum in Bulgaria, Denmark, Malta, the Netherlands, Portugal and Slovakia had greater than two in five chances of obtaining asylum. Italy, Greece's Mediterranean neighbour, granted asylum to more than 38% of all applicants (Eurostat 2010b).

Why do these differences in national recognition rates persist? The short answer is that, despite the increasing Europeanization of asylum policy, national institutions and practices continue to matter. In general, the greater the number of actors involved in asylum decision-making bodies within a particular country, the higher the asylum recognition rate. According to Sicakkan (2008b) asylum decision systems that allow a multiplicity of domestic actors – central authorities, courts, non-governmental organizations (NGOs), asylum boards, etc. – to participate in asylum decisions tend to yield comparatively robust recognition rates. In addition, however, the share of legitimate claims may also differ across different European countries due to asylum-seekers' different countries of origin.

Beyond this headline variation in numbers, a recent report issued by the United Nations High Commissioner for Refugees (UNHCR) highlights the considerable differences between EU member states in how they scrutinize the merits of asylum claims and how vigorously or conscientiously they apply

Table 3.1 EU member state decisions on asylum applications (2009)

Country	Rate of recognition (in %)	
	First instance	Final appeal
Malta	65.7	0.0
Slovakia	56.2	41.7
Portugal	51.1	–
Netherlands	48.3	33.8
Denmark	47.9	29.7
Bulgaria	41.7	21.6
Poland	38.4	92.1
Italy	38.4	12.5
Germany	36.5	34.1
Finland	36.2	80.6
Sweden	29.6	12.9
Lithuania	29.4	9.3
Cyprus	29.3	3.0
EU	27.0	19.2
United Kingdom	26.9	30.0
Luxembourg	23.6	15.3
Austria	21.7	15.0
Hungary	21.5	5.3
Romania	20.8	14.2
Belgium	20.2	3.8
Latvia	19.0	20.0
Czech Republic	18.8	6.0
Estonia	17.4	0.0
Slovenia	15.2	0.0
France	14.3	27.4
Spain	7.8	1.8
Ireland	4.0	7.8
Greece	1.2	2.0

Source: Eurostat (2010b)

the Asylum Procedures Directive. According to the report, the directive (UNHCR 2010: 4)

> has not, based on UNHCR's observations, achieved the harmonization of legal standards or practice across the EU. This is partly due to the wide scope of many provisions, which explicitly permit divergent practice and exceptions and derogations. It is also due, however, to differing interpretations of many articles (including mandatory provisions), and different approaches to their application.

As Anneliese Baldaccini, an expert on EU asylum policies at Amnesty International, has astutely observed, the EU "has a set of common rules... [but they] have been interpreted in different ways by Member States, meaning there is no level playing field" (Earth Times 2009). Instead, differences in national asylum policy regimes across the EU have created a virtual "lottery" for asylum-seekers and potential refugees.

Long-term residency

In conferring authority upon the Community in the policy areas of immigration and asylum, the Treaty of Amsterdam facilitated the introduction of the Long-Term Residents Directive in 2003 which regulates the status of TCNs who are long-term residents, i.e. TCNs who are legally and continuously resident in an EU country for five years. Prior to this period, the rights of TCNs, including access to health services, are almost exclusively defined by national laws and general international human rights instruments (Cholewinski 2005; Huber et al. 2008). The 2003 directive created a single status for long-term residents and guaranteed equal treatment with nationals with regard to access to:

- employment and self-employment;
- education and vocational training;
- recognition of professional diplomas, certificates and other qualifications;
- social security, assistance and protection;
- tax benefits;
- access to goods and services;
- freedom of association, affiliation and membership;
- free movement across the entire territory of the EU.

To obtain long-term resident status, TCNs must prove that they have a stable financial income, as well as, in countries with social health insurance systems, health insurance for themselves and their families. All EU member states, except Denmark, Ireland and the United Kingdom, which have opted out of the common immigration, asylum and civil law policies, must comply with the directive and implement it according to the principle of non-discrimination, pursuant to Article 13 of the 1997 Treaty of Amsterdam and Article 21 of the 2000 Charter of Fundamental Rights. Once a permanent residence permit has been obtained, the right to reside indefinitely in the host country is no longer linked to the original motive for migration. The practical effect of this incremental process is that the longer migrants reside in the host country, the more rights they tend to enjoy, eventually achieving par with those of nationals.

Given these common rights, the key question is how the issuance of long-term residence permits is regulated nationally across the EU. Although the Long-Term Residents Directive seeks to standardize the rules governing long-term residence within the EU and, in so doing, displace national permanent residence permits, the process of transposing the directive has led to the curious outcome that in a number of member states there is both a national permanent residence permit and the EU long-term residence permit. Moreover, the conditions for granting national permanent residence permits frequently vary. Member states may require TCNs to comply with integration requirements, including demonstrating sufficient knowledge of the respective national language. Member states may also refuse to grant long-term resident status on the grounds of public security. Moreover, in some instances, they may prevent equal treatment with nationals with respect to access to employment and education, e.g. by requiring proof of language proficiency. Finally, they may also restrict access to core benefits in the fields of social assistance and protection.

Regardless of the specific situation in a given EU member state, several categories of migrants are automatically excluded from the scope of the Long-Term Residents Directive because their situation is precarious or because they are resident on a short-term basis only. Article 3 of the Long-Term Residents Directive, for example, expressly excludes TCNs who are authorized to reside in a member state on the basis of temporary protection; those who have applied for authorization to reside on the basis of temporary protection and are awaiting a decision on their status; those authorized to reside in a member state on the basis of a subsidiary form of protection; refugees; and those who have applied for recognition as refugees and whose application has not yet been finally decided. The directive also excludes seasonal workers.

To what extent do national policies on long-term residence diverge? By assigning a composite score to each member state on the basis of whether they have "critically unfavourable", "unfavourable", "slightly unfavourable", "halfway to best practice", "slightly favourable", "favourable" or "best practice" policies on access of migrants to long-term residence, Niessen et al. (2007) have illuminated the considerable divide separating the most from the least generous member states. According to this classification, Sweden, Belgium and Spain figure among the most generous member states, while Ireland, Lithuania, Cyprus, France and Luxembourg are the least generous ones. As Table 3.2 indicates, the member states do not cluster together according to the timing of their entry into the EU. Rather, the average score for the 10 countries that joined the EU in 2004 (EU10) (57) is slightly lower than that of the EU15 (61) and the average of all 27 member states (60).

Table 3.2 Quality of migrant access to long-term residence across the EU (2007)

Country	Scores*	Country	Scores*
Sweden	76	Estonia	61
Belgium	74	Greece	60
Norway	72	EU27	60
Spain	70	EU10	57
United Kingdom	67	Austria	55
Portugal	67	Germany	53
Poland	67	Switzerland	51
Italy	67	Slovakia	51
Denmark	67	Latvia	51
Netherlands	66	Hungary	50
Malta	65	Luxembourg	48
Finland	65	France	48
Slovenia	63	Cyprus	47
Czech Republic	63	Lithuania	47
EU15	61	Ireland	39

NOTE: *Scores are on the following scale: 0 (critically unfavourable); 1–20 (unfavourable); 21–40 (slightly unfavourable); 41–59 (halfway to best practice); 60–79 (slightly favourable); 80–99 (favourable); and best practice (100).

Source: Niessen et al. (2007).

According to Niessen et al. (2007), in the most inclusive member states, TCNs are eligible to become long-term residents and full "civic citizens" after five or fewer years of legal residence. They are subjected to fair and transparent procedures; their application can only be refused or their permit withdrawn if they are found guilty of fraud in trying to acquire it; they enjoy the same access to education and vocational training as nationals; and they have the right to accept employment, except where they would have to exercise public authority. Moreover, they are eligible for social security, social assistance, health care, and housing benefit.

Conversely, in the least generous member states, migrants must wait eight years or longer and surmount numerous obstacles in order to become eligible for long-term resident status. They must pass a mandatory integration course and expensive written test in order to prove that they possess a high degree of knowledge of the country's language and culture, plus satisfy stringent employment, income and insurance requirements. Moreover, their status can be withdrawn for numerous reasons, including becoming unemployed. They have little protection against expulsion and, upon retiring, lose the right to reside within the country.

Citizenship

The concept of EU citizenship was formally introduced by the 1992 Maastricht Treaty which specified that "every person holding the nationality of a member state shall be a citizen of the Union" (Article 8, Paragraph 1). According to the Treaty on the Functioning of the European Union (Article 20), "citizenship of the Union shall be additional to and not replace national citizenship" (EU 2008). As such, the concept of EU citizenship specifies a set of rights and obligations, including the right not to be discriminated on the basis of nationality. The 1997 Amsterdam Treaty reaffirmed the principle that EU citizenship is a derivative of national citizenship.

Although TCNs, including asylum-seekers, have acquired "bundles of rights" under the 2007 Lisbon Treaty (EU 2007), and specifically under the EU Charter of Fundamental Rights (Guild 2010), two things have remained unchanged since the Maastricht Treaty. First, it remains primarily within the purview of the member states to decide who is and who is not an EU citizen. Even if residing legally within the Community, a TCN must first acquire the nationality of a member state in order to become an EU citizen. Second, neither Maastricht nor subsequent EU treaties have mandated that national citizenship regimes should be harmonized. This means that the EU still has no competence to regulate national citizenship policies. The requirements for obtaining national citizenship consequently continue to vary, as they have historically, from one member state to the next.

The extent of this variation is illustrated in Table 3.3 which compares national citizenship policies (see also Table 3.4 on naturalization rates). Informed by Howard's (2009) Citizenship Policy Index, the last column in Table 3.3 adds together three inter-related factors linked to citizenship: whether children of non-citizens who are born on a country's territory can acquire national

Table 3.3 Components of citizenship policies across the EU (2008)

Category	Country	Jus soli (0–2)	Naturalization requirements (0–2)	Dual citizenship for immigrants (0–2)	CPI score (0–6)
Restrictive	Austria	0.00	0.00	0.00	0.00
	Denmark	0.00	0.00	0.00	0.00
	Lithuania	0.00	0.00	0.00	0.00
	Slovenia	0.00	0.00	0.00	0.00
	Cyprus	0.00	0.11	0.00	0.11
	Czech Republic	0.00	0.68	0.00	0.68
	Estonia	0.00	0.68	0.00	0.68
	Latvia	0.00	0.68	0.00	0.68
	Poland	0.00	0.68	0.00	0.68
	Romania	0.00	0.68	0.00	0.68
	Greece	0.00	0.00	1.00	1.00
	Hungary	0.00	0.00	1.25	1.25
	Spain	0.50	0.38	0.50	1.38
	Italy	0.00	0.25	1.25	1.50
Medium	Bulgaria	0.00	0.68	1.25	1.93
	Malta	0.00	0.68	1.25	1.93
	Slovakia	0.00	0.68	1.25	1.93
	Germany	0.75	0.54	0.75	2.04
	Luxembourg	1.00	0.00	1.25	2.25
Liberal	Netherlands	1.50	1.22	1.50	4.22
	Finland	1.00	1.32	2.00	4.32
	Portugal	1.75	1.07	1.50	4.32
	Ireland	2.00	1.36	1.50	4.86
	France	1.50	1.47	2.00	4.97
	UK	1.75	1.22	2.00	4.97
	Sweden	1.50	1.72	2.00	5.22
	Belgium	1.50	2.00	2.00	5.50

Source: Howard (2009).

citizenship immediately after birth or automatically after a specified period; the minimum length of a country's residency requirement for naturalization of immigrants and immigrant spouses who are married to citizens; and whether or not naturalized immigrants are allowed to hold dual citizenship. Each factor is scored on a 0–2 scale.

As Table 3.3 indicates, even after the 2007 Lisbon Treaty, the citizenship regimes of some member states (Austria, Denmark, Lithuania and Slovenia) are far more exclusive than those of others (Belgium, France, Sweden and the United Kingdom). Indeed, *jus soli* (whereby citizenship is acquired by birth on the territory of the respective state, unlike *jus sanguinis*, in which citizenship is acquired by descent) currently applies in only 19 of 27 member states, and even where it exists it often does so only in weak form. Moreover, although no EU country grants an automatic right to citizenship to children of undocumented migrants and the policies of member states for obtaining citizenship through *jus soli* converge more than their naturalization or dual citizenship policies, the

Table 3.4 Acquisition of citizenship across the EU (2007–08)

	Citizenships acquired		Citizenships acquired per:	
	2007	2008	1000 inhabitants	1000 foreign residents
Belgium	36,060	NA	NA	NA
Cyprus	2,780	NA	NA	NA
Poland	1540	1800	0.0	48
Czech Republic	2370	1200	0.1	3
Lithuania	370	310	0.1	7
Slovakia	1480	480	0.1	9
Romania	30	5590	0.3	NA
Ireland	4650	3250	0.7	6
Hungary	8440	8100	0.8	43
Slovenia	1550	1690	0.8	24
Bulgaria	5970	7140	0.9	NA
Italy	45,490	53,700	0.9	14
Denmark	3650	6020	1.1	19
Germany	113,030	94,470	1.2	13
Austria	14,010	10,270	1.2	12
Finland	4820	6680	1.3	47
EU27*	707,110	695,880	1.4	23
Greece	3920	16,920	1.5	18
Estonia	4240	2120	1.6	10
Malta	550	640	1.6	36
Netherlands	30,650	28,230	1.7	39
Spain	71,940	84,170	1.8	15
Latvia	8320	4230	1.9	10
France	132,000	137,320	2.1	37
Portugal	NA	22,410	2.1	51
United Kingdom	164,540	129,260	2.1	31
Luxembourg	1240	1220	2.5	6
Sweden	33,630	30,460	3.3	54

NOTES: *Includes estimates for member states for which data are not available;
NA: not available.

Source: Eurostat (2010b)

overall Citizenship Policy Index score varies considerably across member states, from 0.0 to 5.5.

If anything, the EU's enlargements in 2004 and 2007 have only increased the divide between the most and the least liberal citizenship regimes, as the central and eastern European member states are disproportionately represented in the most restrictive group of countries. In practice, this means that in the most inclusive member states TCNs are eligible for nationality after only three years of residence, dual nationality is permitted, and being tied to the country by residence or family are the main criteria for becoming a national. In contrast, in one or more of the most restrictive countries, TCNs must wait up to 10 years to apply for citizenship, are not allowed dual citizenship and must prove they are sufficiently integrated into the host country by passing a mandatory written test about its dominant culture, history, language and society. Moreover, in the most inclusive member state (Belgium) new citizens can only lose their citizenship within a five-year period of gaining it, and only if they have committed fraud in obtaining it. In the least inclusive countries, on the other hand, the state can revoke an immigrant's citizenship on numerous grounds at any time, even if in so doing the affected individual becomes stateless (Niessen et al. 2007).

National models of incorporation

Concerns among EU officials about the challenge of successfully incorporating, or "integrating", migrants into the Community are long-standing. However, although numerous legislative measures in the areas of anti-discrimination, employment policy and social affairs have articulated the goal of facilitating the incorporation of TCNs, it was only relatively recently that the EU, and particularly the European Commission, aspired to establish a common policy framework. At the Tampere European Council in 1999, for example, EU leaders called for the adoption of a common immigration policy, including policies to facilitate the incorporation of TCNs. The aspiration of these new incorporation policies was to allow TCNs to exercise rights and fulfil obligations comparable to those of EU citizens. With regard to exercising rights, the Racial Equality Directive was adopted in 2000 to combat discrimination based on "racial or ethnic origin", prohibiting discrimination in the areas of education, employment and occupation, vocational training, membership of employer and employee organizations, social protection (including social security and health care), and access to goods and services (including housing).

In 2004, the Hague Programme for 2005–2010 broadly reiterated the goal of coordinating migrant incorporation policies by setting out that a shared policy framework, based on common basic principles, should underpin future EU initiatives. Such Common Basic Principles were adopted by the Justice and Home Affairs Council of 19 November 2004 and further refined in the Common Agenda for Integration, which was adopted by the European Commission in 2005.

Following these initiatives, the Lisbon Treaty in 2007 established a new legal foundation for TCN incorporation (EU 2007). According to Article 79.4 of the Treaty,

> the European Parliament and the Council, acting in accordance with the ordinary legislative procedure, may establish measures to provide incentives and support for the action of Member States with a view to promoting the integration of third country nationals residing legally in their territories, excluding any harmonization of the laws and regulations of the Member States.

In 2009, the Stockholm Programme for 2010–2014 (Council of the EU 2009) further specified that the successful incorporation of legally resident TCNs is imperative in order to maximize the benefits of immigration. It stated that the integration policies of member states should be supported through the development of structures for exchanging information and coordinating with other related policy areas, such as employment, education and social inclusion. It invited the Commission to support the integration efforts of member states "through the development of a coordination mechanism using a common reference framework, which should improve structures and tools for European knowledge exchange". It also exhorted the Commission to identify ways of supporting integration efforts of member states and to develop indicators for monitoring the results of integration policies.

Because the Common Basic Principles perceive TCN integration as a two-way process, based on a reciprocal relationship in which migrants have obligations as well as economic, political and social rights, member state governments retain ample authority to establish national integration conditions that migrants must satisfy in order to acquire such rights. As a consequence, most member states continue to pursue something approximating national models of incorporation in confronting the domestic challenges posed by mass immigration and immigrant settlement. According to Rodríguez-García et al. (2007: 15–16), these national incorporation models have tended historically

> to be divided into three types: assimilationist or republican (based on the idea that equality can be achieved through the full adoption of the rules and values of the dominant society and through the avoidance of any considerations of diversity, as in the case of France); multiculturalist or pluralist (based on the respect for and protection of cultural diversity within a framework of shared belonging, as in the cases of Sweden, the Netherlands, the UK, and Canada); and a segregationist or exclusion model [...] characterized by separation between, or fragmentation of, ethnic-cultural communities, and distinguished particularly by its restrictive legal framework regarding access to citizenship, based on the ethno-racial criterion of jus sanguinis, as in the cases of Austria, Germany, and Switzerland.

This said, Freeman (2004: 960) appropriately cautions that:

> rather than anticipating a small number of distinct 'modes of immigrant incorporation' that might characterize the policies of particular countries, we should expect different modes in particular domains – state, market, welfare, culture – within individual states; the overall outcome being a mixed bag not fully assimilationist, pluralist, or multicultural.

Against the backdrop of the continued relevance of national models of migrant incorporation and their uneven applicability across specific domains within the respective member states, a 2007 survey (Niessen et al. 2007) rather predictably discovered considerable national diversity in how well member states incorporate migrants. Based on 140 indicators, including the rights of migrants in the workplace, opportunities for permanent settlement, family reunification policy and the enactment and enforcement of domestic laws to combat racism and prejudice, they reported that Sweden, Portugal, Belgium, the Netherlands and Finland do the most to facilitate migrant incorporation and settlement, while Latvia, Cyprus, Austria, Greece and Slovakia do the least. The five states with the largest immigrant populations at the time of the survey – France, Germany, Italy, Spain and the United Kingdom – ranked in the top half of the group, with Italy performing best. Overall, the study found that only Sweden could be classified as a polity that is wholly favourable to promoting migrant incorporation. While many other member states pursued laudable policies, each fell short in at least one key area. Collectively, they were judged to be doing only half as much as they potentially could.

As Hochschild and Mollenkopf (2009: 17) have observed, "the conditions under which immigrants move into a host country affect the terms and ease with which they can pursue incorporation." It is in this context that Hansen (2008) has underscored the restrictive naturalization policies that have been implemented by many member states in the 2000s. During this period, some member states (Belgium, Germany) have recently made access to citizenship for the second generation somewhat easier, while others (Greece) have restricted such access. Similarly, while some member states (Luxembourg) have facilitated naturalization for first-generation migrants, others (United Kingdom) have erected new barriers, including naturalization tests. In sum, rather than serving as a vehicle for migrant incorporation, as it has historically, many, if not most, member state governments now view naturalization as the culmination of the incorporation process (Hansen 2008).

Not surprisingly, one of the consequences of these disparate national models is that TCN naturalization rates vary greatly across the EU. Table 3.4 shows the acquisition of citizenship in EU member states per 1000 inhabitants and foreign residents in 2007–08. Although these data must be interpreted with caution, as not all TCNs are eligible to naturalize, they illustrate that the naturalization process is much more daunting in some member states than in others. As shown in Table 3.4, Sweden (with 3.3 citizenships granted per 1000 inhabitants), Luxembourg (2.5), France, Portugal and the United Kingdom (all 2.1) granted the highest rates of citizenship per inhabitants in 2007–08. In contrast, fewer than one citizenship per 1000 inhabitants was granted to TCNs in ten member states, with Poland, the Czech Republic, Lithuania and Slovakia allowing the fewest. Of the approximately 696,000 persons who acquired the citizenship of an EU member state in 2008, most originated from Africa (29%), non-EU Europe (22%), Asia (19%) and north and south America (17%).

Conclusions

There is little question that "decisive changes towards the Europeanization of rights for TCNs" have occurred in the 2000s and that "as a result of the new EU directives, the traditional distinction between EU citizens and TCNs in terms of their respective rights" has begun to erode (Rosenow 2009: 134–5). Potentially, the most significant recent advance in this respect is the Stockholm Programme's commitment to grant TCNs staying for at least five years rights and obligations comparable to those of EU citizens by 2014, a pledge which harks back to the Tampere Programme's agenda some ten years earlier. Moreover, as argued above, a European migrant incorporation policy has received a significant boost from the Lisbon Treaty, which gives supranational policy-makers a legal foundation on which to develop measures to "support" national strategies for incorporating migrants.

Yet, several factors obstruct the realization of these goals. First, as we saw above, despite the fact that asylum has increasingly been subsumed under the policy jurisdiction of the EU, national practices continue to vary. Moreover, even after having been granted asylum, refugees tend to be treated differently across member states. Second, member states may continue to refuse to grant long-term resident status to TCNs on the grounds of public security. Moreover, in some instances, they may deny them equal treatment with nationals with respect to access to employment, education and core benefits in social assistance and protection. Third, it remains very much within the purview of member states to decide who is and who is not an EU citizen; neither the Maastricht Treaty nor subsequent EU treaties have mandated that national citizenship policies should be harmonized. Finally, because the Common Basic Principles perceive migrant integration as a reciprocal relationship in which migrants have obligations as well as rights, member state governments retain ample authority to establish national integration conditions that migrants must satisfy in order to acquire significant rights. Consequently, most member states continue to pursue national models of migrant incorporation, which vary in their level of inclusivity.

Why do these persistent national differences matter? Ingleby et al. (2005) have persuasively argued that different national ideologies concerning citizenship and diversity lead to different policy outcomes with regard to migrants' rights; moreover, the degree to which migrants are successfully incorporated plays an important role in health service delivery because good communication and mutual understanding are essential for effective care. It is undoubtedly no coincidence that EU member states, that have been historically reluctant to perceive themselves as countries of immigration (such as Germany), tend not to include indicators of immigration in their national health surveys and, as a consequence, are not well positioned to incorporate the special needs of migrants into their health care systems (Mladovsky 2007; see also Chapter 6 on "Monitoring the health of migrants"). Although, as we have seen above, migrant incorporation regimes are becoming increasingly Europeanized, in the interim the persistence of national differences is likely to contribute to significant variation in the accessibility and quality of health services for migrants across the EU.

References

Chauvin, P., Drouot, N., Parizot, I., Simonnot, N. and Tomasin, A. (2007) *European Survey on Undocumented Migrants' Access to Healthcare.* Paris: Médecins du Monde European Observatory on Access to Health Care.

Cholewinski, R. (2005) *Study on Obstacles to Effective Access of Irregular Migrants to Minimum Social Rights.* Strasbourg: Council of Europe Publishing.

Commission of the European Communities (2005) *A Common Agenda for Integration Framework for the Integration of Third-Country Nationals in the European Union* (http://eur-lex.europa.eu/LexUriServ/LexUriServ.do?uri=COM:2005:0389:FIN:EN:PDF, accessed 15 May 2011).

Council of the EU (2009) *The Stockholm Programme – an open and secure Europe serving and protecting the citizens* (http://www.statewatch.org/news/2009/nov/eu-draft-stockholm-programme-23-11-09-16484-09.pdf, accessed 15 May 2010).

Earth Times (2009) *Brussels seeks end to EU 'asylum lottery'* (http://www.earthtimes.org/articles/news/291181,brussels-seeks-end-to-eu-asylum-lottery.html, accessed 15 May 2011).

EU (1992) *The Maastricht Treaty: Provisions amending the treaty establishing the European Economic Community with a view to establishing the European Community* (http://www.eurotreaties.com/maastrichtec.pdf, accessed 15 May 2011).

EU (1997) *Treaty of Amsterdam amending the Treaty on European Union, the treaties establishing the European Communities and certain related acts.* Luxembourg: Office for Official Publications of the European Communities (http://www.europarl.europa.eu/topics/treaty/pdf/amst-en.pdf, accessed 15 May 2010).

EU (2007) Treaty of Lisbon amending the Treaty on European Union and the Treaty establishing the European Community (2007) *Official Journal of the European Union,* C306 (17.12.2007) (http://eur-lex.europa.eu/JOHtml.do?uri=OJ:C:2007:306:SOM:EN:HTML, accessed 15 May 2010).

EU (2008) Consolidated Version of the Treaty on the Functioning of the European Union, *Official Journal of the European Union,* C115: 48-199 (9.5.2008) (http://eur-lex.europa.eu/LexUriServ/LexUriServ.do?uri=OJ:C:2008:115:0047:0199:EN:PDF, accessed 16 June 2011).

European Council on Refugees and Exiles (2010) *Comments from the European Council on Refugees and Exiles on the European Commission Proposal to recast the Asylum Procedures Directive* (http://www.ecre.org/files/ECRE_Comments_APD_May_2010.pdf, accessed 6 June 2011).

Eurostat (2010a) *Acquisition of citizenship in the EU: EU27 Member States granted citizenship to 696 000 persons in 2008* (http://epp.eurostat.ec.europa.eu/cache/ITY_PUBLIC/3-06072010-AP/EN/3-06072010-AP-EN.PDF, accessed 15 May 2011).

Eurostat (2010b) *Asylum decisions in the EU27: EU Member States granted protection to 78 800 asylum seekers in 2009* (http://epp.eurostat.ec.europa.eu/cache/ITY_PUBLIC/3-18062010-AP/EN/3-18062010-AP-EN.PDF, accessed 15 May 2011).

Freeman, G.P. (2004) Immigrant incorporation in western democracies. *International Migration Review,* 38(3): 945–69.

Guild, E. (2010) *The European Union after the Treaty of Lisbon: Fundamental Rights and EU Citizenship.* Global Jean Monnet/European Community Studies Association World Conference, 25–26 May 2010 (http://www.ceps.eu/system/files/book/2010/07/Guild%20Jean%20Monnet%20speech%20e-version.pdf, accessed 15 May 2011).

Hansen, R. (2008) The poverty of postnationalism: citizenship, immigration, and the new Europe. *Theory and Society,* 38(1): 1–24.

Hochschild, J.L. and Mollenkopf, J.H. (2009) Modeling immigrant political incorporation. In: Hochschild, J.L. and Mollenkopf, J.H. (eds) *Bringing Outsiders In: Transatlantic Perspectives on Immigrant Political Incorporation.* Ithaca, New York: Cornell University Press: 15–30.

Howard, M.M. (2009) *The Politics of Citizenship in Europe.* New York: Cambridge University Press.

Huber, M., Stanicole, A., Bremner, J. and Wahlbeck, K. (2008) *Quality in and Equality of Access to Healthcare Services.* Luxembourg: European Commission Directorate-General for Employment, Social Affairs and Equal Opportunities.

Ingleby, D., Chimienti, M., Hatziprokopiou, P., Ormond, M. and De Freitas, C. (2005) The role of health integration. In: Fonseca, M.L. and Malheiros, J. (eds) *Social Integration and Mobility: Education, Housing and Health.* Lisbon: Centro de Estudos Geográficos: 101–37.

Mladovsky, P. (2007) Migrant health in the EU. *Eurohealth,* 13(1): 9–10.

Münz, R. (2006) Europe: Population and Migration in 2005. *Migration Information Source* (http://www.migrationinformation.org/feature/print.cfm?ID=402, accessed 15 May 2011).

Niessen, J., Huddleston, T., Citron, L., with Geddes, A. and Jacobs, D. (2007) *Migrant Integration Policy Index*. Brussels: British Council and Migration Policy Group.

Nørredam, M., Mygind, A. and Krasnik, A. (2006) Access to health care for asylum seekers in the European Union – a comparative study of country policies. *European Journal of Public Health*, 16(3): 286–90.

Rodríguez-García, D., Biles, J., Winnemore, L. and Michalowski, I. (2007) *Policies and Models of Incorporation. A Transatlantic Perspective: Canada, Germany, France and The Netherlands*. Barcelona: Fundació CIDOB.

Rosenow, K. (2009) The Europeanisation of integration policies. *International Migration*, 47(1): 133–59.

Sicakkan, H.G. (2008a) *Do Our Citizenship Requirements Impede the Protection of Political Asylum Seekers? A Comparative Analysis of European Practices*. Lewiston, New York: The Edward Mellen Press.

Sicakkan, H.G. (2008b). Political asylum and sovereignty-sharing in Europe. *Government and Opposition*, 43(2): 206–29.

UNHCR (2010) *Improving Asylum Procedures: Comparative Analysis and Recommendations for Law and Practice*. Brussels: United Nations High Commissioner for Refugees.

Vasileva, K. (2010) Foreigners living in the EU are diverse and largely younger than the nationals of the EU Member States. *Statistics in Focus*, 45. Luxembourg: Eurostat, European Commission.

Section III

Access to health services

chapter four

The right to health of migrants in Europe

Paola Pace

Introduction

On 19 October 2010, the Secretary-General of the United Nations (UN), Ban Ki-Moon, warned Europe against a new "politics of polarization" (United Nations 2010) in relation to immigration. He told the 27-nation European Parliament in Strasbourg, France, that almost seven years ago, his predecessor, Kofi Annan, had "made an impassioned call for Europe to seize the opportunities presented by immigration and to resist those who demonized these newcomers as 'the other'" (United Nations 2010). Ban Ki-Moon went on: "I wish I could report, today, that the situation in Europe has improved over the intervening years. But as a friend of Europe, I share profound concern" (United Nations 2010). The UN Secretary-General pointed out that none of Europe's largest and wealthiest powers had signed or ratified the International Convention on the Protection of the Rights of All Migrant Workers and Members of Their Families, 20 years after it had been adopted. "In some of the world's most advanced democracies, among nations that take just pride in their long history of social progressiveness, migrants are being denied basic human rights", he said (United Nations 2010).

Indeed, for migrants in Europe, limitations or denials of basic rights are daily occurrences. This can be illustrated by some cases from different European Union (EU) member states in 2009–10. A 32-year-old pregnant asylum-seeker, a mother of three, died in an asylum reception centre with allegations that her medical condition had been neglected and that she was abandoned on a mattress in the hallway, with no attempt to call an ambulance. A detainee certified to be suffering from asthma died the day after his request to be hospitalized was ignored. A 20-year-old asylum-seeker died of a heart attack four weeks into a hunger strike while being held in preventive custody at a police centre. In detention or reception centres throughout Europe, numerous children and young adults have committed suicide and countless others have harmed themselves. Neglect of medical and mental health needs has been cited in the European Race Audit as a contributory factor to these tragedies (European Race Audit 2010).

Each of these stories is unique since migrants have different needs and fall into different categories; they may be asylum-seekers and refugees, victims of human trafficking, reunified family members, students, migrant workers, in a regular or irregular situation, and working in the formal or informal sector. Yet, all have the right to health, which all European countries have a legal obligation to uphold.

This chapter provides an overview of key international, European and national provisions on the right to health and discusses how far these provisions are being implemented in practice. It first discusses the international legal framework by which EU member states are bound. This is followed by an exploration of relevant Council of Europe instruments, as well as EU provisions and national legal obligations.

The international legal framework

All EU member states have formally recognized the right of everyone to the highest attainable standard of physical and mental health. This right has been enshrined in numerous international and European legal instruments, which European countries have agreed to be bound by. There are various international mechanisms available to protect and provide redress in the event of a violation of the right to health, which may be activated once the claimant has exhausted local remedies. In many instances, this obligation to respect the right to health is enshrined in national rules, including in the constitution and other laws (Perruchoud 2007).

All EU member states are also members of the UN and have acceded to most of its core international human rights treaties, including the International Covenant on Economic, Social and Cultural Rights, Article 12 of which sets out "the right of everyone to the enjoyment of the highest attainable standard of physical and mental health", belonging to every human being, irrespective of his or her nationality (United Nations 1966).

However, as Ban Ki-Moon indicated, none of the EU member states has signed, ratified or acceded to the International Convention on the Protection of the Rights of All Migrant Workers and Members of Their Families. During the Universal Periodic Review, a review of the human rights records of all 192 UN member states once every four years, some EU member states noted that they had made progress in extending the legal protection of migrants according to the intention of the Convention, but without formally recognizing it. The Convention provides for the right to equal treatment with regard to access to social and health services for regular migrant workers and members of their families. In addition, Article 28 recognizes the right to emergency medical treatment for all migrant workers and members of their families, regardless of the regularity of their stay or employment (United Nations 1990). However, it is worth pointing out that mere commitment to the provision of emergency care to migrants fails to meet the principle of non-discrimination set out in

Article 2 of the International Covenant on Economic, Social and Cultural Rights. Indeed, Article 81 of the International Convention on the Protection of the Rights of All Migrant Workers and Members of Their Families clarifies that the Convention does not constrain the granting of more favourable rights or freedoms granted to migrant workers and their families by domestic law or any other international treaty, such as the International Covenant on Economic, Social and Cultural Rights.

All EU member states are also parties to the Convention relating to the Status of Refugees. Article 23 of the Convention obliges states to accord "refugees lawfully staying in their territory the same treatment with respect to public relief and assistance as is accorded to their nationals" (United Nations 1951), a provision that is particularly relevant for the protection of refugees' right to health.

As member states of the World Health Organization (WHO), EU member states are bound by its 1946 Constitution that first enunciated the right to health (WHO 1946). Some EU member states have also been instrumental in the adoption of the resolution on the "Health of migrants" by the World Health Assembly in 2008 (World Health Assembly 2008).

As members of the International Labour Organization (ILO), EU member states are also bound by its Constitution, which sets out principles of social justice applicable to all persons in their working environment, including those "in countries other than their own" (ILO 2003). Cyprus, Italy, Portugal and Slovenia are also parties to the two ILO conventions specifically concerned with the protection of migrant workers, the 1949 Migration for Employment Convention (Revised) and Convention No. 143 on Migrant Workers (Supplementary Provisions), adopted in 1975. Sweden has acceded only to ILO Convention No.143, while Belgium, France, Germany, the Netherlands, Spain and the United Kingdom are only party to the Migration for Employment Convention (Revised). Article 1 of Convention No. 143 underlines that all migrant workers have basic human rights, which is understood by the ILO Committee of Experts to encompass economic and social rights. The latter convention, which only applies to lawfully resident migrant workers, specifies with regard to the provision of health services (ILO 1949, Article 5):

> Each Member for which this Convention is in force undertakes to maintain, within its jurisdiction, appropriate medical services responsible for: (a) ascertaining, where necessary, both at the time of departure and on arrival, that migrants for employment and the members of their families authorised to accompany or join them are in reasonable health; and (b) ensuring that migrants for employment and members of their families enjoy adequate medical attention and good hygienic conditions at the time of departure, during the journey and on arrival in the territory of destination.

The bodies supervising implementation of the UN human rights treaties have adopted a number of relevant general comments and recommendations, with the aim of assisting states parties in fulfilling their reporting obligations and providing greater clarity on the intent, meaning and content of international human rights treaties, including their applicability to non-nationals.

In General Comment No. 14, the Committee on Economic, Social and Cultural Rights has clarified that the right to health set out in Article 12 of the

International Covenant on Economic, Social and Cultural Rights implies that governments have to generate conditions in which everybody can be as healthy as possible. Such conditions include not only timely and appropriate health care, but also healthy and safe occupational and environmental conditions, adequate housing, safe water, sanitation, food and nutrition (Committee on Economic, Social and Cultural Rights 2000).

The committee further specified that states must ensure that four elements are present throughout all health facilities, goods and services: availability, accessibility, acceptability and quality. Availability refers to the quantity of sufficient health facilities, goods and services throughout the state. Accessibility refers to the ability of people to actually utilize these health facilities, goods and services, including through ensuring non-discrimination. Acceptability refers to the degree to which health facilities, goods and services are respectful of medical ethics and culturally sensitive to the needs of all patients. Quality refers to the skill of medical personnel as well as the scientific and medical appropriateness of health facilities, goods and services (Committee on Economic, Social and Cultural Rights 2000).

The bodies supervising implementation of the International Covenant on Economic, Social and Cultural Rights and the International Convention on the Elimination of All Forms of Racial Discrimination have noted that states are under a specific legal obligation to ensure access to health care for all persons, including undocumented migrants and asylum-seekers (Committee on Economic, Social and Cultural Rights 2000; Committee on the Elimination of Racial Discrimination 2004).

The Committee on Economic, Social and Cultural Rights has further clarified that the rights set out in the Covenant apply to everyone, including non-nationals, refugees, asylum-seekers, stateless persons, migrant workers and victims of international trafficking, regardless of legal status and documentation. Children without legal status, for example, are still entitled to receive education, adequate food and affordable health care (Committee on Economic, Social and Cultural Rights 2009b).

Monitoring implementation of international treaties relies on the submission of regular state reports and their evaluation by treaty-monitoring bodies. In its concluding observations on the report submitted by the United Kingdom, the Committee on Economic, Social and Cultural Rights stressed that it was "concerned at the low level of support and difficult access to health care for rejected asylum-seekers" (Committee on Economic, Social and Cultural Rights 2009a: 7). It recommended (Committee on Economic, Social and Cultural Rights 2009a)

> that the State party review section 4 of the Immigration and Asylum Act 1999 on support and provision regulating essential services to rejected asylum-seekers, and undocumented migrants, including the availability of HIV/AIDS treatment, when necessary.

The committee monitoring implementation of the Convention on the Elimination of All Forms of Discrimination against Women also paid attention to the health of migrants. In its concluding observations on the report submitted by the Netherlands, the committee expressed (Committee on the Elimination of Discrimination against Women 2010, paragraph 46):

> serious concern that the maternal mortality risk for female asylum-seekers is four times higher than for native Dutch women in the Netherlands and that undocumented female immigrants face great difficulties in accessing the health services to which they are formally entitled, mainly because of a lack of appropriate information provided to them.

The committee urged the Netherlands (Committee on the Elimination of Discrimination against Women 2010, paragraph 47)

> to take immediate measures to reduce the maternal mortality of female asylum-seekers and to provide information to undocumented women on their rights as well as practical information on how they can access health-care services.

At the time of writing (January 2011), it was too early to judge whether these recommendations were being followed. In its latest report presented by Germany, the committee expressed regret with regard to (Committee on the Elimination of Discrimination against Women 2009, paragraph 53)

> the lack of data provided in the State party's report on access to health services for migrants, asylum-seekers and refugee women, as well as on the incidence of abortion, disaggregated by age and ethnic group.

The committee asked Germany to provide disaggregated data on access to health services and the incidence of abortion for migrant, asylum-seeker and refugee women in its next periodic report (Committee on the Elimination of Discrimination against Women 2009).

The "special procedures" of the UN Human Rights Council, concerned with specific countries or thematic issues in all parts of the world, have also addressed issues related to the right to health for those who migrate. In his 2010 report to the Human Rights Council, the UN Special Rapporteur on the human rights of migrants focused on the rights to health and adequate housing in the context of migration (Human Rights Council 2010a).

In the same year, the Working Group on Arbitrary Detention reported to the Council that it has sometimes witnessed substandard conditions of detention in overcrowded facilities that affect the health, including the mental health, of undocumented migrants, asylum-seekers and refugees. The Working Group reported the following about practices in Malta (Human Rights Council 2010b, paragraph 41):

> Vulnerable migrants in an irregular situation, such as families with children, unaccompanied minors, pregnant women, breastfeeding mothers, persons with disabilities, elderly persons, or people with serious and/or chronic physical or mental health problems, are also subjected to mandatory detention when arriving to Malta. They are released from detention under a fast-track procedure once the competent Government agency, the Organisation for the Integration and Welfare of Asylum Seekers, has assessed their situation and determined that they are indeed vulnerable.

According to the Government, 'manifestly vulnerable cases' are referred to the Organisation by the Principal Immigration Officer, whose authorization for release upon recommendation by the Organisation is usually obtained within days.

The Working Group urged the Maltese government to end (Human Rights Council 2010b, paragraph 79):

immigration detention of vulnerable groups of migrants, including unaccompanied minors, families with minor children, pregnant women, breastfeeding mothers, elderly persons, persons with disabilities, people with serious and/or chronic physical or mental health problems.

The ILO Committee of Experts on the Application of Conventions and Recommendations reiterated, in its Individual Observation of 2009 on the application of ILO Convention No. 97 in France, the Concluding Observation of the Committee on Economic, Social and Cultural Rights that migrant workers and persons of immigrant origin "are disproportionately concentrated in poor residential areas characterized by [...] inadequate access to health care facilities" (ILO 2009a).

In its 2009 General Survey on occupational safety and health conventions, the ILO has highlighted as a positive development that countries such as the Czech Republic and Spain have extended coverage of the 1981 Occupational Safety and Health Convention to migrant workers (ILO 2009b).

Council of Europe instruments

As highlighted in a 2010 report on criminalization of migration in Europe that was commissioned and published by the Council of Europe's Commissioner for Human Rights, access to social rights such as health or housing is fundamentally affected by the criminalization of migrants:

When state authorities make a decision that an individual is no longer regularly on the territory the consequences for his or her access to social rights is essentially changed. While foreigners who are lawfully present on the territory and working lawfully enjoy protection under the European Social Charter, those who are in an irregular status in practice generally do not. Thus at the stroke of an administrative pen, authorities can extinguish foreigners' rights and access to social benefits and housing notwithstanding the fact that the foreigners may be working, paying social insurance contributions or have a long record of contributions in the past. (Guild 2010: 25)

The European Court of Human Rights is the body ruling on alleged violations of the European Convention for the Protection of Human Rights and Fundamental Freedoms (hereafter European Convention on Human Rights) to which all EU member states have acceded. The Court has held that social benefits (such as health services) come within the scope of Article 1 of the first Protocol to the European Convention on Human Rights, as a property right, even when the individual has never worked and made contributions. Social benefits may also come within the scope of Article 8 where states make them available to families of their nationals, as the non-discrimination duty set out in Article 14 requires such benefits also to be made available to foreigners with family members who meet the criteria (European Court of Human Rights 1996b, 2003, 2005 and 2009).

The denial of health care to undocumented migrants may also amount to an infringement of Article 3 (the right to be free from inhumane and degrading treatment). Moreover, the threshold for breaching this right may be reached when "irregular migrants cannot afford health care and do not benefit from other sources of support" (Cholewinski 2005: 49). Consequently, in the context of an expulsion procedure of a non-national, the Court has recognized that the state's decision to expel an individual may be considered to be in breach of the afore-mentioned Article 3 of the European Convention on Human Rights where the applicant, critically ill and close to death, could not benefit from any nursing or medical care in their country of origin and has no family there willing or able to care for them or provide them with even a basic level of food, shelter or social support (European Court of Human Rights 1996a). It appears from the European Court of Human Rights' case law that the Court gives particular importance to the right to health of minors. In fact, it has recognized that the states parties, in adopting a decision to expel a migrant and the members of his family and in order to comply with the obligations deriving from Article 8 of the Convention, must take into account the impact of this measure on the children's best interest and give due consideration to the possibility that the expulsion will deteriorate their well-being (European Court of Human Rights 2010).

While the European Convention on Human Rights guarantees mostly civil and political rights, the European Social Charter, adopted in 1961 and revised in 1996, guarantees social and economic rights. The European Committee of Social Rights, which supervises the application of the European Social Charter (and Revised Charter), has held that "legislation or practice which denies entitlement to medical assistance to foreign nationals, within the territory of a State Party, even if they are there illegally, is contrary to the Charter" (European Committee of Social Rights 2004). In 2010, the committee concluded that there was a violation of Articles 16, 19, 30 and 31 of the Revised European Social Charter in a case alleging that the so-called "emergency security measures" and an overall racist and xenophobic discourse in Italy had resulted in unlawful campaigns and evictions leading to homelessness and expulsions, disproportionately targeting Roma and Sinti migrants (European Committee of Social Rights 2010). The case also considered social exclusion in access to health services and sanitary and healthy housing.

The Council of Europe's Commissioner for Human Rights also expressed concerns about the situation of migrants in a number of countries. In his report of his visit to Italy in January 2009, the Commissioner raised concern about the proposal to lift the ban on medical personnel to notify the authorities regarding access to medical services by undocumented migrants (Commissioner for Human Rights 2009b). Although, due to the resistance of health professionals, the proposal was never adopted, various cases of denunciation by health personnel occurred in the political climate that followed the proposal. The commissioner also expressed concerns about the treatment of migrants in Greece. As described in the 2010 report on criminalization of migration in Europe (Guild 2010: 26):

A particularly vulnerable group of migrants in need of effective access to health care [in Greece] are those who become disabled while trying to cross borders, as in the case of maimed migrants who attempt to cross the mined areas of the Greek–Turkish borders in Evros. It is to be noted that treatment accorded by states to this group of persons may raise very serious issues with regard to their right to life (art. 2 ECHR) and their freedom from inhuman or degrading treatment (art. 3 ECHR).

In a 2010 report on the detention of asylum-seekers and irregular migrants in Europe, drawn up for the Parliamentary Assembly of the Council of Europe, the Rapporteur affirmed that (Parliamentary Assembly of the Council of Europe 2010a: paragraph 4):

> prolonged detention, often in wholly inappropriate conditions, can amount to inhuman or degrading treatment and result in the deterioration of an individual's mental and physical health.

The report listed a number of principles and rules that should apply, for the entire period of admission to release of irregular migrants and asylum-seekers at detention centres, including many related to health.

Based on this report, the Parliamentary Assembly adopted Resolution 1707, which called on the member states of the Council of Europe in which asylum-seekers and undocumented migrants are detained to comply fully with their obligations under international human rights and refugee law. The Assembly further encouraged them to put into law, and into practice, 15 rules governing minimum standards of detention conditions for migrants and asylum-seekers to ensure, *inter alia*, that "the detention authorities shall safeguard the health and well-being of all detainees in their care" (Parliamentary Assembly of the Council of Europe 2010b).

European Union law

At the level of the EU, the Lisbon Treaty, which was adopted in December 2007 and entered into force on 1 December 2009, has reiterated that respect for human rights is one of the values on which the EU is founded (EU 2010). Notwithstanding that, the competence of the EU on issues related to health is based on and limited by the principle of subsidiarity. Competence to act in the field of public health and health services is still primarily a national matter, in line with the principle of territoriality. Despite all this, direct EU influence is increasing.

With the Lisbon Treaty, "wellbeing" has become a new objective of the EU, with close links to health, defined in the WHO Constitution as "a state of complete physical, mental and social wellbeing (…)" (WHO 1946: 2). Well-being has also translated into horizontal clauses of "health mainstreaming" under Articles 9 and 168 of the consolidated version of the Treaty on European Union (the Consolidated Treaty), both of which assert that European Commission proposals should always take into account their possible adverse effects on health and that proposals should be changed if found problematic. Article 168 of the Consolidated Treaty, which is concerned with public health, has also strengthened cooperation and coordination between member states with regard to health services, encouraging EU member states to establish guidelines, share best practices, and establish systems for monitoring and evaluation. The article pays particular attention to the complementarity of member states' health services in cross-border areas. Following the Lisbon Treaty, the EU now shares competence with member states where common safety concerns in public health have been identified, and can introduce legally-binding legislation.

Probably most importantly, the Treaty also gives legally binding force to the Charter of Fundamental Rights of the European Union. The Charter sets out the right of everyone to access preventive health care and to benefit from medical treatment. Although this right applies "under the conditions established by national laws and practices" (EU 2000: 16), it needs to be understood in the context of the overall objective of health-related provisions of the Treaty, specifying that "a high level of human health protection shall be ensured in the definition and implementation of all the Union's policies and activities" (EU 2000: 16).

The national legal framework

Finally, there are legal provisions at the national, regional, and local levels of EU member states that are relevant to the right of migrants to health. The constitutions of Belgium, Hungary, Italy, the Netherlands, Portugal and Spain recognize the right to health of everyone living on their territories. In countries whose constitution or legislation does not specifically recognize the right to health, elementary health care issues may be derived from more general human rights provisions, such as in Germany (see, for example, the website of the HUMA (Health for Undocumented Migrants and Asylum seekers) network at http://www.huma-network.org/).

In the EU, there are good examples of national legislation clearly defining entitlements of migrants in regular or irregular situations. In Spain, for instance, all migrants are entitled to the same health care coverage as nationals. The only requirement to obtain an individual health card is to register in the "local civil registry" (*padrón*). However, children and pregnant women do not have to register. In order to register in the civil registry, it is necessary to have a valid passport and provide proof of habitual residence. In addition, registration must be renewed every two years in order to retain the health card. A number of undocumented migrants are unable to obtain health cards because they cannot comply with the registration requirements, particularly with the requirement of proving habitual residence. In response, some regions have developed more welcoming systems, in which undocumented migrants are provided with health cards without prior registration in the civil registry.

In Italy, under Article 34 of the National Migration Act of 1998, foreigners have the obligation to register with the National Health Care Service, after which they are granted equal treatment and have the same rights and duties as any Italian citizen. Health assistance is also granted to dependent minors living in Italy, regardless of legal status. Children of foreigners registered with the National Health Care Service are entitled from birth to the same treatment conferred on any minor of Italian nationality. Under Article 35 of the same act, undocumented migrants are entitled to urgent outpatient and hospital treatment or any other basic urgent treatments, even including long hospitalizations and preventive medicine. Preventive, necessary and urgent treatments are expressly defined by law.

There are also rulings by regional courts, such as that of the Regional Administrative Court of Venice, Italy, that in 2008 declared as illegitimate the denial of a residence permit to a Nigerian woman suffering from chronic renal insufficiency and undergoing regular life-sustaining treatment. The claimant's permit had been previously denied because of her irregular status and a previous expulsion (Regional Administrative Court of Venice 2008).

Conclusions

While there is still a long way to go to secure the right to health for migrants in Europe, there are some encouraging developments with regard to access to health services for undocumented migrants at the national level. In Germany, the *Bundesrat* (Federal Council) decided on 18 September 2009 that health workers and those in charge of the reimbursement of hospitals are not required to denounce undocumented migrants accessing health services (Björngren-Cuadra 2010). In Norway, in spring 2010, there was a joint statement from the Minister of Health and the Minister of Justice that undocumented migrants will be given access to health services. In Sweden, a public enquiry on the right to health for undocumented migrants was presented in 2011 and the government agreed to expand the entitlement of undocumented migrants.

Policy-makers can take a number of steps to improve access of migrants to health services. These include clearly defining entitlements by law, publicizing them to migrants and health care providers, ensuring appropriate implementation measures, not conditioning health care to a person's immigration status, and providing protection and assistance to victims of trafficking regardless of whether they cooperate with law enforcement services.

The authors would like to thank Ryszard Cholewinski for his enlightening suggestions.

References

Björngren-Cuadra, C. (2010) *Policies on Health Care for Undocumented Migrants in EU27: Country Report Germany.* Malmö: Malmö University.

Cholewinski, R. (2005) *Study on Obstacles to Effective Access of Irregular Migrants to Minimum Social Rights.* Strasbourg: Council of Europe Publishing.

Commissioner for Human Rights (2009a) *Report by Thomas Hammarberg, Commissioner for Human Rights of the Council of Europe, following his visit to Greece, 8–10 December 2008.* Strasbourg: Commissioner for Human Rights, Council of Europe.

Commissioner for Human Rights (2009b) *Report by Thomas Hammarberg, Commissioner for Human Rights of the Council of Europe, following his visit to Italy on 13–15 January 2009,* Strasbourg: Commissioner for Human Rights, Council of Europe.

Committee on Economic, Social and Cultural Rights (2000) *General Comment No. 14 The Right to the Highest Attainable Standard of Health*. Geneva: Committee on Economic, Social and Cultural Rights.

Committee on Economic, Social and Cultural Rights (2009a) *Concluding Observations, UK*, E/C.12/GBR/CO/5, 12 June 2009. Geneva: Committee on Economic, Social and Cultural Rights.

Committee on Economic, Social and Cultural Rights (2009b) *General Comment No. 20 on Non-Discrimination in Economic, Social and Cultural Rights*. Geneva: Committee on Economic, Social and Cultural Rights.

Committee on the Elimination of Discrimination against Women (2009) *Concluding Observations, Germany*, CEDAW/C/DEU/CO/6, 12 February 2009. Geneva: Committee on the Elimination of Discrimination against Women.

Committee on the Elimination of Discrimination against Women (2010) *Concluding Observations, Netherlands*. CEDAW/C/NLD/CO/5, 5 February 2010. Geneva: Committee on the Elimination of Discrimination against Women.

Committee on the Elimination of Racial Discrimination (2004) *General Recommendation No. 30 on Discrimination Against Non Citizens*. Geneva: Committee on the Elimination of Racial Discrimination.

European Committee of Social Rights (2004) *FIDH v. France, judgment of 8 September 2004*. Strasbourg: European Committee of Social Rights (http://www.escr-net.org/caselaw/caselaw_show.htm?doc_id=400976, accessed 6 June 2011).

European Committee of Social Rights (2010) *Centre on Housing Rights and Evictions (COHRE) v. Italy, judgment of 25 June 2010*. Strasbourg: European Committee of Social Rights.

European Court of Human Rights (1996a) *D. v. the United Kingdom, Commission's report of 15 October 1996*. Strasbourg: European Court of Human Rights.

European Court of Human Rights (1996b) *Gaygusuz v. Austria, Judgment of 16 September 1996*. Strasbourg, European Court of Human Rights.

European Court of Human Rights (2003) *Koua Poirrez v. France, Judgment of 30 September 2003*. Strasbourg: European Court of Human Rights.

European Court of Human Rights (2005) *Niedzwiecki v. Germany, judgment of 25 October 2005*. Strasbourg: European Court of Human Rights.

European Court of Human Rights (2009) *Andrejeva v. Latvia, Judgment of 18 February 2009*. Strasbourg: European Court of Human Rights.

European Court of Human Rights (2010) *Zakayev and Safanova v. Russia, judgment of 11 February 2010*. Strasbourg: European Court of Human Rights.

European Race Audit (2010) *Briefing Paper No. 4 – October 2010 Accelerated removals: a study of the human cost of EU deportation policies, 2009–2010*. London: Institute of Race Relations.

EU (2000) *Charter of Fundamental Rights of the European Union*, (2000/C 364/01). Brussels: European Union.

EU (2010) *Consolidated versions of the Treaty on European Union and the Treaty on the Functioning of the European Union Charter of Fundamental Rights of the European Union*, (OJ C 83, 30.3.2010). Brussels: European Union.

Guild, E. (2010) *Criminalisation of Migration in Europe: Human Rights Implications*. Issue Paper. Strasbourg: Council of Europe Commissioner for Human Rights.

Human Rights Council (2010a) *Report of the Special Rapporteur on the Human Rights of Migrants, Jorge Bustamante*, A/HRC/14/30, 16 April 2010. Geneva: Human Rights Council.

Human Rights Council (2010b) *Report of the Working Group on Arbitrary Detention*, A/HRC/13/30, 15 January 2010. Geneva: Human Rights Council.

ILO (1949) *Migration for Employment Convention (revised)*. Geneva: International Labour Organization

ILO (2003) *Revised Constitution*. Geneva: International Labour Organization.

ILO (2009a) *Committee of Experts on the Application of Conventions and Recommendations Individual Observation concerning Migration for Employment Convention (revised), 1949 (No. 97) France* (ratification: 1954). Geneva: International Labour Organization.

ILO (2009b) *General Survey concerning the Occupational Safety and Health Convention, 1981 (No. 155), the Occupational Safety and Health Recommendation, 1981 (No. 164), and the Protocol of 2002 to the Occupational Safety and Health Convention, 1981*. Geneva: International Labour Organization.

Parliamentary Assembly of the Council of Europe (2010a) *The detention of asylum seekers and irregular migrants in Europe*. Report, Doc.12105, 11 January 2010. Strasbourg: Parliamentary Assembly of the Council of Europe.

Parliamentary Assembly of the Council of Europe (2010b) *The detention of asylum seekers and irregular migrants in Europe*, Resolution 1707 (2010)1. Strasbourg: Parliamentary Assembly of the Council of Europe.

Perruchoud, R. (2007) Consular protection and assistance. In: Cholewinski, R., Perruchoud, R., MacDonald, E. (eds) *International Migration Law: Developing Paradigms and Key Challenges*. The Hague: Asser Press, International Organization for Migration.

Regional Administrative Court of Venice (2008) *Judgment of 12 May 2008*. Venice: Regional Administrative Court.

United Nations (1951) *Convention relating to the Status of Refugees*. New York: United Nations.

United Nations (1966) *International Covenant on Economic, Social and Cultural Rights*. New York: United Nations.

United Nations (1990) *International Convention on the Protection of the Rights of All Migrant Workers and Members of their Families*. New York: United Nations.

United Nations (2010) *Secretary-General addresses European Parliament on major global challenges, 19 October 2010* (http://www.un.org/News/Press/docs/2010/sgsm13190. doc.htm, accessed 15 May 2011).

WHO (1946) *WHO Constitution*. Geneva: World Health Organization.

World Health Assembly (2008) *Health of Migrants*. Geneva: World Health Assembly.

chapter five

Migrants' access to health services

Marie Nørredam and Allan Krasnik

Why is migrants' access to health services an area of concern?

There are several important reasons for focusing on migrants' access to health services in European health systems. First, migrants form an increasing proportion of the population in Europe, so health professionals, managers and politicians need more knowledge on migrants' health and ability to access care in order to make informed decisions.

Second, illness may impede integration processes in the host countries as ill health affects the ability to engage in education, work and activities in society in general. This may lead to further marginalization and social isolation, which again may affect health in a negative way.

The third argument is legal (as well as moral) and is based on the notion of "the right to the highest attainable health". This right was first described in the WHO Constitution of 1946 (WHO 1946) and then reiterated in the 1978 Alma Ata Declaration (WHO 1978) and in the World Health Declaration of 1998 (WHO 1998). In addition, several international human rights documents recognize the right to health (see Chapter 4 on "The right to health of migrants in Europe"). In addition, the 2008 Resolution of the World Health Assembly on the "Health of migrants" called for a number of steps to improve migrant health, including ensuring equitable access to health services (World Health Assembly 2008).

Fourth, for many European health systems, equity in access to health services is a fundamental objective. Equity concerns fairness, which is differentiated from equality, and concerns differences in a mathematical sense. Horizontal equity implies equal treatment for equal needs, whereas vertical equity implies different treatment for different needs (Oliver and Mossialos 2004). Equitable health care requires that resource allocation and access to health care are determined by health need, irrespective of factors such as ethnicity or migration status. Although equitable health care should not be confused with equity in health, as the latter also depends on factors such as individual health behaviour, housing, occupation, social welfare and environmental conditions, increased equity in access to health care may also increase equity in health.

Conceptualizing and measuring access

Access has been described as the "fit" between patients and the health system (Penchansky and Thomas 1981). More concretely, optimal access has been defined as "providing the right services at the right time in the right place" (Rogers et al. 1999: 866). Inequities in access to care are seen when there are systematic variations in access related to factors such as socioeconomic conditions, migrant status or ethnicity, rather than need. Access is considered equitable if it does not depend on, for example, education, income, migrant status, ethnicity or geographical distance. However, access is difficult to measure directly and has most often been measured by utilization levels.

Comparing utilization between different population groups in order to investigate possible inequity in access requires a means to measure need for care. This is fairly easy when comparing utilization of preventive services such as population-based screening for breast cancer, when need is defined at national or sub-national level on the basis of age and gender (every woman in a certain age group is considered to be in need). Groups of patients with a similar diagnosis (i.e. acute myocardial infarction) are also sometimes compared with regard to their utilization of rehabilitation services or preventive drugs, on the basis of well-defined guidelines. Another measure of need is achieved through surveys collecting information on the prevalence of poor self-reported health, chronic diseases or, ideally, indications for treatment (Sanderson et al. 1997). These measures, however, are to some extent also an effect of contact with the health system (i.e. diagnosis of diabetes) and longitudinal studies are therefore required in order to decide on possible cause-and-effect relationships. Alternatively, surveys might try directly to investigate unmet needs by asking migrants about situations where they experienced health problems without contacting the health system. Unfortunately, such studies are quite rare within migrant health research and often lack validity and comparability across migrant groups (see Chapter 6 on "Monitoring the health of migrants").

Utilization of health services by migrants may differ from that by non-migrants, as both migrants' needs and their access to health care are affected by a number of factors related to the process of migration, including health and socioeconomic status, self-perceived needs, health beliefs, health-seeking behaviour, language barriers, cultural differences, trauma and newness. This is especially true for recently arrived migrants, as newcomers to the receiving countries are less knowledgeable about how to navigate the health system and might have special health needs. Furthermore, communication between health professionals and patients may be more difficult for individuals who do not speak and read the same language and have a different cultural background, which may lead to later diagnosis and less optimal choice of treatment. In addition to investigating utilization patterns, it is therefore important to measure access to care by other indicators, such as delay in diagnosis, treatment and care.

Are there differences in migrants' access to health services compared to non-migrants?

Utilization of preventive services

The bulk of the literature on migrants' access to health care compared to non-migrants concerns utilization patterns. Regarding preventive services, studies focus on uptake of cancer screening programmes and prenatal/maternity services (see Chapter 9 on "Maternal and child health"). In several countries, low referral and attendance for mammography (Atri et al. 1996; Lagerlund et al. 2002; Visser et al. 2005; McCormack et al. 2008; Price et al. 2010) have been found for various groups of migrant women compared to non-migrants. Similarly, migrant women have a lower uptake of cervical (Webb et al. 2004; Moser et al. 2009) and bowel cancer screening (Price et al. 2010).

Higher rates of induced abortions for non-western migrants indicate difficulties in accessing preventive measures related to reproductive health (Rasch et al. 2008). Disparities in utilization have also been identified for prenatal care: migrant women from various geographical origins have less contact with maternity care compared to non-migrants (Hemingway et al. 1997; Choté et al. 2009). Furthermore, more newborns of migrant women are transferred to neonatal care units (Merten et al. 2007), which might be an indicator of poorer access to prenatal care.

With regard to vaccination, a Spanish study showed lower coverage of migrant compared to non-migrant children (Borras et al. 2007), while Dutch (Rondy et al. 2010) and British (Brabin et al. 2008) studies have shown lower rates of uptake of human papilloma virus (HPV) vaccine among ethnic minority girls compared to native-born girls.

Utilization of general practitioners

Several European studies show overall higher use of general practitioners (GPs) among migrants compared to non-migrants, although there are differences with regard to country of origin, age and sex (Smaje and Grand 1997; Cooper et al. 1998; Stronks et al. 2001; Uiters et al. 2006). In general, health needs of migrant women seem to be higher than among men, and this is reflected in a higher utilization of GPs among migrant women as compared to migrant men (Gerritsen and Devillé 2009). The reasons for these differences are unclear, but might be related to easier access to GPs in some countries, the broad range of services in general practice, and the pattern of disease burden among migrants, in particular with regard to psycho-social aspects. Alternative explanations include unclear symptoms and poor communication with migrants, resulting in the need for repeated visits and additional diagnostic activities. The legal status of migrants also seems to be of relevance, with a study in London finding that unstable immigration status was associated with lower utilization of GP services (Aung et al. 2010). It should also be borne in mind that arrangements and functions of GPs or primary care differ across European countries, as do referral systems to higher levels of care.

Utilization of emergency departments

Studies of emergency department use tend to show higher utilization rates among migrants compared to non-migrants (Cots et al. 2007; Dyhr et al. 2007). This is the case both for somatic and psychiatric emergency department use, as has been documented in Switzerland (Lay et al. 2006) and Denmark (Mygind et al. 2008). High rates of emergency department use among migrants have been related to inadequate access to other services. However, the evidence on utilization levels is inconclusive (see Chapter 14 on "Good practice in emergency care"). A German study (David et al. 2006) did not find migrant status to be a predictor of inappropriate emergency department use, while a study in London found lower utilization levels among migrants (Hargreaves et al. 2006).

Hospitalization and specialist care

With regard to hospitalization, the literature also shows contrasting results. Some studies found equal utilization rates by those from different countries of origin (Saxena et al. 2002), while others found patterns of underutilization (Cacciani et al. 2006) or overutilization (Robertson et al. 2003) among migrants compared to non-migrants. Concerning length of hospitalization to somatic wards, a Danish study (Krasnik et al. 2002) showed no overall differences between migrants and non-migrants. Findings for psychiatric admissions generally show lower admission rates for migrants, although hospitalization rates vary markedly with sex, migration status and country of origin (Lay et al. 2006). However, rates of compulsory admission have been found to be consistently higher among migrants than among non-migrants (Lay et al. 2006; Nørredam et al. 2010a; Nørredam et al. 2010b).

Studies of specialist or outpatient care show a general tendency towards underutilization by migrant populations of all ages, except for a few studies that show no differences (Stronks et al. 2001; Saxena et al. 2002).

Other indicators related to access

Apart from utilization patterns, problems of access can be identified by health indicators capturing delay in seeking care, as well as by measures such as mortality or disease severity at presentation. However, as mentioned above, these indicators are much less frequently used for measuring access than utilization patterns.

With regard to disease severity at diagnosis, cancer stage at presentation has been used as a proxy of access to health care, showing longer delays in referral and diagnosis at a later stage among migrants with breast, cervical and colorectal cancer compared to non-migrants (Nørredam et al. 2008; Cuthbertson et al. 2009). Delays in diagnosing disease among migrants have also been shown for diabetic complications (David and Kendrick 2004), as well as for clinical indicators of a broad range of infectious diseases (Fakoya et al. 2008).

Avoidable mortality (deaths that should not occur in the presence of timely and effective care) is another indicator of access to care (Nolte and McKee 2004). A Dutch study showed elevated avoidable mortality for migrants compared to non-migrants for almost all infectious and several chronic diseases (Stirbu et al. 2006). Controlling for demographic and socioeconomic factors explained part, but not all, of the differences in avoidable mortality. It is unclear how far barriers to access among migrants have contributed to these findings, but they indicate room for improvement in access to and quality of diagnosis and treatment of infectious diseases, diabetes, asthma, hypertension, and maternal and neonatal care.

Why are there differences in migrants' access to health services compared to non-migrants?

Formal barriers to access

Factors associated with health policies and the organization of health systems can constitute formal barriers to access. These include legal restrictions on entitlement to health services for certain groups of migrants, as well as financial barriers that may affect migrants. In most countries of the European Union (EU), there are legal restrictions on entitlement to health services for asylum-seekers and undocumented migrants. In most countries, only emergency services are available for undocumented migrants, although some EU member states even restrict access to emergency care (Björngren-Cuadra and Cattacin 2010). In some EU member states, asylum-seekers are entitled to general or specially tailored services (Nørredam et al. 2006; Schoevers et al. 2010). Formal barriers can sometimes include special requirements for referral of asylum-seekers to specialist care. User fees can be seen as a general formal barrier, creating inequity in access for many migrant groups due to their generally lower socioeconomic status compared to non-migrants, or as a specific barrier for some migrant groups who are not yet entitled to subsidies during their initial time of residence (Scheppers et al. 2006). It is also important to recognize that health service provision may be more limited or extensive than envisaged by formal legal entitlements.

Informal barriers to access

Informal barriers to accessing health care can be divided into questions of language, communication, sociocultural factors and "newness". Access will often be affected by a complex interaction between all these factors.

Language barriers include lack of comprehensible information about entitlements, what services are available and difficulties in making appointments with physicians. A lack of skilled interpreters may result in poor communication and consequently poor identification of health problems. Barriers to the use of qualified interpreters include lack of funding, a lack of identified need for interpretation, and gaps in the training of staff, who might then prefer *ad hoc* interpretation by family members and others accompanying the patient. A lack of interpreters creates many problems due to poor translation, the sensitivity of communication and the psycho-social stress for family members, in particular children, who are often used as interpreters in these situations (Bischoff et al. 2003; Bischoff and Hudelson 2010).

Yet, communication goes beyond language. A Dutch study showed that GPs communicate differently with migrants compared to non-migrants: consultations with migrants were shorter, GPs more verbally dominant, and migrants less demanding compared to non-migrants (Meeuwesen et al. 2006). Stigmatization and doctors' biological, psychological and social approaches may present additional barriers hampering patient–staff communication. Less effective communication with migrant patients may lead to misunderstandings and non-adherence to treatment (van Wieringen et al. 2002; Harmsen et al. 2003). In a health system characterized by gate-keeping, poor communication with GPs may also result in inadequate referral to secondary care.

The social marginalization and loss of social networks, which often characterizes migration, may also present barriers to seeking health care, as may institutional and personal discrimination and racism based on ethnicity or religion (Bhopal 2007; Worth et al. 2009).

Finally, being a recently arrived migrant might inhibit access to care, in particular for those migrants who have not received any introduction to the health system of their new host country (Worth et al. 2009).

How can health services contribute to the reduction of inequalities in health related to migration?

As the preceding sections of this chapter have illustrated, there is strong evidence that migrants' access to health care differs from that of non-migrants, although there are significant variations according to country of origin, migrant status and socioeconomic position. Migrants' access is affected differently at different levels of the health system. To improve it, several issues need to be addressed, including: entitlements, health policies, structure and organization of services, and the characteristics of the clinical encounter between health professionals and migrants.

First, all EU member states have acceded to international human rights treaties that recognize the right for everyone to enjoy the highest attainable standard of health (see Chapter 4 on "The right to health of migrants in Europe"). National law should ensure that health care is a de facto respected human right for every member of society. Special attention should be taken to guarantee access by vulnerable migrants such as asylum-seekers and undocumented migrants.

In most EU countries, undocumented migrants do not have any recognized legal status, which in many cases results in minimal access to health care (Björngren-Cuadra and Cattacin 2010).

The second step towards improving migrants' access to health care concerns health policies. Migrants' health and access to health care should be incorporated explicitly into health policy documents at local, regional, national and EU levels, including guidelines on how to overcome financial, geographical, language and cultural barriers in relation to migrants' access to health care. A recent comparative study demonstrated that some European countries are more progressive on this than others (Lorant and Bhopal 2010) (see also Chapter 12 on "Migrant health policies in Europe").

Third, the way in which health systems are organized also has major implications for migrants' possibilities of accessing care. Health systems need to consider whether established ways of delivering services meet the needs of changing demographics. Healy and McKee (2004) have outlined several delivery models in response to population diversity. These models can be divided into two overall approaches: mainstream services for all or separate services for migrants. Separate services imply a higher political profile, empowerment of migrants and more targeted services, but they may lead to anti-migrant sentiments. In contrast, proponents of mainstream provision for all argue that this is non-discriminatory, strengthens social solidarity, and that alternative services can undermine unified national health systems. According to McKee (2002), the question of mainstream or specific services depends on the context and, in particular, the political power of the migrant group and their resulting ability to take charge of the services they receive. To date, most European health systems have not developed specific services for migrants, preferring rather to mainstream provision into existing health care structures (see also Chapter 12 on "Migrant health policies in Europe"). Another issue is that services need to be geographically accessible and sufficient in numbers. Increasing "knowledge-related access" is also important, including through the systematic provision of information on health services to all newcomers. "Linguistic access" can be promoted by ensuring an adequate number of professional interpreters, bilingual staff or cultural mediators, with health education material and awareness campaigns developed for specific ethnic and linguistic groups, taking into account levels of education and literacy.

Finally, it is important to improve the clinical encounter between health personnel and migrant patients. A growing body of literature shows that misunderstandings and unsatisfactory communication are prevalent in encounters with migrant patients, hampering health service provision and outcomes. Access to professional interpretation should be ensured formally, financially and in daily practice for all patients without sufficient language skills in order to enable them to communicate adequately with health professionals. Otherwise, both patients and health workers are confronted with lack of information, the risks of inappropriate diagnostic procedures, and negative effects on adherence and quality of care. Introducing cultural mediators into health care is seen by many as an additional innovation in order to enhance cross-cultural communication and understanding. More informal support and advice might also play a role; this could include migrant networks and associations as well as general patient organizations, such as for patients with cancer or heart disease, which might provide specific services to migrants. Health care staff may have strong stereotypical views, lack cultural awareness and ability, or generally manage patients from diverse backgrounds in an unsuitable manner, which can create barriers and generate resentment. This may be due to insecurity on the side of health workers. More consideration should be given to developing cultural competences among health professionals through including a diversity focus in the curriculum of undergraduate training programmes and as part of in-service training of practitioners (see Chapter 13 on "Differences in language, religious beliefs and culture: the need for culturally responsive health services"). It has been shown that an intervention to increase cultural awareness among health staff increases the acceptance of culturally appropriate approaches to care (Beune et al. 2010). It is also important to increase the number of multicultural staff by providing migrants with access to health training and professional opportunities, and by supporting professional recognition or re-training of migrants who have undergone health training in their countries of origin. Multicultural staff are also important in community settings where health care advisors have proved to be valuable in reaching immigrants, providing them with information about the health and welfare system, and referring them to services (Hesselink et al. 2009).

Conclusions

Ensuring access to health care for the general population has been one of the main achievements of European governments during the last six decades, both in order to ensure a strong and healthy workforce and, in national welfare states, to promote social solidarity. Different public and private sector arrangements have been developed to achieve this goal, often combining complex systems of health care purchasers and providers. Patterns of increasing migration and ethnic diversity have created new challenges to European health systems that had previously been developed in order to meet the needs of "native" populations. Health policies, organizational structures, training programmes and daily routines seem to fail in providing equal access to health care to all migrants and minority groups. Research on migrant health in recent decades has generated accumulating descriptive evidence on disparities in access, but less on factors explaining these findings, and hardly any evidence on innovations that might help to create more equity in health care. Such innovations are potentially beneficial for the health of migrants and ethnic minorities, but also for reducing insecurity and stress among health professionals, and saving resources. Developing more inclusive health systems and documenting the processes involved and their potential outcomes might also benefit other vulnerable groups, reduce the risk of increasing social and ethnic inequalities in health, and help to ensure a sufficiently large and healthy workforce in a European continent characterized by rapidly ageing populations.

References

Atri, J., Falshaw, M., Linvingstone, A. and Robson, J. (1996) Fair shares in health care? Ethnic and socioeconomic influences on recording of preventive care in selected inner London general practices. Healthy Eastenders Project. *BMJ*, 312(7031): 614–17.

Aung, N.C., Rechel, B. and Odermatt, P. (2010) Access to and utilisation of GP services among Burmese migrants in London: a cross-sectional descriptive study. *BMC Health Services Research*, 10: 285.

Beune, E.J., Bindels, P.J., Mohrs, J., Stronks, K. and Haafkens, J.A. (2010) Pilot study evaluating the effects of an intervention to enhance culturally appropriate hypertension education among healthcare providers in a primary care setting. *Implementation Science* 5(1): 35 [Epub ahead of print].

Bhopal, R. (2007) Racism in health and health care in Europe: reality or mirage? *European Journal of Public Health*, 17(3): 238–41.

Bischoff, A., Bovier, P.A., Rrustemi, I., et al. (2003) Language barriers between nurses and asylum seekers: their impact on symptom reporting and referral. *Social Science & Medicine*, 57(3): 503–12.

Bischoff, A. and Hudelson, P. (2010) Access to healthcare interpreter services: where are we and where do we need to go? *International Journal of Environmental Research and Public Health*, 7(7): 2838–44 [Epub 12 July 2010].

Björngren-Cuadra, C. and Cattacin, S. (2010) *Policies on Health Care for Undocumented Migrants in the EU27: Towards a Comparative Framework. Summary Report.* Malmö: Health Care in NowHereland, Malmö University.

Borras, E., Dominguez, A., Batalla, J., et al. (2007) Vaccination coverage in indigenous and immigrant children under 3 years of age in Catalonia (Spain). *Vaccine*, 25(16): 3240–3.

Brabin, L., Roberts, S.A., Stretch, R., et al. (2008) Uptake of first two doses of human papillomavirus vaccine by adolescent schoolgirls in Manchester: prospective cohort study. *BMJ*, 336(7652): 1056–8.

Cacciani, L., Baglio, G., Rossi, L., et al. (2006) Hospitalisation among immigrants in Italy. *Emerging Themes in Epidemiology*, 3: 4.

Choté, A.A., de Groot, C.J., Bruijnzeels, M.A., et al. (2009) Ethnic differences in antenatal care use in a large multi-ethnic urban population in the Netherlands. *Midwifery*, 27(1): 36–41 [Epub 25 Nov 2009].

Cooper, H., Smaje, C. and Arber, S. (1998) Use of health services by children and young people according to ethnicity and social class: secondary analysis of a national survey. *BMJ*, 317(7165): 1047–51.

Cots, F., Castells, X. and Garcia, O., et al. (2007) Impact of immigration on the cost of emergency visits in Barcelona (Spain). *BMC Health Services Research*, 7: 9.

Cuthbertson, S.A., Goyder, E.C. and Poole, J. (2009) Inequalities in breast cancer stage at diagnosis in the Trent region, and implications for the NHS Breast Screening Programme. *Journal of Public Health*, 31(3): 398–405.

David, C. and Kendrick, D. (2004) Differences in the process of diabetic care between south Asian and white patients in inner-city practices in Nottingham, UK. *Health & Social Care in the Community*, 12(3): 186–93.

David, M., Schwartau, I., Anand, P.H. and Borde, T. (2006) Emergency outpatient services in the city of Berlin: factors for appropriate use and predictors for hospital admission. *European Journal of Emergency Medicine*, 13(6): 352–7.

Dyhr, L., Andersen, J.S. and Engholm, G. (2007) The pattern of contact with general practice and casualty departments of immigrants and non-immigrants in Copenhagen, Denmark. *Danish Medical Bulletin*, 54(3): 226–9.

Fakoya, I., Reynolds, R., Caswell, G. and Shiripinda, I. (2008) Barriers to HIV testing for migrant black Africans in Western Europe. *HIV Medicine*, 9(Suppl. 2): 23–5.

Gerritsen, A.A. and Devillé, W. (2009) Gender differences in health and health care use in migrants in the Netherlands. *BMC Public Health*, 9: 109.

Hargreaves, S., Friedland, J.S., Gothard, P., et al. (2006) Impact on and use of health services by international migrants: questionnaire survey of inner city London A&E attenders. *BMC Health Services Research*, 6: 153.

Harmsen, H., Meeuwesen, L., van Wieringen, J., Bernsen, R. and Bruijnzeels, M. (2003) When cultures meet in general practice: intercultural differences between GPs and parents of child patients. *Patient Education and Counseling*, 51(2): 99–106.

Healy, J. and McKee, M. (2004) Delivering health services in diverse societies. In: Healy, J. and McKee, M. (eds) *Accessing Health Care*. Oxford: Oxford University Press: 351–79.

Hemingway, H., Saunders, D. and Parsons, L. (1997) Social class, spoken language and pattern of care as determinants of continuity of carer in maternity services in east London. *Journal of Public Health Medicine*, 19(2): 156–61.

Hesselink, A.E., Verhoeff, A.P. and Stronks, K. (2009) Ethnic health care advisors: a good strategy to improve the access to health care and social welfare services for ethnic minorities? *Journal of Community Health*, 34(5): 419–29.

Krasnik, A., Nørredam, M., Sorensen, TM., et al. (2002) Effect of ethnic background on Danish hospital utilisation patterns. *Social Science & Medicine*, 55(7): 1207–11.

Lagerlund, M., Maxwell, A.E., Bastani, R., et al. (2002) Sociodemographic predictors of non-attendance at invitational mammography screening – a population-based register study (Sweden). *Cancer Causes and Control*, 13(1): 73–82.

Lay, B., Lauber, C., Nordt, C. and Rössler, W. (2006) Patterns of inpatient care for immigrants in Switzerland: a case control study. *Social Psychiatry and Psychiatric Epidemiology*, 41(3): 199–207.

Lorant, V. and Bhopal, R. (2010) Comparing policies to tackle ethnic inequalities in health: Belgium 1 Scotland 4. *European Journal of Public Health*, 21(2): 235–40.

McCormack, V.A., Perry, N., Vinnicombe, S.J. and Silva Idos, S. (2008) Ethnic variations in mammographic density: a British multiethnic longitudinal study. *American Journal of Epidemiology*, 168(4): 412–21.

McKee, M. (2002) What can health services contribute to the reduction of inequalities in health? *Scandinavian Journal of Public Health*, 59(Suppl.): 54–8.

Meeuwesen, L., Harmsen, J.A., Bernsen, R.M. and Bruijnzeels, M.A. (2006) Do Dutch doctors communicate differently with immigrant patients than with Dutch patients? *Social Science & Medicine*, 63(9): 2407–17.

Merten, S., Wyss, C. and Ackermann-Liebrich, U. (2007) Caesarean sections and breastfeeding initiation among migrants in Switzerland. *International Journal of Public Health*, 52(4): 210–22.

Moser, K., Patnick, J. and Beral, V. (2009) Inequalities in reported use of breast and cervical screening in Great Britain: analysis of cross sectional survey data. *BMJ*, 338: b2025.

Mygind, A., Nørredam, M., Nielsen, A.S., Bagger, J. and Krasnik, A. (2008) The effect of patient origin and relevance of contact on patient and caregiver satisfaction in the emergency room. *Scandinavian Journal of Public Health*, 36(1): 76–83.

Nolte, E. and McKee, M. (2004) *Does Healthcare Save Lives? Avoidable Mortality Revisited*. London: Nuffield Trust.

Nørredam, M., Garcia-Lopez, A., Keiding, N. and Krasnik, A. (2010a) Excess use of coercive measures in psychiatry among migrants compared with native Danes. *Acta Psychiatrica Scandinavica*, 121(2): 143–51 [Epub 9 July 2009].

Nørredam, M., Garcia-Lopez, A., Keiding, N. and Krasnik, A. (2010b) Risk of mental disorders in family reunification migrants and native Danes: a register-based historically prospective cohort study. *International Journal of Public Health*, 55(5): 413–19.

Nørredam, M., Krasnik, A., Pipper, C. and Keiding, N. (2008) Differences in stage of disease between migrant women and native Danish women diagnosed with cancer: results from a population-based cohort study. *European Journal of Cancer Prevention*, 17(3): 185–90.

Nørredam, M., Mygind, A. and Krasnik, A. (2006) Access to healthcare for asylum seekers in the European Union – a comparative study of country policies. *European Journal of Public Health*, 16(3): 285–9.

Oliver, A. and Mossialos, E. (2004) Equity of access to health care: outlining the foundations for action. *Journal of Epidemiology & Community Health*, 58(8): 655–8.

Penchansky, R. and Thomas, J.W. (1981) The concept of access: definition and relationship to consumer satisfaction. *Medical Care*, 19(2): 127–40.

Price, C.L., Szczepura, A.K., Gumber, A.K. and Patnick, J. (2010) Comparison of breast and bowel cancer screening uptake patterns in a common cohort of South Asian women in England. *BMC Health Services Research*, 10: 103.

Rasch, V., Gammeltoft, T., Knudsen, L.B., et al. (2008) Induced abortion in Denmark: effect of socio-economic situation and country of birth. *European Journal of Public Health*, 18(2): 144–9.

Robertson, E., Malmstrom, M., Sundquist, J. and Johansson, S.E. (2003) Impact of country of birth on hospital admission for women of childbearing age in Sweden: a five year follow up study. *Journal of Epidemiology & Community Health*, 57(11): 877–82.

Rogers, A., Flowers, J. and Pencheon, D. (1999) Improving access needs a whole systems approach. And will be important in averting crises in the millennium winter. *BMJ*, 319(7214): 866–7.

Rondy, M., van Lier, A., van de Kassteele, J., Rust, L. and de Melker, H. (2010) Determinants for HPV vaccine uptake in the Netherlands: a multilevel study. *Vaccine*, 28(9): 2070–5.

Sanderson, C.F., Hunter, D.J., McKee, M. and Black, N. (1997) Limitations of epidemiologically based needs assessment: the case of prostatectomy. *Medical Care*, 35: 669–85.

Saxena, S., Eliahoo, J. and Majeed, A. (2002) Socioeconomic and ethnic group differences in self reported health status and use of health services by children and young people in England: cross sectional study. *BMJ*, 325(7363): 520.

Scheppers, E., van Dongen, E., Dekker, J., Geertzen, J. and Dekker, J. (2006) Potential barriers to the use of health services among ethnic minorities: a review. *Family Practice*, 23: 325–48.

Schoevers, M.A., Loeffen, M.J., van den Muijsenbergh, M.E. and Lagro-Janssen, A.L. (2010) Health care utilisation and problems in accessing health care of female undocumented immigrants in the Netherlands. *International Journal of Public Health*, 55(5): 421–8.

Smaje, C. and Grand, J.L. (1997) Ethnicity, equity and the use of health services in the British NHS. *Social Science & Medicine*, 45(3): 485–96.

Stirbu, I., Kunst, A.E., Bos, V. and Mackenbach, J.P. (2006) Differences in avoidable mortality between migrants and the native Dutch in The Netherlands. *BMC Public Health*, 6(1): 78–83.

Stronks, K., Ravelli, A.C. and Reijneveld, S.A. (2001) Immigrants in the Netherlands: equal access for equal needs? *Journal of Epidemiology & Community Health*, 55(10): 701–7.

Uiters, E., Deville, W.L., Foets, M. and Groenewegen, P.P. (2006) Use of health care services by ethnic minorities in The Netherlands: do patterns differ? *European Journal of Public Health*, 16(4): 388–93.

Van Wieringen, J.C., Harmsen, J.A. and Bruijnzeels, M.A. (2002) Intercultural communication in general practice. *European Journal of Public Health*, 12(1): 63–8.

Visser, O., van Peppen, A.M., Ory, F.G. and van Leeuwen, F.E. (2005) Results of breast cancer screening in first-generation migrants in Northwest Netherlands. *European Journal of Cancer Prevention*, 14(3): 251–5.

Webb, R., Richardson, J., Esmail, A. and Pickles, A. (2004) Uptake for cervical screening by ethnicity and place-of-birth: a population-based cross-sectional study. *Journal of Public Health (Oxford)*, 26(3): 293–6.

World Health Assembly (2008) *Health of migrants, Resolution of the 61st World Health Assembly.* Geneva: World Health Organization.

WHO (1946) *WHO Constitution.* Geneva: World Health Organization.

WHO (1978) *The Alma Ata Declaration.* Geneva: World Health Organization.

WHO (1998) *World Health Declaration.* Geneva: World Health Organization.

WHO (2002) *25 Questions and Answers on Health and Human Rights.* Geneva: World Health Organization.

Worth, A., Irshad, T., Bhopal, R., et al. (2009) Vulnerability and access to care for South Asian Sikh and Muslim patients with life limiting illness in Scotland: prospective longitudinal qualitative study. *BMJ*, 338: b183.

Section IV

Monitoring migrant health

Monitoring the health of migrants

Bernd Rechel, Philipa Mladovsky and Walter Devillé

Introduction

Accurate data on the health of migrants, including health determinants and health service utilization, are an essential pre-condition for providing appropriate and accessible health services to this population group. Yet in many, if not most, European Union (EU) countries, information on the health of migrants is lacking (Rafnsson and Bhopal 2008; Padilla and Miguel 2009), limiting the possibilities for monitoring and improving migrant health, and for conducting comparative studies on inequalities in health and access to health care (Kraler and Reichel 2010b).

There are a number of reasons for this situation, including the lack of any system for routine collection of data on the health of migrants. In contrast to the situation in Australia, Canada, New Zealand and the United States, most countries in Europe do not routinely collect health data by migrant status. While the Netherlands and the United Kingdom have significant experience in conducting population-based surveys that also contain information on migration status or ethnicity, countries such as Belgium, Germany and Spain have only recently started to include such variables in health surveys. The new EU member states generally do not include variables on migration status in health information systems or surveys. Furthermore, even in those countries that do collect routine health data by migrant status, information on the most vulnerable groups of migrants, such as asylum-seekers or undocumented migrants, is generally lacking.

There are conceptual and methodological challenges in collecting data on migrant health, such as different definitions or understandings of who constitutes a migrant – and how many migrants, however defined, there are in a given country (Aung et al. 2010). This chapter reviews current data information systems and ongoing research activities in the EU and examines how far they make it possible to assess and monitor migrant health.

The collection of data on migration status

The European Commission against Racism and Intolerance (ECRI) of the Council of Europe, an independent human rights monitoring body specializing in combating racism and racial discrimination, has regularly called on countries that are members of the Council of Europe to collect relevant data broken down according to categories such as nationality, national or ethnic origin, language and religion, with due respect for the principles of confidentiality, informed consent and voluntary self-identification of persons as belonging to a particular group (European Commission against Racism and Intolerance 1996).

In the United Kingdom, broader anti-discrimination legislation, in the form of the Race Relations (Amendment) Act of 2000, has been an important driver of efforts to adapt health services to the needs of "black and minority ethnic" (BME) groups (Ingleby 2006). The country now has "a very highly structured system to combat discrimination and promote equality, based on systematic statistical monitoring" (Simon 2007: 47). Yet, across EU member states, discrepancies between data collection practices have increased, despite the passing of EU-wide anti-discrimination directives, in particular the Directive 2000/43/EC on "implementing the principle of equal treatment between persons irrespective of racial or ethnic origin" and Directive 2000/78/EC "establishing a general framework for equal treatment in employment and occupation" (Simon 2007). The types of variables related to ethnicity or migration collected in the member states of the Council of Europe are shown in Table 6.1.

Table 6.1 Information on national or ethnic origin, religion and language and their equivalents collected in official statistics in Council of Europe countries

	Country of birth	Citizenship	Nationality or ethnicity	Religion	Language	Country of birth of parents
Albania	X					
Armenia	X	X	X		X	
Austria	X	X		X	X	
Azerbaijan	X	X	X		X	
Belgium	X	X				
Bulgaria	X	X	X	X	X	
Croatia	X	X	X	X	X	
Cyprus	X	X	X	X	X	X
Czech Republic	X	X	X	X	X	X
Denmark	X	X				X
Estonia	X	X	X	X	X	X
Finland	X	X		X	X	
France	X	X				
Georgia	X	X	X	X	X	

Germany	X	X		X		
Greece	X	X				
Hungary	X	X	X	X	X	
Iceland	X	X		X		
Ireland	X	X	X	X	X	
Italy	X	X				
Latvia			X		X	
Liechtenstein		X		X	X	
Lithuania	X	X	X	X	X	
Luxembourg	X	X				
Malta	X	X			X	
Montenegro	X		X	X	X	
Netherlands	X	X				X
Norway	X	X				X
Poland	X	X	X		X	
Portugal	X	X		X		
Republic of Moldova		X	X	X	X	
Romania	X	X	X	X	X	
Russian Federation	X	X	X	X	X	
Serbia	X		X	X	X	
Slovakia	X	X	X	X	X	
Slovenia	X		X	X	X	
Spain	X	X				
Sweden	X	X				
Switzerland	X	X		X	X	X
The former Yugoslav Republic of Macedonia	X	X	X	X	X	
Turkey	X	X				
Ukraine	X	X	X		X	
United Kingdom	X		X	X		
Total (n = 43)	**40**	**37**	**23**	**25**	**27**	**7**

NOTE: The table contains information on data collected in censuses, but also population registers and statistical data systems combining administrative sources and population registers.

Source: adapted from Simon (2007)

The different categorizations and definitions of migrants, and whether it is deemed acceptable to collect "ethnic" data, mainly reflect different historical contexts, statistical traditions, administrative and political structures, welfare regimes and immigration histories (Kraler and Reichel 2010a). For some countries, ethnicity is a major criterion for describing the groups within a population, while others even refuse to use the concept (Simon 2007) (see Chapter 2 on "Trends in Europe's international migration").

In the United Kingdom, immigrant communities largely established through migration from former colonies after the Second World War are referred to as "black and minority ethnic" (BME) groups, rather than migrants, while asylum-seekers and refugees fall outside this category (Ingleby 2006). Migrants who have settled are not considered migrants any more. In the Netherlands, migrants and ethnic minorities are referred to collectively as *"allochtonen"* (i.e. of foreign origin) (Ingleby 2006). Data are collected on where persons or their parents were born and those with at least one parent born outside the Netherlands are classified as *"allochtonen"*. In contrast to the United Kingdom, the third generation appear in the same category as "native" Dutch (Mladovsky 2009). These two examples illustrate that the categories used are shifting social constructions (Ingleby 2009).

Many countries are resistant to collecting "ethnic" data; this is sometimes due to ideological and ethical aspects and sometimes due to concerns over data protection (Simon 2007; Johnson 2008). In Sweden and many eastern European countries, a focus on "ethnicity" is currently regarded as both unnecessary and undesirable (Ingleby 2009), and in several countries, including Sweden, the collection of "ethnic" data is forbidden.

France has for a long time been disinclined to consider the idea of collecting "ethnic" data. In line with the republican ideology that "all citizens are equal", routine data collection systems such as the national census only refer to nationality and country of birth and do not ask any questions about ethnicity or religion (Ingleby 2009). However, the debate has received new impetus through the introduction of anti-discrimination policies and measures to promote diversity in companies (Simon 2007).

In Germany, few analyses of routine data on the health of migrants have been conducted (Zeeb and Razum 2006), as information on the origin of migrants is lacking in most data sources, although some contain information on nationality (Mladovsky 2007). No "ethnic" data are collected officially. The country is still wary of collecting such data, as that would evoke memories of the categorization of individuals that preceded the Holocaust and give rise to concerns that such data might be misused to incite racism and discrimination. Furthermore, there are concerns about data protection; Germany's Data Protection Act was one of the first to be enacted in Europe (Simon 2007).

Indeed, migrants themselves may be reluctant to reveal information on their migration status or related variables. They may – not without justification (European Union Agency for Fundamental Rights 2010) – fear discrimination, stigmatization, exclusion or, in the case of undocumented migrants, even denunciation and deportation (Ingleby 2009; Gushulak 2010; WHO 2010). After all, much historical research on race and ethnicity in Europe and elsewhere has been racist and unethical (Bhopal 1997). Yet, without information on migration status it is very difficult to monitor and improve migrant health and to combat discrimination (Simon 2007).

Conceptual and methodological challenges of data collection

The need for better data on migrant health has been recognized for some time. As long ago as 1983, a consultation by the World Health Organization (WHO) on health and migration recommended more in-depth studies on differences in mortality and morbidity (Gushulak 2010). This was further underlined by the 2008 resolution on the health of migrants by the World Health Assembly, which called on WHO member states to establish health information systems in order to assess and analyse trends in migrants' health, "disaggregating health information by relevant categories" (World Health Assembly 2008: 2) and the subsequent WHO/IOM Global Consultation on Migrant Health (WHO 2010). Within the EU, a consultation on "Migration Health – Better Health for All" in Lisbon in 2009 identified a number of areas for action, including the establishment of structures to support research and comparable data collection to better identify the health specificities of migrants (IOM 2009). The need for better health information systems on migrants has also been recognized in conclusions of the European Council (Council of the EU 2010) and declarations and recommendations of the Council of Europe (Committee of Ministers 2006; Council of Europe 2007).

Why have these calls for more accurate migrant health data failed to elicit improvements in health information systems in many European countries? Beyond the political issues discussed above, there are complex conceptual, methodological and technical challenges involved.

A fundamental conceptual problem is the lack of a universally agreed definition of what constitutes a migrant (Ingleby 2009). UN Recommendations on Statistics of International Migration (United Nations Department of Economic and Social Affairs 1998) and Regulation (EC) No. 862/2007 on Community Statistics on Migration and International Protection (European Parliament and Council of the EU 2007) aimed to establish a set of common definitions and classifications of migratory movement. However, data collection is still guided by national legislative, administrative and policy needs (IOM 2010), and follows national definitions and classifications (ECDC 2009; Ingleby 2009; Gushulak 2010), just as the determination of citizenship, residency and immigration in the EU remains to a large extent a national responsibility (see Chapter 3 on "Asylum, residency and citizenship policies and models of migrant incorporation"). As such, countries define migrants in many different ways, e.g. by country of birth, nationality, residency, and, less frequently, duration of stay (IOM 2010). This makes it very challenging to measure international migration, not to speak of monitoring migrant health or comparing migrant health across countries.

All the different definitions of migrant status have their limitations (Gushulak 2010). Nationality, ethnicity, citizenship and country of birth, for example, do not account for the time of arrival. Citizenship also fails to account for naturalized migrants, so that country of birth seems to be a better indicator of migration status (Juhasz et al. 2010). Country of birth can be used as an indicator for migrant origin or ethnicity, but, as is illustrated by groups such as Kurds coming from Turkey, it needs to be complemented with additional indicators (Stronks et al. 2009). In some countries, it is also complicated to account for children born to European parents in what were then colonies in Africa or Asia.

Another problem is that the commonly used definitions of migrant status do not distinguish between the many sub-categories of migrants, such as asylum-seekers, undocumented migrants, trafficked persons, regular migrants, and students. In migrant health research this poses a problem because these groups have specific health needs (Loue and Bunce 1999) and may face particular legal or other barriers in accessing health services (Watson 2009). Furthermore, even within distinct categories of migrants, there is bound to be great variation in the problems faced (Gushulak 2010).

The changing dynamics of modern migration (see Chapter 2 on "Trends in Europe's international migration") pose another challenge, with an increase in temporary, return or circular migration. Terminologies or classifications modelled on "traditional", unidirectional migration fail to account for these new types of migration (Gushulak 2010). In addition, the health effects of migration often extend beyond the first generation, with second and third generations facing particular health issues making it desirable to collect data in such a way that can capture this variation (Gushulak 2010).

Migrant health data are also limited by the fact that, until recently, the focus has typically been on specific diseases or conditions, particularly communicable disease (Gushulak 2010). In many of the traditional countries of immigration, health assessments are a routine element of immigration procedures (Gushulak 2010). However, they are frequently limited to specific diseases viewed as a public health threat to the host population, such as tuberculosis (Gushulak 2010). Research on social determinants of health, entitlements to health care, and accessibility and quality of care is still rare (Ingleby 2009).

Another common problem in migrant health research is that the denominator, i.e. the size of the underlying population, is unknown (WHO Regional Office for Europe 2010). Even where information is available, data may be misleading if not adjusted for age, sex and socioeconomic and migrant status. This also raises the question of which groups migrants should be compared to: is it to the host population, other groups of migrants, or the population in the country of origin? The latter comparison has hardly been addressed by research so far, but may yield particularly valuable information on how migration has affected those who have moved from one country to another.

The heterogeneity and relatively small size of some migrant communities is also a factor. As over-sampling is often required in surveys or clinical studies in order to yield statistically relevant information on smaller sub-groups of the population, and as researchers tend to be from the ethnically dominant, "native" population, mainstream medical research has for a long time favoured homogenous samples, excluding migrants and ethnic minorities from clinical trials (Ingleby 2006), although there are exceptions such as the ethnic boost in the 2004 Health Survey for England (Sproston and Mindell 2004).

Access to some populations, such as undocumented migrants, is another obstacle to research on migrant health. Finally, much research on migrant health is confined to the grey literature, not translated into English and is not used to inform future research or policy-making in countries other than where it was undertaken (Ingleby 2009).

Background data

In most countries, general background information on the number and sociodemographic characteristics of migrants is routinely collected by national authorities, typically in censuses. Although census data on citizenship or place of birth have considerable limitations, they can be used to provide rough estimates of the size and demography of migrant populations and to plan health policies (Gushulak 2010).

Regulation (EC) No. 763/2008 of the European Parliament and of the Council of the European Union (9 July 2008) on Community Statistics on Population and Housing Censuses (European Parliament and Council of the EU 2008) obliges member states to submit to the Commission (i.e. Eurostat) data on a range of indicators, including the following which can be related to migration:

- place of usual residence;
- country/place of birth;
- country of citizenship;
- ever resided abroad and year of arrival in the country (from 1980);
- previous place of usual residence and date of arrival in the current place; or place of usual residence one year prior to the census.

It can be hoped that the implementation of this regulation at the national level of EU member states will increase the comparability of statistics on migrants.

Data on mortality and morbidity

Health information systems in most European countries are not designed to identify people by migration status and the information collected in medical files rarely includes information on migration origin or status (Juhasz et al. 2010). However, an exception is the death registers maintained in many countries, which include indicators of migration or ethnicity. A study on the availability of large-scale epidemiological data on cardiovascular diseases and diabetes among migrants and ethnic minorities in the EU found that national death registers that allowed for disaggregation according to ethnicity or migrant status were available in 24 countries. Country of birth was used as an indicator in 15 countries, citizenship in 8 countries, and nationality in 7 countries (some countries used more than one indicator) (Rafnsson and Bhopal 2009). Yet, a complicating factor affecting analysis of mortality data is that migrants often return home when they become old or sick (Ingleby 2009), so that register-based studies may underestimate migrant mortality (Mladovsky 2007). The above-mentioned study on the availability of large-scale epidemiological data on cardiovascular diseases and diabetes found that disease-specific, population-based registers with data on ethnicity or migrant status were available only in Germany, England, Scotland and Sweden (Rafnsson and Bhopal 2009), although, as noted above, Germany and Sweden do not register data on ethnicity, but only on country of birth.

Health care utilization data

Health care utilization data can be an important source of information on migrant health. However, utilization levels cannot be equated with health needs, as migrants may face barriers in accessing care. In addition, the utilization of health services may not always be properly monitored and recorded, in particular where there are multiple providers spanning the private and public sectors and social enterprise organizations (Mindell et al. 2008; Gushulak 2010).

In 2008–09, registry data on health care utilization that allowed for some identification of migrants at national or regional levels were available in only 11 of the 27 EU member states: Austria, Belgium, Denmark, Finland, Greece, Italy, Luxembourg, the Netherlands, Poland, Slovenia and Sweden (Nielsen et al. 2009). In all 11 countries, utilization data were available for hospital care (although with varying detail), while only a few countries collected data on care in outpatient settings.

In England, the collection of data on ethnicity is compulsory in secondary care, except in outpatient care, accident and emergency care, and community settings (Mladovsky 2009). In 2007–08, there was an 86% coverage of ethnicity in hospital episode statistics (Jayaweera 2010).

The different categorizations of migrants in EU countries also affect the information collected in registry data on health care utilization: five of the 11 countries mentioned above collected data on both citizenship and country of birth, one on country of birth only, and five collected data only on citizenship (Nielsen et al. 2009).

Survey data

In addition to data routinely collected on the whole population, many governments commission surveys on representative samples of the population, some of which contain information on migrant status or ethnicity. They include health surveys (including health interview surveys and health examination surveys), as well as surveys concerned with broader issues that also contain some information on health, such as living standard surveys. In Sweden, for example, an annual survey on living conditions also collects information on self-assessed health and country of birth, although it does not ask about ethnicity (Mladovsky 2009). Sometimes, more general surveys are supplemented by targeted surveys aimed at hard-to-reach groups and qualitative investigations (WHO 2010).

Although incomplete, Tables 6.2 and 6.3 present a heterogeneous patchwork of indicators of migrant health included (in many cases only recently) in national or European surveys. The migrant data collected from the surveys typically have serious limitations, such as low response rates and low sample sizes; combined with the definitional weaknesses discussed above this makes it difficult to use these data to measure the health of migrants compared to the "native" population. Exceptions include the Netherlands, Sweden and the United Kingdom, which have undertaken extensive surveys on the health of migrants (Mladovsky 2007; Ingleby 2009). For example, in England, survey data on health disaggregated by ethnic origin and country of birth (including parental country of birth) are collected annually in the Health Survey for England. In 1999 and 2004, as noted above, the survey had a special focus on minority ethnic groups, boosting their numbers in order to draw statistically relevant conclusions (Mladovsky 2009).

The above-mentioned study on the availability of large-scale epidemiological data on cardiovascular diseases and diabetes among migrants and ethnic minorities in Europe could identify relevant health survey data in only six of 27 EU countries; data from nationally representative health examination surveys were available in England, France and Scotland. Nationally representative health

Table 6.2 Examples of health and migration indicators collected through surveys in selected European countries

Country	Measurement tools	Migration indicators
Belgium	1. **National Health Survey**, organized by the Scientific Institute of Public Health	• place of birth • present nationality
Denmark	1. **National Survey on Health and Morbidity**, published by the National Institute of Public Health in 1987, 1994, 2000 and 2005	Since 2005: • country of birth • parents' country of birth
Germany	1. **Children and adolescent health survey**, Robert-Koch-Institute, conducted between 2003–06	• citizenship of respondent and of his/her parents • country of birth (respondent/parents) • duration of residency • migrant status
	2. **Telephonic Federal Health Survey**, conducted since 2002 onwards in several consecutive waves by the Robert-Koch-Institute. The surveys have different foci each year	• country of birth of respondent (not parents) • citizenship (not parents) • year of naturalization • age at migration • duration of stay/residency
	3. **Sexually Transmitted Diseases Sentinel**, conducted by the Robert-Koch-Institute, 2003–05	• country of origin • citizenship • migrant group • age of migration • duration of stay/residency • self-estimated level of command of German
	4. **Microcensus** (Federal Office of Statistics)	New legislation was introduced in January 2005 allowing more precise sampling of data related to migration. Before 2005, only nationality (German vs non-German) was included. Current variables include: • nationality of the respondent • previous nationality (if applicable) • nationality of parents • year of entry
	5. **Socioeconomic panel**	• citizenship • country of birth • nationality • residence status • reason for migration • relatives living abroad

Continued overleaf

Table 6.2   *Continued*

Country	Measurement tools	Migration indicators
Finland	There are no national or regional surveys measuring both health and immigration variables, although occasional health surveys focusing on immigrants only have been commissioned by the government	
France	1. **INSEE (the National Institute of Statistics) population census surveys**	• country of origin • nationality • parental place of birth (only in 1999)
	2. **Survey on Health and Social Protection**, conducted by the National Research Institute, the National Statistics Office and the Institut de Recherche et de Documentation en Économie de la Santé biennially since 1988	2002/03: • country of origin • nationality
Ireland	1. **Survey of Lifestyles, Attitudes, and Nutrition (SLAN)** Cross-sectional survey repeated at 4-yearly intervals 2. **Quarterly National Household Survey**	Since 2006: • place of birth • start of residence in Ireland • ethnic or cultural background • nationality • citizenship
Italy	Occasional surveys conducted by the Italian Institute of Statistics	• citizenship
Netherlands	1. **POLS (Permanent Research Life Situation)** Administered every year; it is a general survey including topics such as health, but also safety, leisure time, and living and working conditions	• country of birth • country of birth mother • country of birth father
	2. The **Local and National Health Monitor** consists of three different monitors: one that monitors *child and youth health*; one that monitors *public health*; and one that monitors *elderly health*	• country of birth • country of birth mother • country of birth father • self-assessed ethnic identity

	3. The **Second Dutch National Survey of General Practice** was organized by the Netherlands Institute for Health Services Research (NIVEL). The last survey was held in 2000–02 (but data are still used) and was combined with registration data of 104 GPs	• country of birth • country of birth mother • country of birth father
Spain	1. **National Health Survey 2003**	Citizenship (since 2003), with the following options: • Spanish citizens • foreign citizens coming from: the EU; other European country; Canada or the USA; other American country; an African country; an Asian country; a country in Oceania
	2. **Regional/municipal health surveys**	Some of the latest waves of the regional health surveys include a question on the citizenship of the interviewed.

	e.g. **Catalan Health Survey 2006**	The Catalan Health Survey 2006 contains more detailed information:
		
		• place of birth with four options:
		  1. municipality of residence
		  2. Catalonia
		  3. Spain
		  4. Foreign-born
		• citizenship: Spanish; North Africa; sub-Saharan Africa; South America and Caribbean Islands; East Asia and the Pacific; South Asia; Middle East; Central and eastern Europe; EU; Other developed countries
		• year of arrival in Spain

Sweden	1. **Annual surveys on living conditions (ULF)**, conducted by Statistics Sweden.	Respondents are categorized as: • born outside the country (first-generation migrant) • born in the country, but with both parents born outside the country (second generation) • born in the country, but with one parent born outside the country (second generation) • born in the country with both parents also born in the country (not migrant)

Continued overleaf

Table 6.2   *Continued*

Country	Measurement tools	Migration indicators
	2. **Survey on public health (*Folkhälsoenkäten*)**, conducted by the Swedish National Institute of Public Health	Respondents are categorized by country of birth: Sweden; other Nordic country; other European country; non-European country
United Kingdom	1. **General Household Survey**, an annual cross-sectional survey conducted by the National Statistics Office	• how many years have you/has(...) lived at this address? • in what country were you/was (...) born? ... • in what year did you (...) first arrive in the United Kingdom? • in what country was your/(...'s) father born? • in what country was your/(...'s) mother born? • what do you consider your national identity to be? • to which of these ethnic groups do you consider you belong?
	2. **British Household Panel Survey**, conducted annually since 1991 by the National Statistics Office	• ethnic group • nationality/country of birth • year of arrival in the United Kingdom
	3. **English Longitudinal Survey of Ageing**, conducted biannually since 1998 by University College London, the Institute of Fiscal Studies and the National Centre for Social Research	• ethnic group • cultural background • country of birth • year of arrival
	4. **1970 British Cohort Study**, conducted by the Centre for Longitudinal Studies. Surveys have been conducted at birth (1970), then again after 10, 16, 26, 29 and 34 years	• ethnicity (based on 2001 census question)
	5. **Millennium Cohort Study**, conducted so far at the age of 9 months, 3, 5 and 7 years	• ethnic group
	6. **Health Surveys for England and Scotland** (annual)	• ethnic origin • country of birth

Source: adapted from Mladovsky (2007)

Table 6.3 Selected European surveys collecting information on health and migration

Survey	Migration indicators
European Community Household Panel (ECHP) This is an annual panel survey based on a representative panel of households and individuals in each country (in the EU15), covering a wide range of topics: income, health, education, housing, demographics and employment characteristics. The survey was running from 1994 to 2001.	• last foreign country of residence before coming to present country • foreign country of birth • citizenship
European Union Statistics on Income and Living Conditions (EU-SILC) This survey aims at collecting timely and comparable cross-sectional and longitudinal multidimensional microdata on income, poverty, social exclusion and living conditions. The survey contains the Minimum European Health Module of the European Health Survey System, an EU initiative to improve the comparability of health survey data in the EU.	• country of birth • citizenship
Survey of Health, Ageing and Retirement in Europe (SHARE) This is a multidisciplinary and cross-national survey on health, socioeconomic status and social and family networks of individuals aged 50 or over.	• country of birth • year came to live in country • citizenship
European Health Interview Survey (ECHI) This survey aims to monitor the health status and health care utilization in EU member states. Its basic survey, the European Core Health Interview Survey, is performed Europe-wide under the responsibility of Eurostat and covers about 130 questions. The first wave of surveys was conducted in a limited number of countries in 2009.	• nationality • country of birth

Source: adapted from Mladovsky (2007) and Juhasz et al. (2010)

interview surveys were conducted in Belgium, Denmark, England, France, Italy, Northern Ireland, Portugal and Wales (Rafnsson and Bhopal 2009).

In the Netherlands, the Permanent Research Life Situation (POLS) survey collects data on the general population that are disaggregated by migrant status; there are also regular surveys on child and adolescent health, public health and the health of older people (Mladovsky 2009). In contrast, countries such as Belgium, France, Germany and Spain have only recently begun to include questions on migration status in health surveys (Table 6.2).

The variation in migration-related indicators used makes it almost impossible to use the national surveys for cross-country comparisons. More comparable data across the EU can be derived from European surveys using the same indicators across countries (Table 6.3).

Of the European surveys, SHARE has the richest information on health, but is confined to the population over 50 years of age and has smaller samples from each country, leading to a limited applicability in migration issues. EU-SILC and ECHP have larger samples and cover all age groups, but contain more subjective indicators on health, based on self-reporting (Juhasz et al. 2010). While survey data in general have the advantage of containing a large number of indicators and not being restricted to specific health outcomes, such as mortality (Juhasz et al. 2010), one of the major challenges with population-based surveys is that, as with health interview surveys, they are often confined to subjective measures of health, such as self-reported health, with major question marks over cross-cultural validity (Ingleby 2009). However, this can be addressed to some extent by the use of anchoring vignettes, in which respondents are asked to indicate the health status they would attribute to a hypothetical person (Salomon and Murray 2004). Another problem is low response rates among migrants (Mladovsky 2009; Juhasz et al. 2010), although response rates improve when participatory research approaches are used (Fenton et al. 2002).

Another source of information comprises clinical studies and disease registers that contain information on migration status or ethnicity. However, these are confronted with the challenge that migrants often face barriers in accessing care and that the overall size of the migrant population is often unknown, making it difficult to interpret prevalence or incidence rates (Ingleby 2009). In 2009, epidemiological studies on cardiovascular disease that allowed for the identification of ethnicity or migrant status, were available in England, Germany, the Netherlands, Sweden and Wales, but only the Dutch National Survey on Morbidity Interventions in General Practice was nationally representative (Rafnsson and Bhopal 2009).

European research projects

A number of projects related to migrant health have been funded by the European Commission in the 2000s, including two specifically aimed at improving the evidence base on migrants and their health status (Samuilova et al. 2010):

- Monitoring the Health Status of Migrants within Europe: Development of Indicators. Migration and Ethnic Health Observatory (MEHO) (led by Erasmus University, Netherlands);
- Promoting Comparative Quantitative Research in the Field of Migration and Integration in Europe (Prominstat) (led by Bristol University, United Kingdom).

Several of the studies quoted in this chapter have been the result of these research initiatives. Yet, while the EU has supported some work and research on migrant health, overall cohesion and direction was sometimes missing, as efforts were fragmented between different agencies of the European Commission, as well as between the research projects it funded and those initiated by International Organization for Migration (IOM), WHO or others

(Ingleby 2009). In addition, findings and results from surveys coordinated by the European Commission are not always easily accessible to the public (Mladovsky et al. 2008; Kraler and Reichel 2010b).

Conclusions

This chapter has reviewed the availability of migrant health data in the EU and some of the challenges involved in data collection. At present, most EU countries do not collect routine data on morbidity and health care utilization by migrants, and those that do use different categorizations and definitions, so that data are not comparable across countries.

Furthermore, available data often refer to health status only. It is imperative to move beyond this disease-based monitoring of migrant health and also collect data on age, sex and social determinants of health, as well as on health-seeking behaviours of migrants, entitlements, provider attitudes, and how health systems perform with regard to health services to migrants (WHO 2010). It is also important to define better those indicators of health directly related to the migration process and to conduct cost–benefit analyses of interventions to improve migrant health.

Many countries need to step up efforts to monitor migrant health if the current lack of data on migrant health is to be overcome. There is a clear need for standardized definitions, and the inclusion of relevant questions on migration and health in existing data collection activities, such as censuses, national statistics and health surveys, as well as in the collection of routine health information (Bischoff and Wanner 2004; Juhasz et al. 2010; WHO 2010). Ideally, this should put minimal additional requirements onto existing data collection systems; allow duration of stay to be assessed; include the descendants of migrants; and be uniform across Europe (Razum 2006). At the same time, these efforts must ensure respect for the principles of confidentiality, informed consent and voluntary self-identification.

However, this chapter has shown that this will not be an easy task, as categorizations and definitions are often related to dominant perceptions of national identity and specific immigration contexts and histories. Apart from stepping up European-wide surveys, the development and implementation of EU guidance or legislation on data collection on migrant health might be one option to improve the standardization of data collection and the comparability of data, in line with the 2008 regulation on community statistics. The EU has funded several projects for improving data collection on migrant health, but there is substantial scope for developing migrant health research further, including through increased collaboration at the European level. An overall European vision on the collection of migrant health data, agreed with other major stakeholders such as the IOM and WHO, would help to ensure a more coherent approach to improving the monitoring of migrant health in Europe.

References

Aung, N., Rechel, B. and Odermatt, P. (2010) Access to and utilisation of GP services among Burmese migrants in London: a cross-sectional descriptive study. *BMC Health Services Research*, 10: 285.

Bhopal, R. (1997) Is research into ethnicity and health racist, unsound, or important science? *BMJ*, 314(7096): 1751–6.

Bischoff, A. and Wanner, P. (2004) *Ein Gesundheitsmonitoring von MigrantInnen: Sinnvoll? Machbar? Realistisch?* Neuchâtel: Swiss Forum for Migration and Population Studies.

Committee of Ministers (2006) *Recommendation Rec(2006)18 of the Committee of Ministers to Member States on health services in a multicultural society.* Strasbourg: Council of Europe.

Council of Europe (2007) *Bratislava Declaration on Health, Human Rights and Migration, 23 November 2007, 8th Conference of European Health Ministers.* Bratislava: Council of Europe.

Council of the EU (2010) *Council Conclusions on Equity and Health in All policies: Solidarity in Health.* 3019th Employment, Social Policy, Health and Consumer Affairs Council meeting, Brussels, 8 June 2010. Brussels: Council of the European Union.

ECDC (2009) *Migrant Health: Background note to the 'ECDC Report on migration and infectious diseases in the EU'.* Technical Report. Stockholm: European Centre for Disease Prevention and Control.

European Commission against Racism and Intolerance (1996) *General Policy Recommendation No. 1.* Strasbourg: Council of Europe.

European Parliament and Council of the EU (2007) Regulation (EC) No 862/2007 of the European Parliament and of the Council of 11 July 2007 on Community statistics on migration and international protection and repealing Council Regulation (EEC) No 311/76 on the compilation of statistics on foreign workers. *Official Journal of the European Union*, L 199/23: EN(31.7.2007).

European Parliament and Council of the EU (2008) Regulation (EC) No 763/2008 of the European Parliament and of the Council of 9 July 2008 on population and housing censuses. *Official Journal of the European Union* L 218/14: EN(13.8.2008).

European Union Agency for Fundamental Rights (2010) *Annual Report 2010.* Vienna: European Union Agency for Fundamental Rights.

Fenton, K., Chinouya, M., Davidson, O., Copas, A. and MAYISHA study team (2002) HIV testing and high risk sexual behaviour among London's migrant African communities: a participatory research study. *Sexually Transmittted Infections*, 78(4): 241–5.

Gushulak, B. (2010) Monitoring migrants' health. In: *Health of Migrants – The Way Forward.* Report of a global consultation, Madrid, Spain, 3–5 March 2010. Geneva: World Health Organization: 28–42.

Ingleby, D. (2006) Getting multicultural health care off the ground: Britain and the Netherlands compared. *International Journal of Migration, Health and Social Care*, 2(3/4): 4–14.

Ingleby, D. (2009) *European Research on Migration and Health.* Background paper developed within the framework of the IOM project "Assisting Migrants and Communities (AMAC): Analysis of social determinants of health and health inequalities". Geneva: International Organization for Migration.

IOM (2009) *Migration Health: Better Health for All in Europe.* Brussels: International Organization for Migration.

IOM (2010) *World Migration Report 2010. The future of migration: Building capacities for change.* Geneva: International Organization for Migration.

Jayaweera, H. (2010) *Health and Access to Health Care of Migrants in the UK.* London: Race Equality Foundation.

Johnson, M.R.D. (2008) Making difference count: ethnic monitoring in health (and social care). *Radical Statistics*, 96: 38–45.

Juhasz, J., Makara, P. and Taller A. (2010) *Possibilities and limitations of comparative research on international migration and health. Promoting Comparative Quantitative Research in the Field of Migration and Integration in Europe (PROMINSTAT).* Working Paper No. 09. Brussels: European Commission.

Kraler, A. and Reichel, D. (2010a) *Quantitative data in the area of migration, integration and discrimination in Europe – an overview. Promoting Comparative Quantitative Research in the Field of Migration and Integration in Europe (PROMINSTAT).* Working Paper No. 01. Brussels: European Commission.

Kraler, A. and Reichel, D. (2010b) *Statistics on Migration, Integration and Discrimination in Europe.* PROMINSTAT Final Report. Brussels: European Commission.

Loue, S. and Bunce, A. (1999) The assessment of immigration status in health research. *Vital and Health Statistics, Series 2,* 127: 1–115.

Mindell, J., Klodawski, E., Fitzpatrick, J. et al. (2008) The impact of private sector provision on equitable utilisation of coronary revascularisation. *Heart,* 94: 1008–11.

Mladovsky, P. (2007) *Research Note: Migration and Health in the EU.* Brussels: European Commission.

Mladovsky, P. (2009) A framework for analysing migrant health policies in Europe. *Health Policy,* 93(1): 55–63.

Mladovsky, P., Mossialos, E. and McKee, M. (2008) Improving access to research data in Europe. *BMJ,* 336: 287–8.

Nielsen, S., Krasnik, A. and Rosano, A. (2009) Registry data for cross-country comparisons of migrants' healthcare utilization in the EU: a survey study of availability and content. *BMC Health Services Research,* 9: 210.

Padilla, B. and Miguel, J.P. (2009) Health and migration in the EU: building a shared vision for action. In: Fernandes, A. and Miguel, J.P. (eds) *Health and Migration in the European Union: Better Health for All in an Inclusive Society.* Lisbon: Instituto Nacional de Saude Doutor Ricardo Jorge: 15–22.

Rafnsson, S.B. and Bhopal, R.S. (2008) Migrant and ethnic health research: report on the European Public Health Association Conference 2007. *European Journal of Public Health,* 122: 532–4.

Rafnsson, S.B. and Bhopal, R.S. (2009) Large-scale epidemiological data on cardiovascular diseases and diabetes in migrant and ethnic minority groups in Europe. *European Journal of Public Health,* 19(5): 484–91.

Razum, O. (2006) Commentary: of salmon and time travellers – musing on the mystery of migrant mortality. *International Journal of Epidemiology,* 35(4): 919–21.

Salomon, J., Tandon, A. and Murray, C. (2004) Comparability of self rated health: cross sectional multi-country survey using anchoring vignettes. *BMJ,* 328(7434): 258.

Samuilova, M., Peiro, M.-J. and Benedict, R. (2010) Access to health care for undocumented migrants in the EU: a first landscape of NowHereland. *Eurohealth,* 16(1): 26–8.

Simon, P. (2007) *'Ethnic' statistics and data protection in the Council of Europe countries.* Study Report. Strasbourg: Council of Europe.

Sproston, K. and Mindell, J. (eds) (2004) *Health Survey for England 2004, Volume 1: The health of minority ethnic groups.* Leeds: The Information Centre.

Stronks, K., Kulu-Glasgow, I. and Agyemang, C. (2009) The utility of 'country of birth' for the classification of ethnic groups in health research: the Dutch experience. *Ethnicity & Health,* 14(3): 255–69.

United Nations Department of Economic and Social Affairs (1998) *Recommendations on Statistics of International Migration, Revision 1.* New York: Statistics Division, UN DESA (Statistical Papers, Series M, No. 58, Rev.1).

Watson, R. (2009) Migrants in Europe are losing out on care they are entitled to. *BMJ,* 339: b3895.

WHO (2010) *Health of Migrants – The Way Forward.* Report of a global consultation, Madrid, Spain, 3–5 March 2010. Geneva: World Health Organization.

WHO Regional Office for Europe (2010) *How Health Systems can Address Health Inequities Linked to Migration and Ethnicity.* Copenhagen: WHO Regional Office for Europe.

World Health Assembly (2008) *Health of Migrants, Resolution 61.17.* Geneva: World Health Organization.

Zeeb, H. and Razum, O. (2006) Epidemiologische Studien in der Migrationsforschung: Ein Überblick. *Bundesgesundheitsblatt Gesundheitsforschung Gesundheitsschutz*, 49(9): 845–52.

Section V

Selected areas of migrant health

chapter seven

Non-communicable diseases

Anton E. Kunst,
Karien Stronks and Charles Agyemang

Introduction

Populations in the European Union (EU) are increasingly diverse. As compared to 10 or 20 years ago, a much larger part of European populations is born in foreign countries, including low- or middle-income countries. Often, the epidemiological profile of these migrants differs from that of local-born residents. As a result, the inflow of migrants may greatly increase the diversity in the health of European populations, including the pattern of non-communicable diseases (NCDs). As will be illustrated in this chapter, numerous reports have shown large differences between migrants and locally born populations in the risk of NCDs. While some diseases, such as diabetes mellitus, occur more frequently among migrant groups, lower risks have been reported for some other NCDs, such as lung and breast cancer. Moreover, studies of specific diseases often report great diversity between different migrant groups, with higher risks for migrants coming from certain countries or regions (e.g. western Africa), compared to lower risks for those born elsewhere (e.g. Latin America).

This diversity in risks is an intriguing phenomenon, especially when compared with the relative homogeneity in inequalities in NCD risk according to socioeconomic status (Mackenbach et al. 2008). Within locally born European populations, people in disadvantaged socioeconomic positions are at an increased risk for all the main NCDs, with the exception of breast cancer. The combined effect of these consistent patterns is a large degree of socioeconomic inequality in general health and life expectancy (Majer et al. 2010). In contrast, for migrants to European countries, the health disadvantage appears to be more linked to specific diseases, and life expectancy is not consistently lower than among locally born residents (Bos et al. 2005).

This situation presents particular challenges to the monitoring of NCD among migrants. Ideally, a fine-grained approach is applied, in which disease occurrence is measured in a systematic way for a broad range of NCDs and for different migrant groups. This would enable identification of those diseases that are more frequent among migrants, and the specific migrant groups that are most affected by these diseases.

This chapter presents an overview of the occurrence of NCD among migrants in Europe. Due to space limitations, it does not provide a systematic overview of every combination of NCD, migrant group and European country, but instead summarizes the scientific literature on the subject and illustrates it with examples from different countries. Most examples come from the Netherlands and England, both countries with a long tradition in research on migrant health.

This chapter addresses NCD risk of people who are residing in a European country but were born in another country. We focus on migrants born in low- and middle-income countries outside of Europe, and use the terms "non-western migrants" and "migrants" to refer to them. We do not systematically address disease in descendants of non-western migrants. In several European countries, the age structure of the second generation is still too young to influence patterns of NCD risk substantially among populations of non-western origin. This chapter does also not discuss asylum-seekers and un-documented migrants, as representative data on the NCD risk of these people are still scant.

Sources of data: potentials and limitations

Different sources of data can be used to describe the occurrence of NCDs in relationship to indicators of migration or ethnicity, such as country of birth, country of origin of (grand)parents, self-identified ethnicity, and more specific features such as language and religious affiliation (Rafnsson and Bhopal 2009; Stronks et al. 2009). Mortality registries at national or local level are the most commonly used data source to describe NCD risk among migrant populations (Courbage and Khlat 1996; Bos et al. 2004; Leinsalu et al. 2004; Albin et al. 2006; Fischbacher et al. 2007; Rafnsson and Bhopal 2009; Regidor et al. 2009). So-called "unlinked" cross-sectional studies utilize information on country of birth as given on the death certificate. Such studies are available for several European countries, including England, France, Italy, Spain, and a few eastern European countries. In longitudinal studies, information on the deceased is obtained by linking deaths records individually to the last population census or to a continuous population register. National longitudinal studies are available for a few countries, such as Belgium, the Netherlands and the Nordic countries. Longitudinal studies at the local level or within national samples are available for a few more countries, such as England, France and Spain. The main advantages of mortality data are that they cover the entire resident population and enable the study of changes over time. Unfortunately, mortality data are not available for a minority of European countries (mostly in the east and south of Europe). Where they are available, the quality of information on migrant populations is often compromised. The main problems relate to differences between death registries and population censuses in the measures that could be used to identify migrants, and undercounting of immigrants who have recently immigrated, who re-migrated and/or who died abroad (see Chapter 6 on "Monitoring the health of migrants").

Data on the clinical incidence and prevalence of NCD among migrant groups can in principle be obtained from health service-based registries, such as those for hospital admissions and general practitioners (GPs) (Lindert et al. 2004; Hedlund et al. 2007; Rafnsson and Bhopal 2009). For diseases such as cancer and congenital anomalies, data may also be available from disease-specific registers. Unfortunately, in most European countries, these data sources do not include information on the country of birth of patients (see Chapter 6 on "Monitoring the health of migrants"). In several countries, however, cancer registries at national or regional level do have information on country of birth of patients with cancer. Studies on the basis of these cancer registries have produced reliable estimates of cancer incidence and mortality for several migrant populations (Hemminki et al. 2002; Visser and van Leeuwen 2007; Spallek et al. 2009; Arnold et al. 2010).

For specific NCDs, such as cardiovascular diseases, information may also be available from epidemiological studies of population samples. Examples include international studies, such as the MONICA (MONItoring of trends and determinants in CArdiovascular disease) study, and comparable studies at national or local level (Hedlund et al. 2007). Unfortunately, in Europe, this type of study has so far generated only limited evidence on NCD risk among migrant populations (see Chapter 6 on "Monitoring the health of migrants").

Finally, information on the prevalence of NCD is in principle available from cross-sectional health interview surveys. However, the evidence from interview surveys may be seriously compromised because of high non-response rates and because of the failure by some respondents to report the diseases they have, due to under-diagnosis. Both problems might affect prevalence estimates for migrant populations to a greater extent than for locally born people (see Chapter 6 on "Monitoring the health of migrants").

Due to these limitations, the published evidence on the incidence and prevalence of NCD among migrant groups is highly fragmentary. Reports are often restricted to one specific disease or migrant group, and usually refer to only one European country or city. Moreover, most data sources cannot be used to stratify migrant populations according to socioeconomic position, length of residence, legal status, or indicators of "culture" and ethnicity.

Cancers: higher risks for locally born Europeans

In several European countries, studies have reported that cancer incidence and mortality is generally lower among migrant groups than among locally born residents. Lower incidence and mortality rates have been observed for nearly every major cancer type, including cancers of the lung, breast, ovary, prostate, colon, kidney and bladder. Typically, migrants have 20–50% lower incidence and mortality rates (Courbage and Khlat 1996; Hemminki et al. 2002; Bos et al. 2004; Stirbu et al. 2006b; Ho and Kunst 2007; Visser and van Leeuwen 2007; Regidor et al. 2008; Harding et al. 2009; Spallek et al. 2009; Arnold et al. 2010). For example, in north Holland in the Netherlands, despite increased risks of several specific cancers, incidence rates for all cancers combined were 20–40% lower for non-western migrants as compared to the population that was born in the Netherlands (Visser and van Leeuwen 2007).

Much larger differences have been observed in rare cases, such as skin cancer. For example, among Turkish migrants to Hamburg, Germany, skin cancer incidence was 60% lower than among non-Turkish men and women (Spallek et al. 2009). Migrants to Amsterdam had about 70% lower rates of skin cancer as compared to the locally born population (Visser and van Leeuwen 2007). While some migrant groups may be protected by darker skin, other migrant groups may reap the benefits of adhering to sunshine-avoiding lifestyles in climates where intensive sunshine is more rare than in their country of origin.

Although the risk of cancer incidence and mortality appears to be low in most or all migrant groups, the precise level of risk varies strongly between different migrant groups. For example, compared to the locally born Dutch population, breast cancer mortality was 53% lower among Moroccan migrants, but only 17% lower among Surinamese migrants (Bos et al. 2004). Such variations reflect differences between migrant groups in the degree of exposure to specific risk factors, such as a lower age at first childbirth among Moroccan as compared to Surinamese women.

Similarly, the relative advantage of migrants over locally born populations has been reported to differ between women and men. A striking gendered pattern is often observed for lung cancer. Among non-western migrants, lung cancer mortality was found to be 50% lower among men and 80% lower among women, when compared to locally born Dutch residents (Bos et al. 2004). Low lung cancer risks of migrant women are also observed in other European countries (Hemminki et al. 2002). This reflects a generalized pattern of low smoking prevalence among women in most non-western societies.

Some cancer types are more common among non-western migrants. Mortality and incidence rates of stomach cancer are generally higher among migrants than among locally born people, with the rate of excess varying from a modest 10% to more than 100% (Arnold et al. 2010). A general explanation is that migrants from low- and middle-income countries are more likely to have been more exposed to the *Helicobacter pylori* bacterium in childhood, which is an important risk factor for developing stomach cancer in later life (Fischbacher et al. 2004).

A common finding of many studies is that some groups of migrants also have much higher incidence and mortality rates for other cancers related to infectious disease, such as nasopharyngeal cancer, hepatic cancer, Kaposi's sarcoma, cervical cancer and some lymphomas (Arnold et al. 2010). Migrants' risks for these cancers often exceed the risks of locally born people to a large extent, and relative risks greater than 3 or 4 are not uncommon. The excess risk of these cancers is widely attributed to infections earlier in life, such as human papilloma virus (HPV) infection in the case of cervical cancer. Typically, incidence rates for these cancers remain increased during the rest of the life course of migrants, including for migrants who migrated to Europe a long time ago or early in life.

Addressing the higher occurrence of cancers with infectious origin could be one of the priorities for policies aimed at improving migrants' health.

However, as already mentioned, overall rates of cancer mortality and incidence are substantially lower among migrant populations than among locally born residents. As this advantage may tend to diminish over time (see below), a key challenge to migrant health policies is to develop strategies to preserve migrants' lower cancer risk.

Cardiovascular disease: large variations among migrant groups

In contrast to cancer, recent European studies do not yield a consistent picture of increased or decreased risk of cardiovascular disease among non-western migrants. Incidence and mortality levels appear to vary substantially between migrants from different countries of origin. In the Netherlands, mortality from all cardiovascular diseases combined was found to be 13% higher among male migrants from Suriname, but 50% lower among male migrants from Morocco (Bos et al. 2004). In a study from Madrid, mortality rates from cardiovascular diseases compared to the population born in Spain were lower among those born in northern Africa and southern America, higher among those born in Asia or the Caribbean, and especially high among migrants from sub-Saharan Africa (Regidor et al. 2009).

A more consistent picture emerges when the two main types of cardiovascular diseases, stroke and coronary heart disease, are distinguished. In the case of stroke, consistently higher mortality and incidence rates have been observed for migrants of west African origin. In England in 1999–2003, stroke mortality was almost 200% higher among male migrants from west Africa, and almost 100% higher among those from the Caribbean (Harding et al. 2009). These findings bear similarities with the high stroke mortality of Surinamese and Antillean-born residents in the Netherlands, and the higher stroke mortality of black people in the United States (Stirbu et al. 2006a; Keppel et al. 2010). This pattern has been attributed to high rates of hypertension among people of western African origin. It is uncertain whether this is mostly due to genetic or environmental factors. A predominant role of the environment is suggested by studies that found a higher prevalence of hypertension of west African migrants compared to people in their countries of origin (Cooper et al. 1997).

Although high stroke rates are not a universal pattern among migrant groups, they seem to be the rule rather than the exception (Stirbu et al. 2006a; Harding et al. 2008; Regidor et al. 2009). Hypertension contributes to the higher risks for many groups, although some have a lower prevalence of hypertension than the locally born population. Increased stroke mortality levels may be partly linked to other factors, such as problems in timely diagnosis and care for patients with hypertension or stroke. Although the evidence on this issue is still inconclusive, there are indications of ethnic differences in the control and treatment of high blood pressure (Cappuccio et al. 1997).

With regard to coronary heart disease (CHD), migrants from non-western countries do not appear to show consistently higher or lower mortality rates than the locally born populations of European countries. In Sweden, for example, the incidence of myocardial infarction was 50% higher among men born in Turkey or south Asia, but 20–30% lower among men born in north Africa and southeast Asia (Hedlund et al. 2007). Similar patterns are observed in other European countries (Razum and Zeeb 2000; Bos et al. 2004; Albin et al. 2006; Fischbacher et al. 2007; Ho et al. 2007; Regidor et al. 2008).

Several English studies have explored the high rates of CHD mortality among residents born on the Indian subcontinent (Bhopal 2000). While the rates of CHD mortality of these migrant groups have declined in recent decades, as in the locally born English population, the gap in CHD risk has persisted or even widened (Harding et al. 2008). The causes of the higher CHD rates are still uncertain, and may in part be related to genetic factors. South Asian migrants have higher rates of overweight, but also a greater CHD risk at similar levels of body mass index. Furthermore, south Asians are less likely than locally born people in England to present themselves with the classic symptoms of CHD, which might hinder timely diagnosis and treatment (Barakat et al. 2003). High rates of CHD may also be related to the high prevalence of diabetes mellitus (DM).

Diabetes mellitus: the epidemic hits migrants most

With few exceptions, DM incidence, prevalence and mortality rates are much higher among migrants than among locally born residents (Deboosere and Gadeyne 2005; Misra and Ganda 2007). The evidence for this is based on both mortality studies and health interview surveys. In the Netherlands, DM is more common among each of the main immigrant groups, i.e. those born in Turkey, Morocco, Suriname or the Antilles. For all of these groups combined, DM prevalence rates were 2 times higher than among the locally born population (Lindert et al. 2004). Even larger differences were observed in terms of DM mortality (i.e. deaths for which DM was identified as the "underlying" cause of death), with 3 times higher rates among migrant men, and 4 times higher rates among migrant women compared to the locally born population. Migrants of Surinamese origin had the highest prevalence and mortality rates (Stirbu et al. 2006a).

These rates are likely to be due primarily to higher DM incidence rates, although differences in case-fatality may also play a role. However, due to a lack of data sources, direct evidence on DM incidence or case-fatality among migrants in Europe is scarce. One of the few examples is an English follow-up study which found that diabetic patients from south Asia had higher diabetes mortality rates than European diabetic patients, especially at younger ages (Mather et al. 1998).

Using mortality data, a European study reviewed the extent to which DM was more common among migrants (Vandenheede et al. 2011). The study considered data on 30 migrant groups in seven European countries. For the majority of migrant groups, DM mortality was found to be much higher than for locally born residents. On average, DM mortality among migrants was 90% higher for men and 120% higher for women. These findings illustrate that, of all NCDs for which sufficient data are available, DM is the only disease which is much more common in virtually all migrant groups.

There are several interacting causes of the increased DM risk of migrants, including genetic predisposition, changing environments and insufficient medical control. A certain susceptibility to insulin resistance and abdominal adiposity, the intrauterine environment and biological imprinting all act synergistically to increase the risk of DM in migrant populations (Ramachandran et al. 2010). Moreover, metabolic control is poor among migrant groups with diabetes, and HbA1c (the amount of glucose that is being carried by the red blood cells in the body) in migrants is generally higher than in the locally born population, increasing the risk of diabetic complications (Lanting et al. 2005).

A more general explanation suggests that migrants' excess DM mortality is due to a dramatic change from a poor to an affluent environment (Misra and Ganda 2007). According to this hypothesis, DM risk is raised because many migrants in non-western countries have been brought up in situations of poverty, and their bodies have been "programmed" to cope with starvation. As a result, later in life, they are especially susceptible to gaining weight in the obesogenic (nutrient-rich and activity-poor) environments of European host countries.

Lifestyle factors that are thought to be involved include both physical inactivity and unhealthy diet. Their joint effect is to raise the prevalence of overweight and obesity in many migrant populations as compared to locally born residents (Misra and Ganda 2007; Agyemang et al. 2009). Obesity may be especially important as a factor contributing to increased insulin concentrations and decreased insulin sensitivity, underlining the need for migrant-sensitive health promotion activities.

The large differences in the prevalence of both DM and overweight are illustrated in Figure 7.1, which is based on a survey conducted in Amsterdam in 1999–2000. The prevalence of self-reported DM was about 4 times higher among

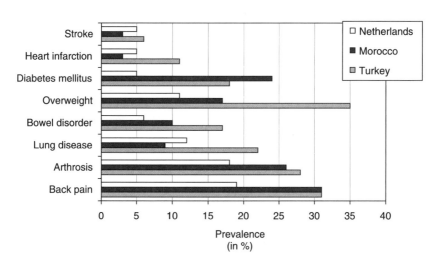

Figure 7.1 Self-reported NCD prevalence in Amsterdam in populations born in the Netherlands, Morocco and Turkey, 1999–2000, men and women combined

Source: unpublished data of the Amsterdam Health Monitor 1999–2000

Turkish and Moroccan migrants than among residents born in the Netherlands. Inequalities were much less pronounced for the prevalence of stroke and heart infarction. However, consistently large inequalities were observed for bowel diseases, arthrosis and back pain.

Other non-communicable diseases: fragmentary evidence on complex patterns

In contrast to the diseases discussed so far, the prevalence of many NCDs among migrants cannot be measured adequately by mortality data alone. As these diseases have a small impact on mortality, their importance mostly derives from their impact on health-related quality of life. However, the scientific literature on the occurrence of these NCDs among migrants is extremely fragmented. Extensive reviews are needed to construct a representative picture of the occurrence of the wide variety of diseases among all migrant groups in Europe. To our knowledge, few such reviews have been undertaken for any European country, let alone for Europe as a whole. This section presents the results of a systematic review that we have made of the relatively abundant Dutch literature (Kunst et al. 2008). Table 7.1 provides an overview of the available data sources for these NCDs.

As shown in Table 7.1, no information was available on the occurrence of dementia, Parkinson's disease and osteoporosis. As many of these diseases are strongly related to old age, the lack of evidence may reflect the young age structure of migrant populations. For most other NCDs, data were available from different sources, but risk estimates were commonly affected by problems of internal and external validity.

Very few studies exist on the occurrence of neurological diseases such as epilepsy among migrants. In one study in the Netherlands, the prevalence was reported to be about 2 times higher than among locally born residents (Lindert et al. 2004).

The occurrence of asthma was found to be higher in some migrant populations in the Netherlands. Mortality data showed important variations between migrant groups: whereas asthma mortality was not higher among Turkish and Moroccan migrants, it was more than 200% higher among Suriname- and Antillean-born migrants than among residents born in the Netherlands (Stirbu et al. 2006a; Misra and Ganda 2007).

For chronic obstructive pulmonary disease (COPD), such as chronic bronchitis, mortality and prevalence studies did not find consistent differences between migrants and locally born populations in the Netherlands. The prevalence of COPD was only higher among older Turkish and Surinamese men (Lindert et al. 2004), which can be attributed to a greater prevalence of cigarette smoking among these migrants than among the locally born population, which contrasts with lower smoking prevalence rates in other migrant groups.

With regard to gastrointestinal diseases, no clear evidence was found of large differences between migrants and locally born people. However, in Amsterdam, prevalence of inflammatory bowel disease was higher among non-western migrants than among Dutch-born residents (see also Figure 7.1).

Table 7.1 Available information on NCDs (other than cancer, heart disease and DM) among migrants, and estimated differences with locally born residents in the Netherlands

Condition	Sources of data	Quality of risk estimates	Relative risk of migrants
Dementia	None	–	–
Parkinson's disease	None	–	–
Multiple sclerosis	None	–	–
Epilepsy	Death, GP	Fair	2.03
Problem of vision	GP	Poor	2.18
Problem of hearing	GP	Poor	0.80
Asthma	Death, Survey	Fair	2.11
Chronic obstructive lung disease	Death, Survey	Fair	0.99
Ulcer of stomach and duodenum	Death	Poor	1.00
Inflammatory bowel disease	Survey	Poor	1.40
Contact eczema	GP	Poor	1.46
Decubitus (pressure ulcer)	None	–	–
Musculoskeletal problems	Survey, GP	Fair	1.52
Osteoporosis	None	–	–
Congenital anomaly of the central nervous system	Death, Register	Good	1.40
Congenital anomaly of heart	Death, Register	Good	1.02
Hip fracture	None	–	–

NOTES: Death = cause-of-death registry; GP = general practitioner registries and surveys; Register = disease-specific register; Survey = interview surveys in general population; the relative risk of migrants is the best estimate of the occurrence among all non-western migrants as compared to the locally born population.

Source: Kunst et al. (2008)

Large differences were observed with regard to the prevalence of musculoskeletal problems, including arthritis and arthrosis. Their prevalence in migrant groups in the Netherlands is about 50% higher than among locally born people (see also Figure 7.1).

Registries of congenital anomalies allow incidence rates between migrant groups and the locally born population to be compared (Anthony et al. 2005). In general, incidence rates were not consistently higher in migrant populations, but there was a general tendency for these anomalies to occur more often among children born to migrants. Notably, congenital heart anomalies occurred about 50% more often among children from parents who were born in Turkey or Morocco than among children born to parents of Dutch origin. This increased incidence is consistent with a higher frequency of consanguineous marriages among Turkish and Moroccan migrants in the Netherlands (see Chapter 9 on "Maternal and child health").

Convergence towards European levels: a slow process

So far, the assessment has been static, with no consideration of trends over time. However, disease occurrence in migrant groups may change considerably. Many authors expect that NCD risk in migrant groups will converge towards the levels of the locally born populations. This relates to the "healthy migrant" effect, which assumes that mainly young and healthy migrants migrate, resulting in low NCD occurrence among migrants in the first period after their arrival in European countries (Razum 2006). Over time, this protective effect may weaken, diminishing the relative advantage of migrants over locally born people. Another reason to expect convergence in NCD risk is that migrants may gradually integrate, or even assimilate, into their host societies. As integration proceeds, with migrants adopting the same lifestyles and facing the same environmental risks as locally born people, the epidemiological profiles of migrants may converge towards those of the host country (Bollini and Siem 1995).

Evidence in support of this convergence hypothesis has come from different types of studies, including "period" studies (comparing different periods in time) and "cohort" studies (comparing cohorts of migrants who differ in terms of acculturation) (Parkin and Khlat 1996).

In "period" studies, the differences between migrant and locally born populations are assessed for subsequent periods of time (Zeeb et al. 2002). Most of these studies observed that the differences between migrants and locally born people in NCD risk tend to change over time. For example, an English study assessed changes in CHD mortality among migrants and locally born residents between 1979 and 2003 (Harding et al. 2008; Harding et al. 2009). An early mortality advantage of migrants from western Africa and the Caribbean was found to diminish strongly over time. Some other migrant groups had higher mortality rates to start with; this mortality excess did not narrow for any of these groups, and even increased for migrants from Pakistan and Bangladesh. A similar pattern of change was observed for stroke. This study illustrates that "convergence upwards" (i.e. from initially low levels up to local levels) is a common phenomenon, while "convergence downwards" (i.e. from initially higher levels down to local levels) is – unfortunately – the exception rather than the rule for NCD.

In "cohort" studies, comparisons are made between sub-groups of migrants who differ in their duration of exposure to the living conditions in the host country. Cohort studies have been applied in particular to cancer incidence and mortality among migrants (Parkin and Khlat 1996). In one type of study, the occurrence of cancer was compared between migrants who had migrated recently and those who had migrated a long time ago (Bos et al. 2007). In another type, the cancer risk of "first-generation migrants" (who have lived in the host country only part of their life) was compared to that of the second generation (who have lived there all their life) (Stirbu et al. 2006b). In an extension of this approach, comparisons can be made within the first generation, between those who migrated at a young age (childhood or adolescence) and those who migrated at older ages (young or late adulthood) (Stirbu et al. 2006b). In each type of study, the observed patterns were consistent with the convergence hypothesis: cancer risk was most in line with that of the locally born populations among those with a longer duration of stay, i.e. among the second generation, and, within the first generation, among those who had migrated during their childhood.

Although "cohort" studies strongly support the convergence hypothesis in the case of cancer, it is important to note that convergence is often a slow process (Parkin and Khlat 1996; Stirbu et al. 2006b; Harding et al. 2009). NCD mortality and incidence rates of migrants differ substantially from locally born residents, even for the second generation and those who migrated a long time ago. For example, Indonesian migrants to the Netherlands have very distinct profiles of mortality according to cause of death, although most have lived in the Netherlands for more than 40 years (Ho et al. 2007). In Sweden, the excess risk of myocardial infarction of men born in the Middle East diminished with increasing length of stay in Sweden, but incidence rates were still 84% higher among those who had migrated more than 20 years ago (Hedlund et al. 2007).

For several NCDs, convergence may not be a likely scenario at all. For diseases such as stroke and stomach cancer, incidence rates may be largely determined by exposures in early life. In these cases, NCD incidence rates are unlikely to converge towards the levels of host countries among those migrants who arrived in adulthood. Genetic factors may also be important, for example, in contributing to the higher prevalence rates of DM among south Asians and higher rates of hypertension among west African migrants, although, as discussed above, the obesogenic environment of host countries also plays a major role. To the extent that genetic factors do play a role, migrants' higher prevalence rates may be encountered in subsequent generations as well.

Finally, in cases of complete convergence, the NCD risk of migrant groups may not move towards the rates observed for the total population of the host country, but towards the rates of people in similar socioeconomic positions. For most NCDs, we might therefore expect occurrence rates ultimately to converge with the increased rates that are characteristic of lower socioeconomic groups (Mackenbach et al. 2008). Given this expectation, the fact that the occurrence of some NCDs, such as the main sorts of cancer, appear to be still far below national levels is even more indicative of the slow pace of convergence.

Countries of origin: another yardstick of comparison for migrants

A limited number of studies have compared NCD risk of migrants not only to the locally born populations of European host countries, but also to the populations of the countries of origin. These comparisons are essential to assess the extent to which the NCD risk of migrants is affected by the migration process and the subsequent life circumstances in Europe, including access to health services. More generally, such comparisons can inform discussions on the extent to which NCD risk in late life is determined by exposures in early life (i.e. in countries of origin) instead of exposures in later life (i.e. in countries of destination). For the migrants themselves, a comparison with countries of origin can tell them how their decision to emigrate has modified their NCD risk in comparison to those who stayed behind.

This section will provide four examples of studies that extended within-country analyses to a comparison between countries, and how these studies

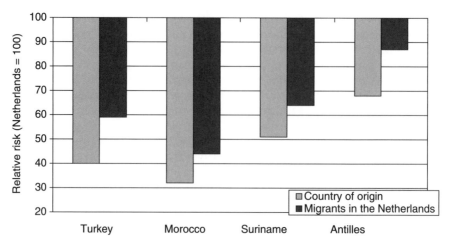

Figure 7.2 Cancer incidence in migrant groups and the respective countries of origin compared to the locally born Dutch population (set at 100), 1996–2002, men and women combined

NOTE: relative risks were estimated on the basis of incidence rates of four cancer sites (lung, breast, colon, prostate) combined.

Source: Kunst and Stirbu (2006)

have contributed to a better understanding of the occurrence of NCD in migrant populations. The most common type of comparison starts by assessing the occurrence of NCD in countries of origin (Parkin and Khlat 1996). Figure 7.2 illustrates this type of study for the Netherlands. In this figure, estimates of cancer incidence in the Antilles, Morocco, Surinam and Turkey are compared to the cancer risk of those who migrated from these countries to the Netherlands (Kunst and Stirbu 2006). Without exception, the cancer incidence rates of migrants were between the rates of the countries of origin and those of the Netherlands. As this case illustrates, the occurrence of NCD in specific migrant groups reflects to some extent the occurrence rates in their countries of origin. This yields further support to the convergence hypothesis. Especially cancer studies suggest strongly that convergence is a very likely, although slow, process (Parkin and Khlat 1996).

A similar approach has been applied to the study of other NCDs and their risk factors, such as DM and overweight. Unlike studies on cancer incidence, some studies observed large differences between migrants and their countries of origin. For example, in a study on the prevalence of overweight among Ghanaian migrants in the Netherlands, overweight was found to be 10 times more common among those living in Amsterdam compared to those living in rural Ghana (Agyemang et al. 2009). The evidence of this and similar studies suggests that migration is associated with a substantial increase in the risk of obesity and DM, most likely through drastic changes in lifestyle and environment (Misra and Ganda 2007).

When measures of NCD risk are not directly available for the countries of origin, attempts could be made to measure characteristics of these countries that might affect NCD risk over the life-course. One study assessed mortality from DM among 30 migrant groups in seven European countries (Vandenheede et al. 2011). When comparing DM mortality levels of migrants with the general characteristics of the countries of origin, a strong relationship was found with the overall level of socioeconomic development, as measured by the gross domestic product (GDP). Compared to locally born European populations, DM mortality was more than 200% higher among migrants from low-income countries, compared to a 100% higher rate for migrants from middle-income countries. This pattern supports the hypothesis that the high DM mortality levels of migrants are related to the transition from living in a poverty-ridden rural environment in early life to living in an obesogenic urban environment in later life, although available data do not allow firm conclusions to be drawn.

A final way of analysing the role of countries of origin is to compare migrants who come from the same country, but now live in different European countries. This methodology has been used in a series of studies comparing migrants of south Asian origin in England and the Netherlands (Agyemang et al. 2010a; Agyemang et al. 2010b). A study on smoking prevalence observed large differences between migrants who had moved to the Netherlands, as compared to those who had moved to England. Those who lived in the Netherlands had generally higher smoking prevalence rates, due to higher rates of smoking initiation and lower rates of smoking cessation. These differences reflected a similar pattern between locally born residents of England and the Netherlands (Agyemang et al. 2010b). These findings suggest that the particular conditions in the host country, such as the ways in which anti-smoking policies have been implemented, may strongly modify the NCD risk of migrants living in these countries. To migrants, it does not only matter where they come from, but also where they migrate to.

Burden of disease among migrants: NCDs have a major share

While the previous sections discussed the NCD risk of migrants in comparison to locally born populations or to those who remained in the countries of origin, such comparisons may not be the most relevant to migrants themselves. For them, rather than knowing about relative rates, it may be more important to learn about the absolute burden of individual diseases, and to know which of these diseases are most likely to cause discomfort, disability and early death.

To assess the absolute burden of disease, it is essential to have a measure against which the impact of different types of diseases can be assessed. In a Dutch study, we compared the different diseases in terms of disability-adjusted life years (DALYs), which are an integral measure combining the effects of diseases on the length of life and on the health-related quality of life within a population (Ezzati et al. 2002). DALY estimates were made for migrant populations living in the Netherlands by taking DALYs for the Dutch population at large and combining them with information on relative differences between migrant and locally born populations in the occurrence of diseases (such as shown in Table 7.1). The 53 conditions with the highest burden of disease in the total Dutch population were included in the evaluation (Kunst et al. 2008).

Table 7.2 Rank order of conditions posing the greatest burden of disease among non-western migrants in the Netherlands, 2005, compared to the rank order for the locally born population

Condition	Rank order among migrants	Rank order among locally born	% of migrants in total disease burden
Anxiety disorder	1	6	10.9
Diabetes	2	4	8.5
Depression	3	10	10.5
Coronary heart disease	4	1	2.1
Stroke	5	2	2.6
Injury around the house	6	11	6.0
Asthma	7	26	26.7
Traffic injury	8	19	8.3
Rheumatoid arthritis	9	17	5.6
Mental handicap	10	22	15.4
Arthrosis	11	7	2.5
Infection of lower respiratory tract	12	14	4.4
COPD	13	5	2.3
Alcohol dependency	14	16	4.6
Suicide	15	21	10.8
Contact eczema	16	28	16.0
Back pain	17	23	10.5
Problems of vision	18	9	2.5
Congenital anomaly of central nervous system	19	35	24.4
Murder and manslaughter	20	47	61.8
Schizophrenia	21	31	18.6
Breast cancer	22	18	2.4
Infection of digestive system	23	41	26.9
Epilepsy	24	37	19.8
Congenital anomaly of heart	25	39	21.1

NOTE: the percentage of migrants in the total disease burden was calculated as the total amount of the burden of disease among all non-western migrants divided by the amount in the total Dutch population, as captured by health statistics.

Source: Kunst et al. (2008)

The first column of Table 7.2 shows the 25 diseases with the highest burden of disease in non-western migrant populations in the Netherlands. Several NCDs are found among the 10 most important diseases, including diabetes, CHD, stroke, asthma and rheumatoid arthritis. Lower down the list are other important NCDs, such as COPD, arthrosis, and dorsopathy.

Some NCDs have about the same rank among migrants as in the locally born population in the Netherlands. However, there are many exceptions. NCDs with a higher rank among migrants include DM, asthma and some musculoskeletal diseases, such as back pain. The opposite pattern, with a greater burden among the locally born population, can be observed for various diseases, including COPD, problems of vision, lung cancer and dementia. Moreover, cancers are not in the top 20 of migrants, whereas they rank highly in the locally born population, a finding in line with the relatively low incidence and prevalence rates of main cancers in migrant populations. The higher rank of DM, on the other hand, is due to the high rates of DM mortality and prevalence among non-western migrants.

It is also important to note that migrant populations in the Netherlands have a relatively young age structure, so that "young age" diseases (e.g. asthma) can be more important among migrants, whereas "old age" diseases (e.g. dementia, COPD) tend to be more important among locally born populations. The relatively young age structure also explains the relatively high impact among migrant populations of anxiety disorder, depression, traffic injuries, home injuries, and murder and manslaughter.

Interestingly, the 25 diseases with the highest impact among migrants do not include infectious diseases typically related to migrant origin (such as tuberculosis or HIV/AIDS) or cancer types related to infectious diseases (such as hepatic cancer). In relative terms, these diseases do occur much more frequently among migrants than among locally born people, with relative risks exceeding 5 for some diseases (see Chapter 8 on "Communicable diseases"). However, even among migrants, the impact of these diseases on general health and survival is small when compared to other diseases. Infectious diseases contribute only little to the total burden of disease among migrants in the Netherlands, with a much greater impact of non-communicable diseases (together with mental disorders and injuries).

Similar patterns could be observed for each migrant group in the Netherlands, and for men and women alike. Although these estimates cannot simply be extrapolated to other European countries, it is likely that NCDs have the greatest impact on the general health and survival of migrant populations in Europe.

Conclusions

We have found that the risk of NCD does not seem to be consistently higher in migrant groups when compared to the locally born population in Europe. Cancers related to "western" lifestyles generally occur less often in migrant groups. For many other NCDs, incidence, prevalence or mortality rates are higher in some migrant groups, but lower in others. However, some NCDs tend to occur more often among non-western migrants in general, such as stomach cancer, cervical cancer, stroke and DM. Other examples may include asthma and musculoskeletal problems, although the evidence on these diseases is still very fragmentary. Diseases that are important contributors to the total burden of disease in migrant populations obviously deserve special attention in policies aimed at improving the health situation of migrants.

Explanations of the diverse patterns of NCD risk are necessarily complex. Socioeconomic status is likely to play an important role (Stronks and Kunst 2009). Moreover, this role is likely to increase in the future for migrant groups that will integrate more into European societies but still not succeed in climbing the social ladder. However, socioeconomic factors alone cannot account for the great diversity of relationships that are observed now (Bos et al. 2005; Hedlund et al. 2007). For example, migrants' lower risk of the main cancer types is not observed among deprived socioeconomic groups within locally born populations (Menvielle et al. 2008). Similarly, although both migrants and lower socioeconomic groups have an increased risk of DM, the excess risk seems larger for migrants than for disadvantaged groups in the locally born population (Espelt et al. 2008). In these cases, the explanation needs to go beyond socioeconomic factors.

The role of health care is as yet relatively under-researched. In most European countries, in which the financing and structure of health care ensures equal access to different social groups, no gross ethnic inequalities in access to and utilization of health services are observed (Atri et al. 1996; Cooper et al. 1998; Hjern et al. 2001). Nonetheless, elevated mortality levels of some NCDs among migrant groups present a challenge to the health system. Particular attention should be given to the detection, control and timely and appropriate treatment of diabetes, hypertension and asthma. Although the observed inequalities in NCD may not only be attributable to unequal access to detection and treatment, these inequalities can partly be addressed by improving health services and public health measures for patients from specific migrant groups.

Migrants' risk of NCD is subject to considerable change. As a general rule, when the occurrence of NCD in migrants is relatively low, as with most cancers, their rates tend to converge over time towards the higher rates of locally born residents. Although this convergence may not be surprising, it is less easy to predict how fast it will occur, as the observed changes were often slow. Some studies found that even migrants with a long duration of stay or an early age of immigration differed considerably in their NCD risk from locally born residents. These cases of slow convergence imply that migrant populations may retain a different profile of NCD risk in the near future. Full convergence may take decades, or another generation, especially if the NCD risk is determined by exposures in early life or by lifestyles that are learned in early life. Convergence will take even longer where genetic factors are involved, in particular when health systems fail to respond to differences in risk.

Cross-national comparisons illustrate that the NCD risk of migrants needs to be seen in relation to their countries of origin. Examples of relevant factors include genetic endowment, living conditions in childhood (including poverty, poor sanitary conditions, dietary factors and infections), and cultural norms and lifestyles that are retained in adult life. Conditions related to the country of origin appear to have a large protective effect on most cancers, but no such protective effect is observed in many studies on DM and obesity.

An important avenue of future research is to compare the NCD risk of migrants to that of those living in the countries of origin. While such cross-national comparisons have often been carried out for cancer, they are more rare for other NCDs. Such comparisons are not only relevant for aetiological purposes, but also from the perspective of migrants themselves. Another "yardstick" is to compare migrants who come from the same country of origin but now live in different European countries. Such cross-national comparisons show how the NCD risk is modified by the choice between moving to, say, either England or France.

A major challenge is to explain the difference in NCD risk between migrant and locally born populations. Longitudinal studies should aim to demonstrate and quantify the contribution of different types of factors, including genetic factors, early living conditions, behavioural factors, health and integration policies, and their interactions. For example, in Amsterdam, the Healthy Life in an Urban Setting (HELIUS) study was started in 2011 with the baseline measurement of a cohort of about 60,000 residents representing five migrant groups as well as locally born residents. The ultimate aim of this longitudinal study is to identify factors that contribute to ethnic differences in different diseases, including cardiovascular diseases and mental disorders. Similar longitudinal studies in other European countries could yield rich dividends and allow comparisons between different settings.

The monitoring of NCDs among migrants in Europe faces multiple tasks. First, given the diversity of patterns observed so far, a fine-grained monitoring system is required that includes different migrant groups and a broad range of NCDs. Second, the reporting should not only present relative measures based on comparisons with the locally born population, but also absolute measures that express the importance of NCD in terms of the overall burden of disease. Third, changes should be monitored using both "period" approaches (i.e. repeated measurements for subsequent years) and "cohort" approaches (i.e. measurement of variations according to generation, age at migration, or duration of residence). Finally, if possible, comparable data should be obtained on the NCD occurrence in countries of origin, and among migrants who have moved to other European countries.

Note

All figures cited in this chapter on differences in NCD risk between migrants and locally born populations control for differences in the age structures of these populations.

References

Agyemang, C., Kunst, A., Bhopal, R., et al. (2010a) A cross-national comparative study of blood pressure and hypertension between English and Dutch South-Asian- and African-origin populations: the role of national context. *American Journal of Hypertension*, 23(6): 639–48.

Agyemang, C., Owusu-Dabo, E., de Jonge A., et al. (2009) Overweight and obesity among Ghanaian residents in The Netherlands: how do they weigh against their urban and rural counterparts in Ghana? *Public Health Nutrition*, 12(7): 909–16.

Agyemang, C., Stronks, K., Tromp, N., et al. (2010b) A cross-national comparative study of smoking prevalence and cessation between English and Dutch South Asian and African origin populations: the role of national context. *Nicotine & Tobacco Research*, 12(6): 557–66.

Albin, B., Hjelm, K., Ekberg, J. and Elmstahl, S. (2006) Higher mortality and different pattern of causes of death among foreign-born compared to native Swedes 1970–1999. *Journal of Immigrant and Minority Health*, 8(2): 101–13.

Anthony, S., Kateman, H., Brand, R., et al. (2005) Ethnic differences in congenital malformations in the Netherlands: analyses of a 5-year birth cohort. *Paediatric and Perinatal Epidemiology*, 19(2): 135–44.

Arnold, M., Razum, O. and Coebergh, J.W. (2010) Cancer risk diversity in non-western migrants to Europe: an overview of the literature. *European Journal of Cancer*, 46(14): 2647–59.

Atri, J., Falshaw, M., Linvingstone, A. and Robson, J. (1996) Fair shares in health care? Ethnic and socioeconomic influences on recording of preventive care in selected inner London general practices. Healthy Eastenders Project. *BMJ*, 312(7031): 614–17.

Barakat, K., Wells, Z., Ramdhany, S., Mills, P.G. and Timmis, A.D. (2003) Bangladeshi patients present with non-classic features of acute myocardial infarction and are treated less aggressively in east London, UK. *Heart*, 89(3): 276–9.

Bhopal, R. (2000) What is the risk of coronary heart disease in South Asians? A review of UK research. *Journal of Public Health Medicine*, 22(3): 375–85.

Bollini, P. and Siem, H. (1995) No real progress towards equity: health of migrants and ethnic minorities on the eve of the year 2000. *Social Science & Medicine*, 41(6): 819–28.

Bos, V., Kunst, A.E., Garssen, J. and Mackenbach, J.P. (2005) Socioeconomic inequalities in mortality within ethnic groups in the Netherlands, 1995–2000. *Journal of Epidemiology & Community Health*, 59(4): 329–35.

Bos, V., Kunst, A.E., Garssen, J. and Mackenbach, J.P. (2007) Duration of residence was not consistently related to immigrant mortality. *Journal of Clinical Epidemiology*, 60(6): 585–92.

Bos, V., Kunst, A.E., Keij-Deerenberg, I.M., Garssen, J. and Mackenbach, J.P. (2004) Ethnic inequalities in age- and cause-specific mortality in The Netherlands. *International Journal of Epidemiology*, 33(5): 1112–19.

Cappuccio, F.P., Cook, D.G., Atkinson, R.W. and Strazzullo, P. (1997) Prevalence, detection, and management of cardiovascular risk factors in different ethnic groups in south London. *Heart*, 78(6): 555–63.

Cooper, H., Smaje, C. and Arber, S. (1998) Use of health services by children and young people according to ethnicity and social class: secondary analysis of a national survey. *BMJ*, 317(7165): 1047–51.

Cooper, R., Rotimi, C., Ataman, S., et al. (1997) The prevalence of hypertension in seven populations of west African origin. *American Journal of Public Health*, 87(2): 160–8.

Courbage, Y. and Khlat, M. (1996) Mortality and causes of death of Moroccans in France, 1979–91. *Population*, 8: 59–94.

Deboosere, P. and Gadeyne, S. (2005) Adult migrant mortality advantage in Belgium: evidence using census and register data. *Population*, 60: 655–98.

Espelt, A., Borrell, C., Roskam, A.J., et al. (2008) Socioeconomic inequalities in diabetes mellitus across Europe at the beginning of the 21st century. *Diabetologia*, 51(11): 1971–9.

Ezzati, M., Lopez, A.D., Rodgers, A., Vander, H.S. and Murray, C.J. (2002) Selected major risk factors and global and regional burden of disease. *Lancet*, 360(9343): 1347–60.

Fischbacher, C.M., Blackwell, C.C., Bhopal, R., et al. (2004) Serological evidence of Helicobacter pylori infection in UK South Asian and European populations: implications for gastric cancer and coronary heart disease. *Journal of Infection*, 48(2): 168–74.

Fischbacher, C.M., Steiner, M., Bhopal, R., et al. (2007) Variations in all cause and cardiovascular mortality by country of birth in Scotland, 1997–2003. *Scottish Medical Journal*, 52(4): 5–10.

Harding, S., Rosato, M. and Teyhan, A. (2008) Trends for coronary heart disease and stroke mortality among migrants in England and Wales, 1979–2003: slow declines notable for some groups. *Heart*, 94(4): 463–70.

Harding, S., Rosato, M. and Teyhan, A. (2009) Trends in cancer mortality among migrants in England and Wales, 1979–2003. *European Journal of Cancer*, 45(12): 2168–79.

Hedlund, E., Lange, A. and Hammar, N. (2007) Acute myocardial infarction incidence in immigrants to Sweden. Country of birth, time since immigration, and time trends over 20 years. *European Journal of Epidemiology*, 22(8): 493–503.

Hemminki, K., Li, X. and Czene, K. (2002) Cancer risks in first-generation immigrants to Sweden. *International Journal of Cancer*, 99(2): 218–28.

Hjern, A., Haglund, B., Persson, G. and Rosen, M. (2001) Is there equity in access to health services for ethnic minorities in Sweden? *European Journal of Public Health*, 11(2): 147–52.

Ho, L., Bos, V. and Kunst, A.E. (2007) Differences in cause-of-death patterns between the native Dutch and persons of Indonesian descent in the Netherlands. *American Journal of Public Health*, 97(9): 1616–18.

Keppel, K.G., Pearcy, J.N. and Heron, M.P. (2010) Is there progress toward eliminating racial/ethnic disparities in the leading causes of death? *Public Health Reports*, 125(5): 689–97.

Kunst, A.E. and Stirbu, I. (2006) Aantallen nu en in de toekomst. In: *Allochtonen en kanker: sociaal-culturele en epidemiologische aspecten.* [Numbers now and in the future. In: *Allochtonous people and cancer: social-cultural and epidemiological aspect*]. Amsterdam: KWF [Cancer Foundation]: 35–90.

Kunst, A.E., Mackenbach, J.P., Lamkaddem, M., Rademakers, J. and Devillé, W. (2008) *Overzicht en evaluatie van resultaten van wetenschappelijk onderzoek naar etnische verschillen in gezondheid, gezondheidsrisico's en zorggebruik in Nederland. [Overview and evaluation of results of scientific research on ethnic differences in health, health risks, and health care use in the Netherlands].* Rotterdam / Utrecht: Erasmus MC/NIVEL.

Lanting, L.C., Joung, I.M., Mackenbach, J.P., Lamberts, S.W. and Bootsma, A.H. (2005) Ethnic differences in mortality, end-stage complications, and quality of care among diabetic patients: a review. *Diabetes Care*, 28(9): 2280–8.

Leinsalu, M., Vagero, D. and Kunst, A.E. (2004) Increasing ethnic differences in mortality in Estonia after the collapse of the Soviet Union. *Journal of Epidemiology & Community Health*, 58(7): 583–9.

Lindert, H. van, Droomers, M. and Westert, G.P. (2004) *Tweede Nationale Studie naar ziekten en verrichtingen in de huisartspraktijk. Een kwestie van verschil: verschillen in zelfgerapporteerde leefstijl, gezondheid en zorggebruik. [Second National Study on Diseases and Treatments in General Practitioner Practices. A matter of difference: differences in self-reported lifestyle, and health care].* Utrecht: NIVEL.

Mackenbach, J.P., Stirbu, I., Roskam, A.J., et al. (2008) Socioeconomic inequalities in health in 22 European countries. *New England Journal of Medicine*, 358(23): 2468–81.

Majer, I.M., Nusselder, W.J., Mackenbach, J.P. and Kunst, A.E. (2010) Socioeconomic inequalities in life and health expectancies around official retirement age in 10 Western-European countries. *Journal of Epidemiology & Community Health*, 23 Nov 2010 [Epub ahead of print].

Mather, H.M., Chaturvedi, N. and Fuller, J.H. (1998) Mortality and morbidity from diabetes in South Asians and Europeans: 11-year follow-up of the Southall Diabetes Survey, London, UK. *Diabetic Medicine*, 15(1): 53–9.

Menvielle, G., Kunst, A.E., Stirbu, I., et al. (2008) Educational differences in cancer mortality among women and men: a gender pattern that differs across Europe. *British Journal of Cancer*, 98(5): 1012–19.

Misra, A. and Ganda, O.P. (2007) Migration and its impact on adiposity and type 2 diabetes. *Nutrition*, 23(9): 696–708.

Parkin, D.M. and Khlat, M. (1996) Studies of cancer in migrants: rationale and methodology. *European Journal of Cancer*, 32A(5): 761–71.

Rafnsson, S.B. and Bhopal, R.S. (2009) Large-scale epidemiological data on cardiovascular diseases and diabetes in migrant and ethnic minority groups in Europe. *European Journal of Public Health*, 19(5): 484–91.

Ramachandran, A., Ma, R.C. and Snehalatha, C. (2010) Diabetes in Asia. *Lancet*, 375(9712): 408–18.

Razum, O. (2006) Commentary: of salmon and time travellers – musing on the mystery of migrant mortality. *International Journal of Epidemiology*, 35(4): 919–21.

Razum, O. and Zeeb, H. (2000) Risk of coronary heart disease among Turkish migrants to Germany: further epidemiological evidence. *Atherosclerosis*, 150(2): 439–40.

Regidor, E., de La Fuente. L., Martinez, D.J, Calle, M.E. and Dominguez, V. (2008) Heterogeneity in cause-specific mortality according to birthplace in immigrant men residing in Madrid, Spain. *Annals of Epidemiology*, 18(8): 605–13.

Regidor, E., Ronda, E., Pascual, C., et al. (2009) Mortalidad por enfermedades cardiovasculares en inmigrantes residentes en la Comunidad de Madrid [Mortality from cardiovascular diseases in immigrants residing in Madrid]. *Medicina Clinica (Barcelona)*, 132(16): 621–4.

Spallek, J., Arnold, M., Hentschel, S. and Razum, O. (2009) Cancer incidence rate ratios of Turkish immigrants in Hamburg, Germany: a registry based study. *Cancer Epidemiology*, 33(6): 413–18.

Stirbu, I., Kunst, A.E., Bos, V. and Mackenbach, J.P. (2006a) Differences in avoidable mortality between migrants and the native Dutch in The Netherlands. *BMC Public Health*, 6: 78.

Stirbu, I., Kunst, A.E., Vlems, F.A., et al. (2006b) Cancer mortality rates among first and second generation migrants in the Netherlands: convergence toward the rates of the native Dutch population. *International Journal of Cancer*, 119(11): 2665–72.

Stronks, K. and Kunst, A.E. (2009) The complex interrelationship between ethnic and socio-economic inequalities in health. *Journal of Public Health (Oxford)*, 31(3): 324–5.

Stronks, K., Kulu-Glasgow, I. and Agyemang, C. (2009) The utility of 'country of birth' for the classification of ethnic groups in health research: the Dutch experience. *Ethnicity & Health*, 14(3): 255–69.

Vandenheede, H., Deboosere, P., Stirbu, I., et al. (2011) Migrant mortality from diabetes mellitus across Europe: the importance of socio-economic change. *European Journal of Epidemiology* [under review].

Visser, O. and van Leeuwen, F.E. (2007) Cancer risk in first generation migrants in North-Holland/Flevoland, The Netherlands, 1995–2004. *European Journal of Cancer*, 43(5): 901–8.

Zeeb, H., Razum, O., Blettner, M. and Stegmaier, C. (2002) Transition in cancer patterns among Turks residing in Germany. *European Journal of Cancer*, 38(5): 705–11.

eight

Communicable diseases

Tanja Wörmann and Alexander Krämer

Introduction

Until the early twentieth century, communicable diseases were the main cause of morbidity and mortality in north America, Australia and Europe. The introduction of antibiotics, the implementation of immunization programmes, and a general improvement in hygiene and living standards led to a decrease of infectious diseases so that non-communicable diseases became the predominant causes of morbidity and premature mortality. As a consequence of what is commonly described as the "epidemiological transition" (Omran et al. 1971), infectious disease mortality declined sharply in most European countries. In Italy, for example, mortality from infectious disease declined 6-fold between 1969 and 1994 (Angeletti et al. 2004).

However, despite these changes, communicable diseases continue to be responsible for a considerable burden of disease. According to World Health Organization (WHO) estimates, they accounted for 9% of the disease burden in the WHO European Region in 2002, half of which was related to the human immunodeficiency virus (HIV) and tuberculosis (TB), both of which have experienced an upsurge in several European countries in recent decades (WHO Regional Office for Europe 2005). The incidence of sexually transmitted infections (STIs) has also increased in some countries, while new infectious diseases, such as swine flu (caused by the H1N1 virus), have appeared.

Migration has been discussed as a driver of infectious disease in northern and western European countries, in particular in those countries which receive immigrants from places with a much higher prevalence of infectious diseases than in Europe. National surveillance systems indicate higher incidence and prevalence rates of certain infectious diseases among migrants, such as HIV, TB and hepatitis, findings confirmed by more detailed studies. This chapter presents the available evidence on communicable diseases among migrants in Europe and discusses the range of policies adopted in European countries in respect of screening migrants for communicable diseases.

The available evidence on communicable diseases among migrants in Europe

Tuberculosis

It has been estimated that one third of the world's population currently has latent TB infection (WHO 2010). TB is considered a disease of poverty. People who live in communities characterized by low levels of education, poor nutrition, inadequate or overcrowded housing and with poor access to preventive and curative medical services are the most vulnerable to infection. Improvements in these conditions in western Europe after the Second World War have contributed to the substantial decline in TB. However, since 2004, the downward trend has been interrupted by the re-emergence of TB among vulnerable populations, including migrants from countries where TB is less well controlled. Many studies from different European countries show that migrants represent an increasing proportion of new cases.

The total number of new TB cases in the WHO European Region in 2008 was 461,645 (52.2 per 100,000 population), with the highest rates in countries of the former Soviet Union. Worldwide, the Russian Federation is the country with the eleventh highest TB burden. Within the European Union (EU), TB incidence in 2008 was 16.7 per 100,000 population, with the highest rates in Romania (115.1), Lithuania (66.8), Latvia (47.1), Bulgaria (41.2) and Estonia (33.1) (ECDC 2010).

According to the European Centre for Disease Prevention and Control (ECDC 2010), 22.4% of all reported cases in the countries of the European Economic Area in 2008 occurred in persons of foreign origin, mainly from Asia or Africa. If data from Romania and Bulgaria are excluded, the proportion of TB cases among persons of foreign origin increases to 33.8%. Since 2001, TB cases among native-born people have declined steadily, while cases among foreign-born people have increased.

In 17 out of 28 countries of the WHO European Region where surveillance data include information on the migrant status of individuals with active TB, the percentage of all cases that are in people of foreign origin in 2008 was over 20%. In the Czech Republic, Greece, Ireland, Slovenia and Spain, these figures were in the range of 20–40%, whereas in Belgium, France, Germany and Italy, 30–40% of all cases were among people of foreign origin. In Denmark, Iceland, the Netherlands and the United Kingdom, the corresponding figures were 60–70%, while in Cyprus, Malta, Norway and Sweden they were more than 70%, reaching almost 90% in Cyprus (ECDC 2010). Interestingly, in five low-incidence countries (the Netherlands, France, Italy, Spain and the United Kingdom), the percentage of children newly infected with TB was higher among native-born than among foreign-born children, although it is likely that some of these children, although born in low-burden countries, have parents who have migrated from high-burden countries and are therefore at higher risk.

In Germany, almost 46% of all newly reported cases in 2004 were born outside of Germany and 35% had a foreign citizenship. Many of those born outside of Germany had migrated from countries of the former Soviet Union, mostly from the Russian Federation (12.4%) and Kazakhstan (8.7%). In 2004, children with foreign citizenship had 7 times higher risk of TB infection than those with German citizenship (Brodhun et al. 2006). Similarly, in France, the 2002 incidence of TB was 11 times higher in children from migrant families compared to those who were not from migrant families (Gaudelus and De Pontual 2005). A study from Switzerland reported how undocumented migrants were at particularly high risk (Wolff et al. 2010).

TB infection tends to occur at younger ages in those from high-burden countries and those infected are more likely to default on treatment and have a poor outcome (Brodhun et al. 2006). Migrants from high-burden countries (particularly the former Soviet Union) contribute disproportionately to cases of multidrug-resistant and extensively drug-resistant TB. However, it should be noted that poor socioeconomic conditions, social exclusion and limited access to health services appear to be far more important determinants of TB infection than purely country of origin. Furthermore, evidence from epidemiological studies indicates that the risk of transmission from migrants to the general population is low, underlining further that TB among migrants is primarily an issue of access to appropriate diagnosis, care and treatment (ECDC 2009).

Viral hepatitis infections

Hepatitis is an inflammation of the liver, most often caused by infection with one of the five main hepatitis viruses (HAV, HBV, HCV, HDV, HEV). While faecal–oral transmitted infections with HAV and HEV usually do not become chronic, infections with HBV, HCV and HDV are transmitted parentally or sexually and have a higher risk of chronic infection, in some cases resulting in cirrhosis or cancer of the liver.

Most evidence on the role of migration in the epidemiology of viral hepatitis in Europe relates to hepatitis B (HBV). The incidence of hepatitis B in the countries of the European Economic Area (except Bulgaria, Liechtenstein and Romania) declined substantially between 1995 and 2005, from 6.7 to 1.5 cases per 100,000. The lowest incidence rates were reported from France (0.2 cases per 100,000 population), Denmark (0.5) and the United Kingdom (0.7), while the highest rates were reported from Austria (7.0), Latvia (7.4) and Iceland (11.2) (Rantala and van de Laar 2008).

The prevalence of chronic HBV (defined as the presence of the hepatitis B surface antigen (HBsAg) for more than 6 months) also shows significant variations, both worldwide and within Europe (Figure 8.1). HBV is most common in China, other parts of Asia, sub-Saharan Africa and the Amazon region, where more than 8% of the population is chronically infected with the virus. Within Europe, intermediate to high prevalence rates are found in Bulgaria, Latvia, Romania and Turkey, whereas lower prevalence rates are found in the Netherlands, Germany, the United Kingdom and the Scandinavian countries.

A number of studies indicate that migration into the EU from countries with intermediate or high prevalence of HBV contributes materially to prevalence rates, especially in countries where infection rates are low. For example, at

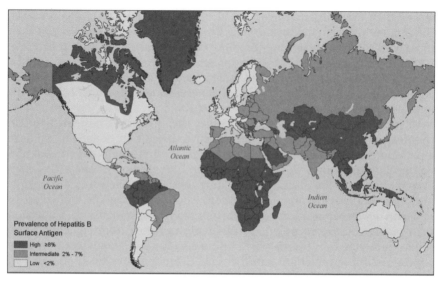

Figure 8.1 Map of global prevalence of chronic HBV infections, 2006
Source: CDC (2010)

a conservative estimate, 42% of all chronic carriers of HBV in Germany had a migrant background, although migrants represented only 12.7% of the adult German population (Marschall et al. 2005). The risk of becoming chronically infected was 7.1 times higher for resettlers (*"Aussiedler"*; persons of German descent returning to Germany from eastern Europe) and 4.3 times higher for foreign citizens than for the "native" German population (Marschall et al. 2005). Similar results were found in the Netherlands, where the overall HBV prevalence was estimated to be 0.32–0.51%, whereas the HBV prevalence in migrants was 3.77% (Marschall et al. 2008). Both studies showed that the prevalence of chronic hepatitis B was underestimated by national sero-surveillance studies, due to inadequate inclusion of migrants.

Studies in Denmark, Greece, Italy, Spain, Sweden and the United Kingdom also showed higher prevalences of chronic hepatitis B in the migrant compared to the non-migrant population. In Denmark, the prevalence of HBsAg carriers in the "native" population decreased from 0.15% in 1970 to 0.03% in 2001, but the overall national prevalence rate has remained unchanged, due to immigration of new HBsAg carriers from developing countries (Gjørup et al. 2003). In a Swedish study conducted in Gothenburg, a slight increase in HBV carriage rates was observed between 1980 and 1990. Of all hepatitis B carriers, 76% were immigrants from areas with intermediate or high HBsAg prevalence, mainly from the Middle East and southeast Asia, and only 19% were native Swedes (Lindh et al. 1993). In a survey on the prevalence of chronic viral hepatitis in 4998 people of South Asian origin living in England and attending community centres, the prevalence of chronic HBV was 1.2%, with the highest rates among people born in Bangladesh (1.5%) and Pakistan (1.8%), and lower rates among those born in India (0.1%) and the United Kingdom (0.2%) (Uddin et al. 2010). These findings confirmed the results of an earlier study, which found that chronic HBV infections were mostly associated with immigration (Hahne et al. 2004). A study in Italy also found a significantly higher prevalence of chronic HBV infections in immigrants compared to non-migrants (6.4% in immigrants vs 0.8% in non-migrants; $P = 0.01$) (Fabris et al. 2008). Another Italian study on immigrants who had arrived in the previous 6 months showed a high (9.3%) prevalence of chronic HBV infection. Interestingly, chronic infection was only found in men, the majority of whom came from Africa (62.6%), with fewer numbers from Asia (21.6%) and eastern Europe (16.8%) (Palumbo et al. 2008). Two studies from Spain showed high HBsAg prevalences in immigrants from sub-Saharan Africa. One found an HBsAg prevalence of 9.8% in this group, while the second, conducted among healthy immigrants who had lived in the EU for less than 5 years, found an HBsAg prevalence of 18.2% among those from sub-Saharan Africa (Valerio et al. 2008; Monge-Maillo et al. 2009). A study on chronic HBV infections in pregnant women in Greece ($n = 749$) found an overall HBsAg prevalence of 4.1%, with the highest rates among women who had immigrated from Albania (12%), followed by women from eastern European countries (2.1%), as compared to a prevalence among women of Greek origin of 0.8% (Elefsiniotis et al. 2009). Another study from Greece, comparing two population-based sero-prevalence surveys carried out in 1992–1994 and 1998–2006, showed a decline in the prevalence of chronic HBV in both the "native" and the immigrant population. Yet, the percentage of HBsAg carriers was still high in the 1998–2006 survey among the population of Turkish origin (8.2% in adults and 2% in children/adolescents) and among immigrants from the former Soviet Union (4.3% and 1.1%, respectively). Both groups had a significantly higher prevalence compared to the "native" population (3.4% and 0.6%, respectively; $P <0.005$) (Zacharakis et al. 2009).

There is very little information on the impact of migration on other viral hepatitis infections. As with HBV, the prevalence of co- or super-infections with hepatitis delta virus (HDV) varies considerably among different geographical areas (WHO 2001). A substantial decline in the prevalence of HDV in Europe was observed until the late 1990s. This has been attributed to the introduction of HBV vaccinations for children and young adults in many European countries, as well as in other parts of the world. Since then, however, prevalence rates have remained stable. There is some evidence that the epidemiology of HDV in Europe is driven by two specific population groups. One comprises those who survived the peak of the hepatitis D epidemic in the 1970s and 1980s. The other group comprises young people infected with HDV who migrated to Europe from areas where it is still highly endemic (Rizzetto 2009). Studies in Germany and the United Kingdom support this view. A retrospective analysis of HBV-infected adult patients at a hospital in south London found HDV in 8.5%, most of whom were born in endemic regions for HDV, such as southern or eastern Europe (28.1%), Africa (26.8%) or the Middle East (7.3%) (Cross et al. 2008). Similarly, in a German study, only 19% of HDV-infected patients were born in Germany, while most were either migrants from Turkey (26%) or from eastern Europe and countries of the former Soviet Union (28%) (Wedemeyer et al. 2007).

In some European countries, the prevalence of antibodies to hepatitis A (HAV) and hepatitis E (HEV) also seems to be higher among migrants. In a community-based survey in London, the sero-prevalence of antibodies was 45.1% for HAV and 3.9% for HEV among UK-born people, and 69.7% and 8.8% among those born abroad (Bernal et al. 1996). A study from Germany showed that 43.6% of all reported HAV cases in 2007–08 were acquired abroad, with an over-representation of male patients and children. A migration background was reported in 42.2% of cases, with most migrants coming from Turkey (48.5%), the former Yugoslavia (11.9%), south and southeast Asia (9.7%), and the former Soviet Union (8.8%) (Faber et al. 2009). The study suggested that children of migrants who return frequently to their countries of origin to visit friends and family members seem to be at special risk of becoming infected with HAV, a finding confirmed by a study from the Netherlands (Richardus et al. 2004). Active vaccination of children against HAV seems to be the easiest and most effective way of preventing further infections. With regard to hepatitis C (HCV), a Spanish study showed especially high rates of antibodies among recent migrants from eastern Europe (19.6%) and south Asia (14.9%) (Valerio et al. 2008).

HIV/AIDS

As with TB and hepatitis, the incidence and prevalence of HIV/AIDS varies considerably, not only worldwide, but also within Europe. The extent to which migration has impacted on the overall burden of HIV/AIDS in Europe is not entirely clear. The most important transmission routes for HIV in Europe are unsafe sex among men who have sex with men and unsafe injecting drug use, two risk-groups in which migrants are not highly represented.

However, when considering heterosexual transmission, the influence of migration becomes obvious: 43% of all heterosexually transmitted HIV infections reported in western Europe in 2006 occurred among migrants from high-prevalence countries (EuroHIV 2007). Data from 12 western European countries (Belgium, Denmark, Finland, Germany, Greece, Iceland, Ireland, Luxembourg, Norway, Sweden, Switzerland, and the United Kingdom) showed that of all heterosexually acquired HIV infections diagnosed in 1997–2002, two-thirds were among people from countries with generalized HIV epidemics (Hamers et al. 2004). However, the proportion of heterosexually acquired HIV infections among migrants from countries where HIV is endemic differed across Europe, ranging from 21% in Portugal to 65% in Sweden and Norway (EuroHIV 2007).

Overall, migrants seem to be particularly highly represented in the HIV statistics from Belgium, Cyprus, France, Ireland, Luxembourg, Malta, Sweden and the United Kingdom. In these countries, only 13–38% of all reported cases in 2006 were reported among people who were born in or had the nationality of the respective country (EuroHIV 2007). Migrants from Africa seemed to be the main group at risk. In the WHO European Region, 16.4% of all reported HIV cases in 2006 originated from sub-Saharan Africa, increasing to 19.1% when only considering EU countries. The highest proportions of sub-Saharan migrants among newly infected HIV cases were reported from Norway (39.5%), Iceland (36.4%), Cyprus (35.3%), Sweden (35.3%), Malta (34.5%) and Ireland (32.2%) (EuroHIV 2007). The majority of HIV infections diagnosed in migrants seemed to have been acquired within their countries of origin (Hamers et al. 2004).

In addition to national surveillance statistics, studies from different European countries can be used to illustrate the possible impact of migration on HIV/ AIDS in Europe. For example, one Greek study found that around 12% of all HIV cases reported in 1989–2003 occurred among migrants. Most originated from sub-Saharan Africa (32.4%) and central and eastern Europe (almost 20%) (Nikolopoulos et al. 2005).

A large Spanish survey, in which 8861 people with and without migration background were tested for HIV, also showed a high proportion of HIV infections among migrants (34.7%). Over half of these infections were among female sex workers originating from Latin America. The HIV prevalence in non-migrant subjects differed significantly from that in migrants from sub-Saharan Africa (1.8% vs 8.4%; P <0.001) (Castilla et al. 2002).

In a study in Italy, 3003 undocumented adult migrants were tested for HIV. Twenty-nine (0.97%) of them were HIV-positive, with an estimated prevalence in the national population of 0.4%. Information on the time of infection was available for 27 of these persons, six of whom (22.2%) acquired their infection after arriving in Italy, illustrating the importance of migrant-specific health education programmes and free access to HIV testing and care for (undocumented) migrants. The main risk factors identified were practising commercial or unsafe sex and being from sub-Saharan Africa (Pezzoli et al. 2009). The HIV incidence rate was also high among regular migrants in Italy, with an estimated rate that was 11 times higher than that for native-born Italians in 2007 (Pezzoli et al. 2009). An earlier Italian study showed a marked increase of the proportion of new HIV infections among people with another country of origin than Italy, increasing from 2.4% in 1997–2000 to 17.6% in 2001–04. Of those, 71.4% originated from sub-Saharan Africa (Madeddu et al. 2007).

These patterns are also manifest in studies of deaths from AIDS, with especially high rates in those from sub-Saharan Africa (Del Amo et al. 2004). A study in Portugal on mortality from infectious disease among African migrants found higher mortality from AIDS in migrants than in those born in Portugal (Williamson et al. 2009). Mortality from AIDS among men from Cape Verde was more than twice that of men born in Portugal. That study also found that death rates from AIDS among Africans in Portugal (87.7 male deaths per 100,000 population and 22.2 female deaths per 100,000) were much higher than those among Africans in England and Wales (10.7 male deaths per 100,000 and 11.6 female deaths per 100,000) (Williamson et al. 2009). According to Williamson et al. (2009), a possible explanation for these differences is that, in Portugal, African migrants were mainly from Cape Verde, Mozambique and Angola, whereas those in the United Kingdom were mainly from Ghana and Nigeria. In the latter countries, the prevalence of HIV is much lower than in the former. This underlines the importance of not only studying the continent, but also the country of origin in studies on migrants. Higher rates of AIDS and AIDS deaths in migrants can, at least in part, be attributed to the high frequency of late diagnosis (e.g. diagnosis with an AIDS-defining illness). This reflects the presence of many different barriers, such as access to testing and care, fear of disease and death, fear of discrimination in the community and (mainly unfounded) fear of deportation (Fakoya et al. 2008).

Childhood diseases

Many communicable diseases occurring during childhood, such as measles, mumps, rubella and polio, are preventable by immunization and their incidence is now low in most developed countries. However, other common childhood diseases, such as gastroenteritis and acute respiratory infections, are not notifiable and, even if they are, migration status is rarely recorded. In addition, data on vaccination coverage of children generally do not include information on migration background.

One of the few studies on this topic analysed routine surveillance data of 32 European countries on measles for 2006–07 (Muscat et al. 2009). Within this period, 12,132 measles cases were reported, 85% of them from Germany, Italy, Romania, Switzerland and the United Kingdom. Where data were available, the study analysed whether measles cases were of indigenous origin or imported from another country, finding substantial differences across countries. In total, 210 cases were imported in 2006 and 2007. In Bulgaria, Croatia, Cyprus, Finland, Hungary, Iceland, Portugal, Slovakia and Slovenia, all reported measles cases seemed to be imported (Muscat et al. 2009). A recent study from Italy suggested that at least one of the two measles outbreaks which took place in 2006 and 2007 seemed to be due to imported cases from Romania (Curtale et al. 2010).

According to one German study, children of parents with non-German nationality had a lower immunization rate for measles, mumps and rubella (MMR) (Markuzzi et al. 1997). Studies in Greenland and Belgium also identified migration as a risk factor for low immunization coverage (Hansen et al. 2003; Vandermeulen et al. 2008). Another German study explored whether there was an association between immunization coverage of pre-school children and their acculturation, i.e. the process of cultural adaption to their new host country. While the study did not find any difference in immunization status for the MMR vaccine, lower acculturation was associated with incomplete immunization with the multi-dose vaccine against HBV, but the "native" population was more likely to forego vaccination altogether (Mikolajczyk et al. 2008).

The practice of screening migrants for infectious diseases

Discussions of migration and communicable disease often revolve around the practice of screening migrants at entry. However, the value of screening incoming migrants for infectious diseases is highly contested and there is no consistent policy across Europe. There are countries that have established screening programmes for immigrants and others that have none. Furthermore, countries with existing screening programmes can be differentiated according to the following characteristics:

- the types of infectious diseases migrants are screened for;
- the migrant groups that are being screened (e.g. people from countries with a high prevalence of a specific infectious disease; only migrants with high-risk behaviour; all migrants; only those who are intending to stay);
- the place and time at which migrants should be screened;
- the type of screening method (e.g. radiography, tuberculin test);
- whether screening is taking place according to national guidelines;
- whether screening is a legal requirement for entering the country.

Several studies of screening practices for communicable diseases in Europe have been undertaken, most focussing on screening for TB.

Screening for TB

At least 13 of the 27 EU countries (Belgium, Czech Republic, Denmark, Finland, France, Germany, Greece, Ireland, Latvia, Malta, the Netherlands, Portugal and the United Kingdom) as well as Iceland, Norway and Switzerland have TB screening programmes specifically for migrants. Seven other EU countries and four countries from the rest of Europe are known not to have TB screening programmes specifically for migrants (Albania, Austria, Bulgaria, Croatia, Hungary, Italy, Republic of Moldova, Poland, Romania, Spain and Turkey) (Rieder et al. 1994; Coker et al. 2004; Carballo 2007). We were unable to obtain information on practice in other European countries.

In all countries with TB screening programmes, except four (Belgium, Denmark, Greece and Portugal), some system of screening is a legal requirement. The migrant groups which are being screened for TB vary. In almost all countries for which information is available on the target groups for screening, asylum-seekers and refugees are screened. However, screening of all incoming migrants, or at least of those who are coming from countries with intermediate or high TB prevalence, is also common. In France, for example, in addition to asylum-seekers and refugees, all foreigners who are planning to stay for more than four months are screened for TB. The United Kingdom screens migrants from high prevalence countries. In Greece, TB screening is compulsory for migrants who apply for or want to renew a permanent residence permit. In the Netherlands, migrants from high-prevalence countries, including foreign students who are planning to stay for more than three months, must undergo periodic screening for TB. Similarly, in Switzerland, all migrants from outside the EU, the European Free Trade Association, north America, New Zealand and Australia are screened for TB (Table 8.1).

Apart from the diversity of target groups, there are also variations in the timing and location of TB screening. Possible locations include the port of arrival or entry, specific reception or holding centres within the community and hospitals or chest units. Most migrants are screened at reception or holding centres, but screening in the community after arrival is also common. In the

Table 8.1 Target groups of TB screening in selected European countries

Country	Screened migrant groups					
	Foreign workers (staying for....)	Asylum-seekers	Refugees	All incoming migrants (staying for....)	Migrants from high endemic countries	Others* (staying for....)
Belgium	X	X	X			
Czech Republic		X	X	X		
Denmark		X	X			
Finland	X (>4 months)	X				
France	X (>3 months)	X	X	X (>3 months)		
Germany	X	X (aged >15 years)	X (aged >15 years)			X
Greece	X	X	X	X†		
Iceland		X	X	X		
Ireland		X		X		
Latvia		X	X			
Malta		X	X			X
Netherlands	X (>3 months)	X	X		X	
Norway		X	X	X (>3 months)		X (>3 months)
Portugal	X	X	X			
Sweden	X	X				
Switzerland	X	X	X	X		
United Kingdom	X (>6 months)		X	X (>6 months)		X

NOTE: *other migrant groups are for example students, undocumented migrants, adopted children and, in Germany, "resettlers"; †who apply for or renew a permanent residence permit.

Sources: Rieder et al. (1994); Coker et al. (2004); Feil et al. (2004); Carballo (2007)

Czech Republic, France, Greece and Portugal, all targeted migrant groups are screened at or shortly after arrival, at reception or holding centres. Iceland and Latvia screen migrants after arrival in the community. In Ireland, screening seems to be undertaken only at the port of entry. In Denmark, migrants are screened at the port of arrival or in reception or holding centres. In the Netherlands and Norway, migrants are either screened at reception or holding centres or in the community. Switzerland and the United Kingdom conduct screening at the port of entry and in the community. In Belgium, screening is possible in three locations: the port of entry, reception or holding centres and within the community.

In some countries, screening locations vary according to the migrant groups concerned. In Greece, for example, refugees are screened in hospitals, whereas asylum-seekers are screened at reception or holding centres (Coker et al. 2004). Information on the methods used for TB screening and age-specific formalities is summarized in Table 8.2.

As noted above, the individual and public health benefit as well as the cost-effectiveness of screening migrants for TB is highly contested and practice often depends on the lead ministry, which is not always the Ministry of Health. Although many countries use chest radiography to detect active TB in migrants, a study from Dasgupta and Menzies (2005) showed that radiographic screening for active TB at entry has only a small impact and is not cost-effective because the prevalence of active TB is very low, as is the positive predictive value of this test. If screening at entry is offered, it usually takes place only once at the time of initial entry. This can be seen as a further limitation of screening migrants, because some of them will make frequent return visits and are therefore at higher risk of getting infected with TB during returns to their countries of origin. Additional screening tests for such migrants are not performed, leading to low rates of treatment and follow-up (Hargreaves et al. 2009; Klinkenberg et al. 2009). Furthermore, in the Netherlands, it has been found that most active TB infections appear after immigration, so that screening would not affect onward transmission (Van Burg et al. 2003).

Where screening programmes identify latent TB among migrants, preventive treatment is given in most, but not all, European countries (Coker et al., 2004). This indicates that screening cannot be seen in isolation from access to health care and treatment for migrants. Indeed, research in Australia has challenged whether screening brings any benefits to certain migrants at all, given the lack of follow-up (Gray et al. 2008). Comprehensive contact tracing within foreign-born communities may be an alternative (Dasgupta and Menzies 2005; Mulder et al. 2009).

It is particularly important to have mechanisms that will allow undocumented migrants to access uninterrupted care. A European Working Group recently proposed that authorities should ensure easy access to low-threshold facilities where undocumented migrants who suspect they may have TB can be diagnosed and treated without giving their names and without fear of being reported to the police or migration officials. Governments should ensure that undocumented migrants with TB are not deported until completion of treatment, and both authorities and non-governmental actors should raise awareness among undocumented migrants about TB, emphasizing that diagnosis and treatment

Table 8.2 Type of TB screening methods targeting migrants in selected European countries

Country	Screening method used					Specifics
	CXR	Mantoux tuberculin skin test	Clinical history	Physical examination	BCG check	
Belgium	X	X	X[1]	X[1]	X[2]	TST <5 years and pregnant woman
						CXR >5 years
Czech Republic	X	X	X			TST for <15 years
						CXR for those >1 year
Denmark	X		X	X[3]	X	CXR if clinical suspicion
Finland	X					
France	X		X	X	X	BCG scar checked
Germany	X	X				TST in children
Greece	X	X	X	X		TST in those with symptoms and signs in reception centres or positives
						CXR in hospitals
						CXR for all in hospitals >18 years
Iceland	X	X				TST (Mantoux) <35 years
						CXR >34 years
Ireland	X	X				
Latvia	X	X				TST (Mantoux) <14 years
						CXR ≥15 years
Malta	X	X	X[4]	X[4]	X[5]	CXR >10 years

Country						
Netherlands	X	X			X	CXR >12 years <12 years if BCG scar then CXR; if no BCG scar, then TST
Norway	X	X	X^6		X	TST (Pirquet)
Portugal	X	X	X	X		TST for <15 years
Sweden	X	X				
Switzerland	X					
United Kingdom (England)	X^7	X^8				
United Kingdom (Northern Ireland)	X^9	X^{10}		X		

NOTES: BCG = Bacillus Calmette-Guérin immunization; CXR = chest X-ray; TST = tuberculin skin test.
[1] In those with abnormal CXR or positive TST; [2] checked in weakly positive TST; [3] = offered; [4] = only those with abnormal CXR; [5] BCG checked if TST positive; [6] for those with symptoms or history of TB; [7] at port of entry; [8] in community, TST (Heaf); if strongly positive TST (Heaf 2–4 in <16 years, 3–4 >16), then CXR; [9] if suspicious symptoms and/or positive TST; [10] if suspicious symptoms and/or positive TST.

Source: Authors' compilation, based on Rieder et al. (1994) and Coker et al. (2004)

should be free of charge and wholly independent of migration status (Heldal et al. 2008).

Screening for HIV

In three eastern European countries (Belarus, Republic of Moldova, Russian Federation), screening of migrants and asylum-seekers for HIV is compulsory. In some other European countries (Bulgaria, Cyprus, Czech Republic, Germany, Malta, Norway and Slovakia), HIV tests are also required or routinely performed on migrants. Although migrants have the formal right to refuse HIV testing in some of these countries, in practice, most entrants are subjected to testing. Other countries generally offer or recommend HIV testing for migrants (Mounier-Jack et al. 2008). At least in the Republic of Moldova and the Russian Federation, immigration is prohibited if migrants are infected with HIV or suffer from diseases that can represent a threat to the health of the population. In those countries where HIV testing is not a legal requirement, anonymous screening with appropriate counselling may be offered in order to enable direct access to any necessary treatment and to prevent further infections; denial of entry is not intended.

Conclusions

The findings presented in this chapter are to some degree limited by the fact that most of the available evidence is derived from registration data and does not take account of potential confounding factors, such as socioeconomic disadvantage. Furthermore, definitions of migrants vary greatly and data on disease incidence and prevalence among migrants are sketchy (see Chapter 6 on "Monitoring the health of migrants").

Throughout Europe, some migrants from outside the EU seem to be at particular risk of communicable diseases, particularly TB, heterosexually transmitted HIV infections, and viral hepatitis. However, it would be mistaken to perceive migrants primarily as infectious disease threats to the non-migrant population. Moreover, the individual and public health benefits, as well as the cost-effectiveness, of screening for specific infectious diseases in all incoming migrants, or at least those from high-endemic countries, remain open to considerable doubt. Of particular concern are the human rights of migrants and access to timely, effective and uninterrupted curative and preventive interventions.

Infections which are acquired within the new host countries can be due to poor living conditions of migrants (e.g. in the case of TB infections) or insufficient information about the importance of preventive measures (e.g. incomplete vaccination in migrated children). Improving the living conditions of migrants and their access to appropriate health services, including the provision of migrant-specific prevention programmes and information materials, is likely to bring about both a reduction of the number and better management of communicable diseases in migrants and a decrease in the incidence and prevalence of infectious diseases in Europe in general. At the same time, priority must be given to improving the global control of communicable diseases and reducing the incidence and prevalence of these diseases in highly endemic countries.

References

Angeletti, C., Piselli, P., Bidoli, E., et al. (2004) Analisi della mortalità per malattie infettive in Italia [Analysis of infectious disease mortality in Italy]. *Le Infezioni in Medicina*,12(3): 174–80.

Bernal, W., Smith, H.M. and Williams, R. (1996) A community prevalence study of antibodies to hepatitis A and E in inner-city London. *Journal of Medical Virology*, 49(3): 230–4.

Brodhun, B., Kunitz, F., Altmann, D., Loddenkemper, R. and Haas, W.H. (2006) Epidemiologie der Tuberkulose in Deutschland und weltweit. *Pneumologe*, 3: 257–65.

Carballo, M. (2007) Communicable diseases. In: EpiSouth (ed.) *Challenges for Health in the Age of Migration* (www.episouth.org/doc/r_documents/Challenges_for_Health_in_ the_age_of_Migration.pdf, accessed 30 May 2011).

Castilla, J., Sobrino, P., del Amo, J.; the EPI-VIH Study Group (2002) HIV infection among people of foreign origin voluntarily tested in Spain. A comparison with national subjects. *Sexually Transmitted Infections*, 78: 250–4.

CDC (2010) Hepatitis B. In: *Yellow book. Chapter 2: The pre-travel consultation/Travel-related vaccine-preventable diseases*. Atlanta: Centers for Disease Control and Prevention (http:// wwwnc.cdc.gov/travel/yellowbook/2010/chapter-2/hepatitis-b.aspx, accessed 30 May 2011).

Coker, R.J., Bell, A., Pitman, R., Hayward, A. and Watson, J. (2004) Screening programmes for tuberculosis in new entrants across Europe. *International Journal of Tuberculosis and Lung Disease*, 8(8): 1022–6.

Cross, T.J., Rizzi, P., Horner, M., et al. (2008) The increasing prevalence of hepatitis delta virus (HDV) infection in South London. *Journal of Medical Virology*, 80(2): 277–82.

Curtale, F., Perrelli, F., Mantovani, J., et al. (2010) Description of two measles outbreaks in the Lazio Region, Italy (2006–2007). Importance of pockets of low vaccine coverage in sustaining the infection. *BMC Infectious Diseases*, 10: 62.

Dasgupta, K. and Menzies, D. (2005) Cost-effectiveness of tuberculosis control strategies among immigrants and refugees. *European Respiratory Journal*, 25(6): 1107–16.

Del Amo, J., Bröring, G., Hamers, F.F., Infuso, A. and Fenton, K. (2004) Monitoring HIV/ AIDS in Europe's migrant communities and ethnic minorities. *AIDS*, 18(14): 1867–73.

ECDC (2009) *Migrant Health: Background note to the 'ECDC Report on migration and infectious diseases in the EU'*. Technical Report. Stockholm: European Centre for Disease Prevention and Control.

ECDC/WHO Regional Office for Europe (2010) *Tuberculosis Surveillance in Europe 2008*. Stockholm: European Centre for Disease Prevention and Control.

Elefsiniotis, I.S., Glynou, I., Zorou, I., et al. (2009) Surveillance for hepatitis B virus infection in pregnant woman in Greece shows high rates of chronic infection among immigrants and low vaccination-induced protection rates: preliminary results of a single center study. *Eurosurveillance*, 14(9) (http://www.eurosurveillance.org/ ViewArticle.aspx?ArticleId=19132, accessed 9 June 2011).

EuroHIV (2007) *HIV/AIDS Surveillance in Europe. End-year report 2006, No. 75*. Saint-Maurice: Institut de Veille Sanitaire.

Faber, M.S., Stark, K., Behnke, S., Schreier, E. and Frank, C. (2009) Epidemiology of hepatitis A virus infections, Germany, 2007–2008. *Emerging Infectious Diseases*, 15(11): 1760–8.

Fabris, P., Baldo, V., Baldovin, T., et al. (2008) Changing epidemiology of HCV and HBV infections in Northern Italy: a survey in the general population. *Journal of Clinical Gastroenterology*, 42(5): 527–32.

Fakoya, I., Reynolds, R., Caswell, G. and Shiripinda, I. (2008) Barriers to HIV testing for migrant black Africans in Western Europe. *HIV Medicine*, 9(Suppl. 2): 23–5.

Feil, F., Dreesman, J. and Steffens, I. (2004) Tuberculosis screening of Aussiedler at the Friedland border immigration centre, Germany. *Eurosurveillance*, 8(18) (http://www.eurosurveillance.org/ViewArticle.aspx?ArticleId=2457, accessed 30 May 2011).

Gaudelus, J. and De Pontual, L. (2005) Épidémiologie de la tuberculose en France. *Archives de Pédiatrie*, 12(Suppl. 2): 83–7.

Gjørup, I.E., Smith, E., Borgwardt, L. and Skinhøj, P. (2003) Twenty-year survey of the epidemiology of hepatitis B in Denmark: effect of immigration. *Scandinavian Journal of Infectious Diseases*, 35(4): 260–4.

Gray, N.J., Hansen-Knarhoi, M. and Krause, V.L. (2008) Tuberculosis in illegal foreign fishermen: whose public health are we protecting? *Medical Journal of Australia*, 188(3): 144–7.

Hahne, S., Ramsey, M., Balogun, K., Edmunds, W.J. and Mortimer, P. (2004) Incidence and routes of transmission of hepatitis B virus in England and Wales, 1995–2000: implication for immunisation policy. *Journal of Clinical Virology*, 29: 211–20.

Hamers, F. and Downs, A.M. (2004) The changing face of the HIV epidemic in western Europe: what are the implications for public health policies? *Lancet*, 364(9428): 83–94.

Hansen, C.H., Koch, A., Wohlfahrt, J. and Melbye, M. (2003) A population-based register study of vaccine coverage among children in Greenland. *Vaccine*, 21(15): 1704–9.

Hargreaves, S., Carballo, M. and Friedland, J.S. (2009) Screening migrants for tuberculosis: where next? *Lancet Infectious Diseases*, 9(3): 139–40.

Heldal, E., Kuyvenhoven, J.V., Wares, F., et al. (2008) Diagnosis and treatment of tuberculosis in undocumented migrants in low- or intermediate-incidence countries. *International Journal of Tuberculosis & Lung Disease*, 12(8): 878–88.

Klinkenberg, E., Manissero, D., Semenza, J.C. and Verver, S. (2009) Migrant tuberculosis screening in the EU/EEA: yield, coverage and limitations. *European Respiratory Journal*, 34(5): 1180–9.

Lindh, M., Norkrans, G., Stenqvist, K., Eriksson, K. and Taranger, J. (1993) Hepatitis B carriers in Sweden – effects of immigration. *Scandinavian Journal of Infectious Diseases*, 25(4): 411–16.

Madeddu, G., Calia, G.M., Lovigu, C., et al. (2007) The changing face of the HIV epidemic in Northern Sardinia: increased diagnosis among pregnant woman. *Infection*, 35(1): 19–21.

Markuzzi, A., Schlipköter, U., Weitkunat, R. and Meyer, G. (1997) Masern-, Mumps- und Rötelnimpfstatus bei Münchner Schulanfängern. *Sozial und Präventivmedizin*, 42(3): 133–43.

Marschall, T., Kretzschmar, M., Mangen, M.J.J. and Schalm, S. (2008) High impact of migration on the prevalence of chronic hepatitis B in the Netherlands. *European Journal of Gastroenterology and Hepatology*, 20(12): 1214–25.

Marschall, T., Prüfer-Krämer, L., Mikolajczyk, R., Kretzschmar, M. and Krämer, A. (2005) Erhöhen Migrationen aus hohen und mittleren Endemiegebieten die Hepatitis-B-Prävalenz in Deutschland? *Deutsche Medizinische Wochenschrift*, 130: 2753–8.

Mikolajczyk, R., Akmatov, M., Stich, H., Krämer, A. and Kretzschmar, M. (2008) Association between acculturation and childhood vaccination coverage in migrant populations: a population based study from a rural region in Bavaria, Germany. *International Journal of Public Health*, 53: 180–7.

Monge-Maillo, B., Jiménez, B.C. and Pérez-Molina, J.A. (2009) Imported infectious diseases in mobile populations, Spain. *Emerging Infectious Diseases*, 15(11): 1745–52.

Mounier-Jack, S., Nielsen, S. and Coker, R.J. (2008) HIV testing strategies across European countries. *HIV Medicine*, 9(Suppl. 2): 13–19.

Mulder, C., Klinkenberg, E., Manissero, D. (2009) Effectiveness of tuberculosis contact tracing among migrants and the foreign-born population. *Eurosurveillance*, 19: 14(11) (http://www.eurosurveillance.org/viewarticle.aspx?articleid=19153, accessed 9 June 2011).

Muscat, M., Bang, H., Wohlfahrt, J., Glismann, S., Molbak, K., for the EUVAC.NET group. (2009) Measles in Europe: an epidemiological assessment. *Lancet*, 373(9661): 383–9.

Nikolopoulos, G., Arvanitis, M., Masgala, A. and Paraskeva, D. (2005) Migration and HIV epidemic in Greece. *European Journal of Public Health*, 15(3): 296–9.

Omran, A.R. (1971) The epidemiologic transition: a theory of the epidemiology of population change. *Milbank Quarterly*, 49 (No.4, Pt.1): 509–38.

Palumbo, E., Scotto, G., Cibelli, D.C., et al. (2008) Immigration and hepatitis B virus: epidemiological, clinical and therapeutic aspects. *Eastern Mediterranean Health Journal*, 14(4): 784–90.

Pezzoli, M.C., El Hamad, I., Scarcella, C., et al. (2009) HIV infection among illegal migrants, Italy, 2004–2007. *Emerging Infectious Diseases*, 15(11): 1802–4.

Rantala, M. and van de Laar, M.J.W. (2008) Surveillance and epidemiology of hepatitis B and C in Europe – a review. *Eurosurveillance*, 13(21) (http://www.eurosurveillance.org/ViewArticle.aspx?ArticleId=18880, accessed 30 May 2011).

Richardus, J.H., Vos, D., Veldhuijzen, I.K. and Groen, J. (2004) Seroprevalence of hepatitis A virus antibodies in Turkish and Moroccan children in Rotterdam. *Journal of Medical Virology*, 72(2): 197–202.

Rieder, H.L, Zellweger, J.P., Raviglione, M.C., Keizer, S.T. and Migliori, G.B. (1994) Tuberculosis control in Europe and international migration. Report of a European Task Force. *European Respiratory Journal*, 7(8): 1545–53.

Rizzetto M. (2009) Hepatitis D: the comeback? *Liver International*, 29(Suppl. 1): 140–2.

Uddin, G., Shoeb, D., Solaiman, S., et al. (2010) Prevalence of chronic viral hepatitis in people of south Asian ethnicity living in England: the prevalence cannot necessarily be predicted from the prevalence in the country of origin. *Journal Viral Hepatitis*, 17(5): 327–35.

Valerio, L., Barro, S., Pérez, B., et al. (2008) Seroprevalencia de marcadores de hepatitis crónica vírica en 791 inmigrantes recientes en Cataluña, España. Recomendaciones de cribado y de vacunación contra La hepatitis B. [Seroprevalence of chronic viral hepatitis markers in 791 recent immigrants in Catalonia, Spain. Screening and vaccination against hepatitis B recommendations.] *Revista Clinica Espanola*, 208(9): 426–31.

Van Burg, J.L., Verver, S. and Borgdorff, M.W. The epidemiology of tuberculosis among asylum seekers in the Netherlands: implications for screening. *International Journal of Tuberculosis and Lung Disease*, 2003; 7: 139–44.

Vandermeulen, C., Roelants, M., Theeten, H., Van Damme, P. and Hoppenbrouwers, K. (2008) Vaccination coverage and sociodemographic determinants of measles-mumps-rubella vaccination in three different age groups. *European Journal of Pediatrics*, 167: 1161–8.

Wedemeyer, H., Heidrich, B. and Manns, M.P. (2007) Hepatitis D virus infection – not a vanishing disease in Europe! *Hepatology*, 45(5): 1331–2.

WHO (2001) *Hepatitis Delta*. Geneva: World Health Organization (http://www.who.int/csr/disease/hepatitis/HepatitisD_whocdscsrncs2001_1.pdf, accessed 30 May 2011).

WHO Regional Office for Europe (2005) *The European Health Report 2005: Public Health Action for Healthier Children and Population*. Copenhagen: WHO Regional Office for Europe (http://www.euro.who.int/__data/assets/pdf_file/0004/82435/E87325.pdf, accessed 30 May 2011).

WHO Regional Office for Europe (2010) *Tuberculosis: Basic facts on tuberculosis (TB) in the WHO European Region*. Copenhagen: WHO Regional Office for Europe (http://www. euro.who.int/en/what-we-do/health-topics/diseases-and-conditions/tuberculosis/ facts-and-figures, accessed 30 May 2011).

Williamson, L.M., Rosato, M., Teyhan, A., Santana, P. and Harding, S. (2009) AIDS mortality in African migrants living in Portugal: evidence of large social inequalities. *Sexually Transmitted Infections*, 85(6): 427–31.

Wolff, H., Janssens, J.P., Bodenmann, P., et al. (2010) Undocumented migrants in Switzerland: geographical origin versus legal status as risk factor for tuberculosis. *Journal of Immigrant and Minority Health*, 12(1): 18–23.

Zacharakis, G., Kotsiou, S., Papoutselis, M., et al. (2009) Changes in the epidemiology of hepatitis B virus infection following the implementation of immunisation programmes in northeastern Greece. *Eurosurveillance*, 14(32) (http://www.eurosurveillance.org/ ViweArticle.aspx?ArticleId=19297, accessed 6 June 2011).

nine

Maternal and child health – from conception to first birthday

Anna Reeske and Oliver Razum

Introduction

Pregnant women and children, especially those in their first year of life, belong to the most vulnerable groups of society and are susceptible to a broad spectrum of health risks. Health differentials during pregnancy, birth, the neonatal period and the first year of life are sensitive indicators of social inequalities. If a group such as migrants experiences higher rates of maternal and child morbidity or mortality, it is usually an indication that they are socially disadvantaged.

This chapter reviews the available evidence on the maternal and child health of migrants in Europe. The focus is on the antenatal period and the first year of life, with particular consideration of unfavourable birth outcomes that are at least partly avoidable. In addition to stillbirths, neonatal and infant mortality, these are low birth weight, preterm birth and malformations. We assess how these indicators are distributed, which modifiable risk factors have been identified, and what conclusions can be drawn for policies aiming to reduce health inequalities.

We do not offer comparisons of maternal mortality ratios between migrants and other population groups. This cause of death has become rare in countries of the European Union (EU), and observed differences are heavily influenced by chance effects, giving rise to methodological problems in assessing differences. The chapter also does not provide an overview of evidence-based interventions to improve perinatal health among migrants, since a sound evidence base for interventions in migrant populations using randomized controlled designs is currently lacking.

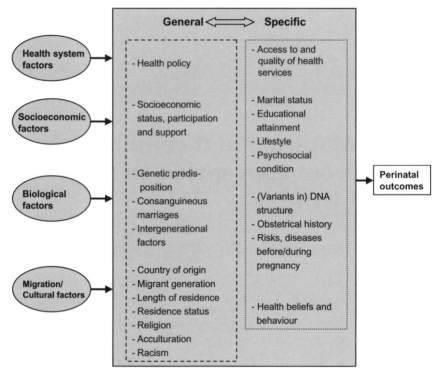

Figure 9.1 Factors influencing perinatal outcomes among migrants

Source: Authors' compilation

A number of factors can be distinguished that determine differences in perinatal outcomes between migrants and non-migrants (Figure 9.1). Apart from characteristics of the countries of origin and destination as well as possible genetic factors, the more specific factors include:

- access to, and uptake of, antenatal care;
- the quality of services offered, including the ability of health services to cater for the needs of a diverse clientele;
- social factors, such as the mother's marital status and educational attainment.

As there is only little knowledge concerning the role of genetic factors in the pathways leading to differences in perinatal outcomes (but see below), it is these three factors that this chapter will focus on.

Perinatal and infant mortality

Throughout Europe, perinatal and infant mortality rates vary by social and ethnic group. Migrants tend to be disadvantaged: among immigrant women in the Netherlands (van Enk et al. 1998; Schulpen et al. 2001; Troe et al. 2006; Troe et al. 2007a; Alderliesten et al. 2008), Denmark (Villadsen et al. 2009), Finland

(Malin and Gissler 2009) and Germany (David et al. 2006; Sievers and Hellmeier 2007), perinatal and infant mortality rates are higher than those among women of the respective majority populations.

In a recent systematic literature review by Gissler et al. (2009) on the topic of stillbirth, neonatal mortality and infant mortality among migrants in Europe, over half of the 55 studies reviewed reported worse mortality outcomes for migrants compared to the respective non-migratory population, approximately one-third of the studies found no difference, and only 13% reported better outcomes. Babies born to migrant women, in particular from the non-western countries of Turkey, Morocco, Pakistan and Somalia, have a higher mortality risk. Refugees are an especially vulnerable group, often having higher rates of stillbirth and neonatal and perinatal mortality compared to the respective majority population. There are however migrant groups, particularly from eastern Europe, who experience a lower risk or one similar to that of the non-migratory population (Gissler et al. 2009).

In the Netherlands, infant mortality rates also differ across generations (Troe et al. 2007a). Data from Statistics Netherlands for 1995–2000 show that infant mortality among offspring of women of Turkish origin increased with time in the Netherlands; for Turkish women who immigrated after their 16th birthday, infant mortality averaged 5.5 per 1000 live births. This rate increased to 6.4 for women who immigrated before their 16th birthday, and was highest (6.8) for women of Turkish origin born in the Netherlands. Among women from Suriname, the trend was reversed, with infant mortality lowest (5.5) among those migrants born in the Netherlands. Furthermore, the risk of infant death due to malformations or perinatal causes increases with decreasing age of the Turkish mother at migration, while for women from Suriname the risk decreases with decreasing age at migration (Troe et al. 2007a).

Possible determinants of differentials in infant mortality

Explaining disparities in mortality in the context of migration requires a multifaceted approach. Due to the heterogeneity in the definition of migration status (i.e. country of birth, self-reported ethnicity, nationality), few studies from different European countries are comparable methodologically.

An important finding is that infants born into families who have migrated are at greater risk of dying due to perinatal causes (e.g. conditions relating to short gestation). In some migrant groups, higher infant mortality can be attributed entirely to higher rates of preterm birth (Schulpen et al. 2001; Alderliesten et al. 2008). This is, for example, the case in the Netherlands (Schulpen et al. 2001), where the perinatal mortality of infants born between 1990 and 1993 to black women was more than 2 times higher than that of "native" women, while the risk of infants born to West-Indian Asians from Suriname and the Netherlands Antilles was 1.4 times higher. Among migrant women from non-western countries (in particular Ghana), a higher preterm birth rate compared to native Dutch women appears to be the primary reason for the higher rate of perinatal mortality (Alderliesten et al. 2008). In contrast, in the group of migrants from Mediterranean countries, higher risks of perinatal mortality were attributed to a higher proportion of teenage pregnancies and multiparity rather than to higher preterm birth rates (Schulpen et al. 2001). However, findings on this topic are inconsistent.

Higher infant mortality among migrants is also linked to a higher frequency of congenital malformations, particularly among newborns of Turkish, Pakistani, Somali and Moroccan migrants in the Netherlands and Denmark, as well as among Pakistani or Bangladeshi migrants in England and Wales (Schulpen et al. 2001; Troe et al. 2006; Villadsen et al. 2009). In the Netherlands, the risk of infant mortality among Turkish and Moroccan migrants is 1.3 times higher than among "native" women, particularly in the post-neonatal period and in connection with congenital malformations (Troe et al. 2006). In Denmark, risks are higher for stillbirth and infant mortality among Turkish (risk ratio (RR): 1.28 and 1.41, respectively), Pakistani (RR: 1.62 and 1.88, respectively) and Somali migrants (RR: 2.11 and 1.39, respectively) compared to Danish women. These children are at higher risk of death due to malformations, although this excess mortality disappears after adjusting for household income and/or maternal education. For migrants from Lebanon and the former Yugoslavia, the risk of death is comparable to that of the non-migrant population (Villadsen et al. 2009).

A significant risk factor for malformations is consanguineous marriage: the risk of neonatal death or severe malformation is markedly higher for infants of related parents compared to infants of non-related parents (Bittles et al. 1991). An increased rate of malformations in some migrant groups (such as from Pakistan) can be explained, at least partially, by a high prevalence of next-of-kin marriages (Terry et al. 1985; Stoltenberg et al. 1997). The highest rates of consanguineous marriages have been reported in Arab countries (about 20–50% of all marriages; especially in Egypt, Iraq, the Libyan Arab Jamahiriya, Oman, Saudi Arabia) (Tadmouri et al. 2009). In Turkey and among Muslim populations of India and Pakistan, marriages between relatives are also common (Bittles et al. 1991; Stöckler-Ipsiroglu et al. 2005). Consanguinity rates seem to differ within countries, with a trend to higher rates in rural settings compared to urban areas (Tadmouri et al. 2009). Migrants to western Europe, many of whom originate in these rural areas, show a tendency to marry close relatives when residing in the host country (Bittles et al. 1991).

Consanguineous marriages lead to an increased risk for offspring to be born with (rare) hereditary diseases and illnesses with multifactorial aetiologies that often result in a life of suffering or, in some cases, a reduced life expectancy.

It is within this context that Stoltenberg et al. (1997) studied the effect of consanguinity and educational level of parents on the occurrence of congenital malformations among Pakistani (based on the country of origin) migrants to Norway and the general Norwegian population. Among Pakistani migrants (both parents from Pakistan), 40% of parents were related, whereas among the Norwegian sample (both parents from Norway), only 1% were related. The proportion of children born with malformations was highest among those in which both parents originated from Pakistan (3.0% vs 1.5% among Norwegians). Vangen et al. (1999) confirmed these findings: the risk of malformations among infants born to non-related parents was similar across all groups investigated in Norway, independent of country of origin and educational level. In contrast, children of related parents, across all groups, were nearly twice as likely to be born with malformations. In the group of Pakistani migrants, consanguinity was a significant risk factor for the occurrence of malformations, accounting for 30% of all cases. While the likelihood of next-of-kin marriage decreases with increasing education, there appears to be no independent effect of social status on the risk of malformations (Stoltenberg et al. 1997).

Somewhat surprisingly, socioeconomic and demographic factors do not appear to play a significant role in perinatal mortality risk among migrants (Schulpen et al. 2001; Villadsen et al. 2009). In the Netherlands (Troe et al. 2006), socioeconomic and demographic factors (such as marital status and maternal age) only partially explain the higher infant mortality among migrants compared to non-migrant women, although an earlier study suggested that employment status and not country of birth was the main explanatory factor for increased perinatal mortality (Lumey and Reijneveld 1995).

Refugees, asylum-seekers and undocumented migrants

Migrants who lack legal residence status or whose position is uncertain, as well as those who have been politically persecuted in their home country, are at particularly high risk of unfavourable perinatal health outcomes. Gissler et al. (2009) reviewed data from Ireland, the Netherlands, Norway and Sweden, showing that registered refugees had higher stillbirth, early neonatal mortality and perinatal mortality rates compared to non-refugee women from the host countries. In Ireland and Sweden, the refugees were primarily from Africa (in Sweden, especially from Somalia). Data from Croatia and Serbia indicate that displaced women from countries of the former Yugoslavia have less favourable perinatal mortality outcomes. They experience higher early neonatal and perinatal mortality rates than non-displaced women in Croatia and Serbia.

In the United Kingdom, asylum-seekers from Somalia had less favourable demographic and obstetric characteristics (e.g. higher number of children) than British-born women. These risk factors, however, seemed to have little effect on obstetric and foetal outcomes (Yoong et al. 2005), and there were no major differences in mode of delivery and birth outcomes (e.g. preterm birth, birthweight, caesarean section, instrumental delivery) between asylum-seekers and non-migrants. The authors explained these findings as reflecting an increased vigilance by health professionals in a multiethnic society, as well as a (self-)selection of migrant women who are at low obstetric risk.

Undocumented migrants are believed to be at particularly high risk, due to their uncertain situation and additional legal barriers in obtaining health services, although some EU member states have introduced special regulations for pregnant women and early childhood. In Italy, for example, undocumented pregnant women are granted full access to the health system until 6 months after childbirth. In Germany, pregnant women are exempted from deportation.

The few studies addressing undocumented migrants indicate that they are exposed to poor housing and nutrition, psychological pressure, and a higher prevalence of tuberculosis and other infectious diseases (Lindert 2003), which is likely to have an impact on perinatal and infant health.

Although undocumented migrants may encounter particular difficulties in accessing antenatal care, some studies have found that undocumented migrant women have pregnancy risks that are comparable to those of women from the host country. A study in Geneva (Switzerland) suggested that some birth outcomes among undocumented migrants were even more favourable, which might be explained by a lower risk profile in terms of lifestyle-related factors (e.g. lower rates of smoking or alcohol consumption) (Wolff et al. 2008). Nevertheless, pregnancies among undocumented migrant women should normally be considered "high risk pregnancies" and be carefully monitored. Wolff et al. (2008) also emphasize the high prevalence of unintended pregnancies and violence during pregnancy among undocumented migrants. When treating such populations, health practitioners should keep this additional risk factor for both children and mothers in mind.

Low birth weight and preterm birth

In comparison to developing countries, the frequency of low birth weight and preterm birth in Europe is relatively low. However, due to its potentially serious consequences, even at this low rate it is considered an important public health problem. Newborns born prematurely or with low birth weight are at high risk of perinatal and neonatal mortality, as well as short- and long-term morbidity (Wilcox and Russell 1983). Particularly problematic is the underdevelopment of the organ systems and their functions. There is a likely association between these adverse birth outcomes and an increased risk for chronic illnesses among adults (Barker 1998).

Studies on associations between migration background and low birth weight or preterm birth are inconsistent. Although, as mentioned above, higher infant mortality can be attributed entirely to higher rates of preterm birth in some migrant groups, a recent systematic review of the literature (Gagnon et al. 2009) identified a total of 133 publications from 1995 to 2008, of which 23 were included in the review. Over half of the studies found either no difference between migrants and non-migrants regarding low birth weight and preterm birth, or better outcomes for migrants. However, due to the heterogeneity of study designs, including definitions of migrants and confounders considered, results should be interpreted with caution.

Low birth weight

Two large population-based cohort studies from the United Kingdom (Kelly et al. 2009) and the Netherlands (Troe et al. 2007b) demonstrate that children with a migration background have a significantly lower birth weight than the non-migrant population. In the Netherlands, shorter gestational age and lower parental height constitute strong determinants for lower birth weight in the non-Dutch population. It is assumed that the influence of parental height is due to a mixture of genetic and environmental factors. Further studies are needed to clarify the impact of these factors.

The authors also attribute differences in birth weight to socioeconomic factors (Kelly et al. 2009), although this conflicts with other studies in which socioeconomic factors were either not at all or only weakly associated with differences in risk (Teitler et al. 2007). In contrast to earlier studies, Kelly et al. used more indicators of socioeconomic status (e.g. household income, lone parent household, highest academic qualification) and found that they had an influence on birth weight in black Caribbean, black African, Bangladeshi and Pakistani infants, whereas maternal factors had a stronger influence in other migrant groups (Indian and Bangladeshi infants). Despite the associations with socioeconomic status, however, the specific pathways leading to lower birth weight are still unclear and much of the difference remains unexplained.

The hypothesis that health risks and behaviours undergo change between migrants and their descendants does not appear to apply to mean birth weight or the incidence of low birth weight, at least in the United Kingdom, where these two parameters differ only minimally between migrants and their UK-born offspring (Harding et al. 2004). This finding might be surprising, because socioeconomic conditions often improve from one generation to the next and health care in the new host country tends to be better than in the country of origin. However, a number of studies have shown that health behaviours, such as smoking, and health outcomes can worsen over generations or with extended residency (Harding 2003; Hosper et al. 2007; Reeske et al. 2009).

Despite worse concomitant circumstances, such as increased psychological and medical risk factors and low utilization of antenatal services, the risk for low-birth-weight babies among migrants to Germany from eastern Europe and the Mediterranean (Reime et al. 2006; Koller et al. 2009) is similar to that of native women. Non-migrant single mothers and unemployed women, as well as women with lower occupational status, were found to have a higher risk of low-birth-weight babies. This can be partially explained by a higher prevalence of smoking, lower utilization of antenatal services and greater levels of psychosocial stress. Since migrants often tend to occupy lower socioeconomic strata, migration status cannot be excluded as a risk factor and must be studied more closely, in order to develop targeted measures.

In France and Belgium, women of north African origin are less likely than non-migrant women to deliver a low-birth-weight or preterm baby (Guendelman et al. 1999), despite the fact that utilization of antenatal care is much lower. However, as argued by Troe et al. (2007b), these observations fail to explain the differences in low birth weight and preterm birth between migrants and non-migrants. Alternative explanations include the protective effect of culturally-based healthier lifestyles among these migrant women, and a (self-)selection of relatively healthy migrant women with fewer risk factors and accordingly lower pregnancy and delivery complications (the "healthy migrant effect").

Preterm birth

The risk of preterm birth among migrant women varies according to country of origin and birth. In general, women of African and Asian origin have an elevated risk of preterm birth (Rasmussen et al. 1995; Aveyard et al. 2002; Zeitlin et al. 2004; Goedhart et al. 2008).

In a population-based cohort study in Amsterdam (Goedhart et al. 2008), the greater risk of preterm birth among migrants could to some extent be explained by cumulative risk factors, such as previous stillbirth or preterm birth, obesity, low level of education, single motherhood, depression or unpaid work. Migrant women from sub-Saharan Africa and French Overseas Territories were found to have a significantly higher risk of both natural preterm birth (particularly preterm birth before the 33rd week of pregnancy) and induced preterm birth, compared to women from metropolitan France (Zeitlin et al. 2004). This has been attributed to higher rates of hypertension among these migrant women, while factors such as delayed utilization of antenatal care and low health insurance coverage had virtually no impact on the risk of preterm birth. Migrants from southern Europe, north Africa and Asia, on the other hand, were found to have a risk of preterm delivery that was comparable to the non-migrant population.

In Germany and the Netherlands, migrants of Turkish and Moroccan backgrounds, despite having a more adverse risk profile, are not at significantly greater risk of preterm birth than the respective non-migrant populations (David et al. 2006; Goedhart et al. 2008). The extent to which environmental or genetic factors influence these favourable outcomes is, to a large degree, unclear and warrants further research.

The close correlation between migration background and lower socioeconomic status makes it difficult to identify which of the two factors has a greater effect on risk of preterm birth. Although a number of studies have demonstrated a clear association between preterm birth and socioeconomic factors (Parker et al. 1994; Olsen et al. 1995; Peacock et al. 1995), the precise nature of the connection between the two parameters often remains elusive. Kramer et al. present a comprehensive overview of possible causal pathways and mechanisms to explain the connection. In particular, they emphasize the role of intermediary steps, such as increased chronic and acute stress, lower intake of folic acid and a greater incidence of genital infections (Kramer et al. 2001). Against this backdrop, Aveyard et al. (2002), in the United Kingdom, demonstrated that variations in the risk of preterm birth between the ethnic groups under study could be largely explained by adverse socioeconomic factors, such as material deprivation and marital status. It is therefore likely that the pathways described by Kramer et al. (2001) also play a role in explaining the difference in risk of preterm birth between various migrant groups and the respective non-migrant population.

Genetic factors

The causal pathways leading to many of the perinatal outcomes discussed above are not yet fully understood or are subjects of debate. In addition to lifestyle-related factors, the role of genetic factors must be considered, particularly when investigating ethnic disparities in perinatal outcomes. Several aetiological studies have suggested the possibility of gene–gene as well as gene–environment interactions (e.g. Nesin 2007; Macones et al. 2001; Simhan et al. 2003; Fortunato et al. 2008). Within this context, a genetic predisposition for unfavourable birth outcomes such as preterm birth among certain ethnic groups has been identified, most notably among black women in the United States. Recurrent preterm births have been found to be associated with a lower frequency of a particular DNA sequence, the interleukin-1β + 3953 T allele. Additionally, an association has been observed between the tumour necrosis factor-α-308 A allele and preterm birth, as well as differences in cytokine and toll-like receptor polymorphisms (Varner and Esplin 2005). Evidence for the contribution of genetic factors to more unfavourable perinatal outcomes in some ethnic groups is still weak, especially for migrant populations in Europe. Nevertheless, genetic influences must be taken into account when examining and interpreting disparities in perinatal health outcomes.

Utilization of antenatal care

Pregnancy and birth outcomes are influenced by both adequate utilization of antenatal care and the quality of services provided. Over the past few decades, Europe has seen a growing number of programmes and initiatives aimed at promoting the utilization of antenatal care, although the organization and content of services vary from country to country. As a consequence, women in Europe are seeking antenatal care more frequently and earlier than, for example, women in the United States (Buekens et al. 1993; Miller 1993). At the same time, barriers to accessing antenatal care still exist in many European countries. The organization of antenatal services, as well as the existence of cultural barriers, including those related to language, make access particularly difficult for migrants. In addition to unmarried and uninsured women, foreign-born women have a notably higher risk of inadequate care (Delvaux et al. 2001).

Number and timing of antenatal care visits

Although opinions differ on the appropriate number of antenatal care visits, experts agree that early and continuous antenatal care helps to prevent pregnancy and delivery complications (Villar et al. 2001). Migrant women tend to begin antenatal visits later in their pregnancy and make fewer visits compared to non-migrant women. A literature review on social class, ethnicity and utilization of antenatal services in the United Kingdom found that, in three of five studies, women from lower social classes tended to wait longer before their first visit and kept overall fewer appointments. Furthermore, women of Asian origin attended their first antenatal appointment later than white women of British origin (Rowe and Garcia 2003). Petrou et al. (2001) found that Pakistani and Indian women kept far fewer antenatal appointments than did white British women.

   In Germany, too, migrant women attend their first antenatal appointment significantly later (on average after the 14th week of gestation) than non-migrant women (between the 8th and 9th week). On average, migrant women attend 10–12 antenatal appointments, minimally fewer than non-migrant women, who attend 11–13 (David et al. 2006). While migrant women in

Germany are more likely to have no pregnancy risks recorded in their medical files, indicating a lower need for additional appointments, it is also possible that the lack of recording indicates disparities in the quality of antenatal care.

In other European countries, foreign-born single women and women from eastern Europe and Mediterranean countries are at greatest risk of inadequate utilization of antenatal services (Simoes et al. 2003; Koller et al. 2009). In Finland, birth outcomes differ greatly by ethnic group, despite the fact that migrant women attend prenatal appointments as frequently as non-migrant women. Among migrant women, only 0.2% used no antenatal services, and just 0.3% attended only one or two visits. It seems that how services are provided is more important than the number and timing of visits (Malin and Gissler 2009).

Data from a large prospective cohort in Amsterdam (2003–04) showed that women born abroad begin antenatal care later than women born in the Netherlands (Alderliesten et al. 2007). Among women immigrating from non-western countries (Turkey, Ghana, Morocco), late utilization of services may be explained by lack of interpreting services and information about available health services, migrants' low levels of education, multiparity and unwanted pregnancies. Over 40% of migrant women from Turkey and Ghana had only minimal Dutch language knowledge, making it difficult to communicate with the attending physician and to obtain information on the topic of pregnancy.

Quality of care

To ensure optimal pregnancy and birth outcomes, continuous participation in and strong adherence to an antenatal programme must be combined with appropriate quality of care. Studies from Denmark, the Netherlands, Norway, Sweden, the United Kingdom and the United States show evidence of suboptimal antenatal care in 25–30% of perinatal mortality cases, indicating that these deaths might have been preventable (Langhoff-Roos et al. 1996; Miranda et al. 1996; Essen et al. 2002; Richardus et al. 2003). Results from retrospective studies in Greece and in Switzerland showed significantly higher rates of caesarean delivery for migrant women (Machado et al. 2009). When services fail to address the needs of people with migrant backgrounds adequately, such as through the provision of interpretation services or cultural mediation, this results in considerable barriers to service delivery (Borde 2008).

However, quality of care is difficult to measure and the use of process indicators or proxy variables is common. In Germany, the completeness of the "maternity log", filled out by the treating physician, has over the years served as a proxy indicator for quality of care (Tadesse et al. 1999), despite the fact that the quality of the documentation is low, irrespective of a woman's country of origin. However, the documentation of foreign-born women is much less complete than that of German-born women. This applies to medical history, documentation of a high-risk pregnancy, cancer screening, pregnancy risks and risk counselling, raising the concern that doctors may be collecting incomplete information from their foreign-born patients, thus compromising the quality of their maternity care. The possibility cannot be excluded that such deficits may have an impact on the pregnancy and birth outcomes of migrant women.

Attitudes and expectations of medical personnel also have an impact. Providers of antenatal care in the United Kingdom find it easier to treat descendants of migrants, mainly because the limited English language skills of migrants complicate the provision of care (Puthussery et al. 2008). However, medical personnel also find the descendants of migrants with close family ties, in particular Muslim women, to be more traditional, less informed, and less assertive, compared to women with higher levels of education who live with their partner rather than an extended family. Medical personnel typecast migrants according to country of origin, style of dress, accent, knowledge about pregnancy, and timing and type of utilization of antenatal classes and care. As this typecasting can be assumed to have an impact on delivery of care, it is vital to support health workers in their cultural competence, for example, through training in communication skills, active listening and encouragement of self-reflection (see Chapter 13 on "Differences in language, religious beliefs and culture: the need for culturally responsive health services").

Conclusions

Throughout Europe, perinatal and infant mortality rates and risks vary by migrant groups and may differ from one generation to the next. Possible determinants of differences in risk between infants of diverse backgrounds suggest that each migrant group faces different barriers and problems, and each has developed different acculturation and integration strategies. The (self-) selection of very healthy women at migration (the "healthy migrant effect") may also vary markedly between groups, contributing to differences in health status.

Medical and sociodemographic risk factors for birth outcomes also vary by migrant group. In general, migrant women face more risk factors than non-migrant women, including previous miscarriage or preterm birth, obesity, hypertension, smoking, low levels of education, low occupational status, single mother status and depression. The cumulative effect of these risk factors appears to contribute to differences in pregnancy and birth outcomes between migrants and non-migrants.

Although improvements have been made concerning the perinatal health situation of migrants and their utilization of antenatal care, this chapter suggests that there are persisting differences in perinatal outcomes between migrants and non-migrants in Europe. Factors contributing to these differences include inequities in access to, uptake of, and quality of antenatal care. Several avenues of action could help to address these inequities, including:

- the training of medical staff to better acknowledge the barriers and needs of heterogeneous migrant populations;
- the development and implementation of migrant-sensitive guidelines for health care in antenatal and prenatal settings;
- the facilitation of health promotion and prevention programmes for pregnant women with diverse levels of education and migration background, based on prior participatory pilot projects and rigorous monitoring and evaluation.

Crucially, future programmes designed to prevent adverse birth outcomes should be tailored according to the needs of individual migrant groups (dependent on country of origin and residence status), and take into account a variety of medical and sociodemographic risk factors.

References

Alderliesten, M.E., Stronks, K., van Lith, J.M., et al. (2008) Ethnic differences in perinatal mortality. A perinatal audit on the role of substandard care. *European Journal of Obstetrics & Gynecology and Reproductive Biology*, 138(2): 164–70.

Alderliesten, M.E., Vrijkotte, T.G., van der Wal, M.F. and Bonsel, G.J. (2007) Late start of antenatal care among ethnic minorities in a large cohort of pregnant women. *BJOG*, 114(10): 1232–9.

Aveyard, P., Cheng, K.K., Manaseki, S. and Gardosi, J. (2002) The risk of preterm delivery in women from different ethnic groups. *BJOG*, 109(8): 894–9.

Barker, D.J.P. (1998) *Mothers, Babies and Health in Later Life*. Edinburgh: Churchill Livingstone.

Bittles, A.H., Mason, W.M., Greene, J. and Rao, N.A. (1991) Reproductive behavior and health in consanguineous marriages. *Science*, 252(5007): 789–94.

Borde, T. (2008) Migrants, access to health care. In: *Encyclopedia Public Health*. Berlin: Springer.

Buekens, P., Kotelchuck, M., Blondel, B., et al. (1993) A comparison of prenatal care use in the United States and Europe. *American Journal of Public Health*, 83(1): 31–6.

David, M., Pachaly, J., and Vetter, K. (2006) Perinatal outcome in Berlin (Germany) among immigrants from Turkey. *Archives of Gynecology and Obstetrics*, 274(5): 271–8.

Delvaux, T., Buekens, P., Godin, I. and Boutsen, M. (2001) Barriers to prenatal care in Europe. *American Journal of Preventive Medicine*, 21(1): 52–9.

Essen, B., Bodker, B., Sjoberg, N.O., et al. (2002) Are some perinatal deaths in immigrant groups linked to suboptimal perinatal care services? *BJOG*, 109(6): 677–82.

Fortunato, S.J., Menon, R., Velez, D.R., Thorsen, P. and Williams, S.M. (2008) Racial disparity in maternal–fetal genetic epistasis in spontaneous preterm birth. *American Journal of Obstetrics & Gynecology*, 198(6): 666–9.

Gagnon, A.J., Zimbeck, M., Zeitlin, J., et al. (2009) Migration to western industrialised countries and perinatal health: a systematic review. *Social Science & Medicine*, 69(6): 934–46.

Gissler, M., Alexander, S., Macfarlane, A., et al. (2009) Stillbirths and infant deaths among migrants in industrialized countries. *Acta Obstetrica et Gynecologica Scandinavica*, 88(2): 134–48.

Goedhart, G., van Eijsden, M., van der Wal, M.F. and Bonsel, G.J. (2008) Ethnic differences in preterm birth and its subtypes: the effect of a cumulative risk profile. *BJOG*, 115(6): 710–19.

Guendelman, S., Buekens, P., Blondel, B., et al. (1999) Birth outcomes of immigrant women in the United States, France, and Belgium. *Maternal and Child Health Journal*, 3(4): 177–87.

Harding, S. (2003) Mortality of migrants from the Indian subcontinent to England and Wales: effect of duration of residence. *Epidemiology*, 14(3): 287–92.

Harding, S., Rosato, M.G. and Cruickshank, J.K. (2004) Lack of change in birthweights of infants by generational status among Indian, Pakistani, Bangladeshi, Black Caribbean, and Black African mothers in a British cohort study. *International Journal of Epidemiology*, 33(6): 1279–85.

Hosper, K., Nierkens, V., Nicolaou, M. and Stronks, K. (2007) Behavioural risk factors in two generations of non-Western migrants: do trends converge towards the host population? *European Journal of Epidemiology*, 22(3): 163–72.

Kelly, Y., Panico, L., Bartley, M., et al. (2009) Why does birthweight vary among ethnic groups in the UK? Findings from the Millennium Cohort Study. *Journal of Public Health (Oxford)*, 31(1): 131–7.

Koller, D., Lack, N. and Mielck, A. (2009) Soziale Unterschiede bei der Inanspruchnahme der Schwangerschafts-Vorsorgeuntersuchungen, beim Rauchen der Mutter während der Schwangerschaft und beim Geburtsgewicht des Neugeborenen. Empirische Analyse auf Basis der Bayerischen Perinatal-Studie. *Gesundheitswesen*, 71: 10–18.

Kramer, M.S., Goulet, L., Lydon, J., et al. (2001) Socio-economic disparities in preterm birth: causal pathways and mechanisms. *Paediatric and Perinatal Epidemiology*, 15(Suppl. 2): 104–23.

Langhoff-Roos, J., Borch-Christensen, H., Larsen, S., Lindberg, B. and Wennergren, M. (1996) Potentially avoidable perinatal deaths in Denmark and Sweden 1991. *Acta Obstetrica et Gynecologica Scandinavica*, 75(9): 820–5.

Lindert, J. (2003) Krankheit kennt keine Papiere. In: Bundesweiter Arbeitskreis Migration und öffentliche Gesundheit: Gesunde Integration. Dokumentation der Fachtagung am 20. und 21. Februar 2003 in Berlin. Herausgegeben von der Beauftragte der Bundesregierung für Migration, Fluchtlinge und Integration. Berlin and Bonn: 143–7.

Lumey, L.H. and Reijneveld, S.A. (1995) Perinatal mortality in a first generation immigrant population and its relation to unemployment in The Netherlands. *Journal of Epidemiology & Community Health*, 49(5): 454–9.

Macones, G., Parry, S., Marder, S., et al. (2001) Evidence of a gene–environment interaction in the etiology of spontaneous preterm birth [abstract]. *American Journal of Obstetrics & Gynecology*, 184: 53.

Machado, M.C., Fernandes, A., Padilla, B., et al. (2009) *Maternal and Child Healthcare for Immigrant Populations*. Background Paper. Geneva: International Organization for Migration (http://www.migrant-health-europe.org/files/Maternal%20and%20 Child%20Care_Background%20Paper(1).pdf, accessed 19 May 2011).

Malin, M. and Gissler, M. (2009) Maternal care and birth outcomes among ethnic minority women in Finland. *BMC Public Health*, 9: 84.

Miller, C.A. (1993) Maternal and infant care: comparisons between Western Europe and the United States. *International Journal of Health Services*, 23(4): 655–64.

Miranda, J.A., Herruzo, A.J., Mozas, J., et al. (1996) Influence of obstetric and perinatal care on perinatal mortality. *European Journal of Obstetrics & Gynecology Reproductive Biology*, 67(2): 103–7.

Nesin, M. (2007) Genetic basis of preterm birth. *Frontiers in Bioscience*, 12: 115–24.

Olsen, P., Laara, E., Rantakallio, P., et al. (1995) Epidemiology of preterm delivery in two birth cohorts with an interval of 20 years. *American Journal of Epidemiology*, 142(11): 1184–93.

Parker, J.D., Schoendorf, K.C. and Kiely, J.L. (1994) Associations between measures of socioeconomic status and low birth weight, small for gestational age, and premature delivery in the United States. *Annals of Epidemiology*, 4(4): 271–8.

Peacock, J.L., Bland, J.M. and Anderson, H.R. (1995) Preterm delivery: effects of socioeconomic factors, psychological stress, smoking, alcohol, and caffeine. *BMJ*, 311(7004): 531–5.

Petrou, S., Kupek, E., Vause, S. and Maresh, M. (2001) Clinical, provider and sociodemographic determinants of the number of antenatal visits in England and Wales. *Social Science & Medicine*, 52(7): 1123–34.

Puthussery, S., Twamley, K., Harding, S., et al. 2008, 'They're more like ordinary stroppy British women': attitudes and expectations of maternity care professionals to UK-born ethnic minority women. *Journal of Health Services Research & Policy*, 13(4): 195–201.

Rasmussen, F., Oldenburg, C.E., Ericson, A. and Gunnarskog, J. (1995) Preterm birth and low birthweight among children of Swedish and immigrant women between 1978 and 1990. *Paediatric and Perinatal Epidemiology*, 9(4): 441–54.

Reeske, A., Spallek, J. and Razum, O. (2009) Changes in smoking prevalence among first- and second-generation Turkish migrants in Germany – an analysis of the 2005 Microcensus. *International Journal for Equity in Health*, 8: 26.

Reime, B., Ratner, P.A., Tomaselli-Reime, S.N., et al. (2006) The role of mediating factors in the association between social deprivation and low birth weight in Germany. *Social Science & Medicine*, 629(7): 1731–44.

Richardus, J.H., Graafmans, W.C., Verloove-Vanhorick, S.P. and Mackenbach, J.P. (2003) Differences in perinatal mortality and suboptimal care between 10 European regions: results of an international audit. *BJOG*, 110(2): 97–105.

Rowe, R.E. and Garcia, J. (2003) Social class, ethnicity and attendance for antenatal care in the United Kingdom: a systematic review. *Journal of Public Health Medicine*, 25(2): 113–19.

Schulpen, T.W., van Steenbergen, J.E. and van Driel, H.F. (2001) Influences of ethnicity on perinatal and child mortality in the Netherlands. *Archives of Disease in Childhood*, 84(3): 222–6.

Simhan, H.N., Caritis, S.N., Krohn, M.A. and Hillier, S.L. (2003) Elevated vaginal pH and neutrophils are associated strongly with early spontaneous preterm birth. *American Journal of Obstetrics & Gynecology*, 189(4): 1150–4.

Simoes, E., Kunz, S., Bosing-Schwenkglenks, M., Schwoerer, P. and Schmahl, F.W. (2003) Inanspruchnahme der Schwangerschaftsvorsorge – ein Spiegel gesellschaftlicher Entwicklungen und Aspekte der Effizienz. Untersuchung auf Basis der Perinatalerhebung Baden-Württemberg 1998–2001. *Geburtshilfe und Frauenheilkunde*, 61: 538–45.

Stöckler-Ipsiroglu, S., Herle, M., Nennstiel, U., et al. (2005) Angeborene Stoffwechselerkrankungen. Besonderheiten in der Betreuung von Kindern aus Migrantenfamilien. *Monatsschrift Kinderheilkunde*, 153: 22–8.

Stoltenberg, C., Magnus, P., Lie, R.T., Daltveit, A.K. and Irgens, L.M. (1997) Birth defects and parental consanguinity in Norway. *American Journal of Epidemiology*, 145(5): 439–48.

Tadesse, R., Jahn, A. and Razum, O. (1999) How well do doctors document their findings in antenatal care – and are there differences between women of German and non-German nationality? 5. *Arbeitstagung der FIDE* [Personal Communication].

Tadmouri, G.O., Nair, P., Obeid, T., et al. (2009) Consanguinity and reproductive health among Arabs. *Reproductive Health*, 6: 17.

Teitler, J.O., Reichman, N.E., Nepomnyaschy, L. and Martinson, M. (2007) A cross-national comparison of racial and ethnic disparities in low birthweight in the United States and England. *Pediatrics*, 120(5): e1182–9.

Terry, P.B., Bissenden, J.G., Condie, R.G. and Mathew, P.M. (1985) Ethnic differences in congenital malformations. *Archives of Disease in Childhood*, 60(9): 866–8.

Troe, E.J., Bos, V., Deerenberg, I.M., Mackenbach, J.P. and Joung, I.M. (2006) Ethnic differences in total and cause-specific infant mortality in The Netherlands. *Paediatric and Perinatal Epidemiology*, 20(2): 140–7.

Troe, E.J., Kunst, A.E., Bos, V., et al. (2007a) The effect of age at immigration and generational status of the mother on infant mortality in ethnic minority populations in The Netherlands. *European Journal of Public Health*, 17(2): 134–8.

Troe, E.J., Raat, H., Jaddoe, V.W., et al. (2007b) Explaining differences in birthweight between ethnic populations. The Generation R Study. *BJOG*, 114(12): 1557–65.

van Enk, A., Buitendijk, S.E., van der Pal, K.M., van Enk, W.J. and Schulpen, T.W. (1998) Perinatal death in ethnic minorities in The Netherlands. *Journal of Epidemiology & Community Health*, 52(11): 735–9.

Vangen, S., Stoltenberg, C. and Stray-Pedersen, B. (1999) Complaints and complications in pregnancy: a study of ethnic Norwegian and ethnic Pakistani women in Oslo. *Ethnicity & Health*, 4(1–2): 19–28.

Varner, M.W. and Esplin, M.S. (2005) Current understanding of genetic factors in preterm birth. *BJOG*, 112(Suppl. 1): 28–31.

Villadsen, S.F., Mortensen, L.H. and Andersen, A.M. (2009) Ethnic disparity in stillbirth and infant mortality in Denmark 1981–2003. *Journal of Epidemiology & Community Health*, 63(2): 106–12.

Villadsen, S. F., Sievers, E., Andersen, A.M., Arntzen, A., Audard-Mariller, M., Martens, G., Ascher, H. and Hjern, A. (2010) Cross-country variation in stillbirth and neonatal mortality in offspring of Turkish migrants in northern Europe. *European Journal of Public Health*, 20(5): 530–5.

Villar, J., Carroli, G., Khan-Neelofur, D., Piaggio, G. and Gulmezoglu, M. (2001) Patterns of routine antenatal care for low-risk pregnancy. *Cochrane Database Syst Rev*, 4: CD000934.

Wilcox, A.J. and Russell, I.T. (1983) Birthweight and perinatal mortality: II. On weight-specific mortality. *International Journal of Epidemiology*, 12(3): 319–25.

Wolff, H., Epiney, M., Lourenco, A.P., et al. (2008) Undocumented migrants lack access to pregnancy care and prevention. *BMC Public Health*, 8: 93.

Yoong, W., Kolhe, S., Karoshi, M., Ullah, M. and Nauta, M. (2005) The obstetric performance of United Kingdom asylum seekers from Somalia: a case-control study and literature review. *International Journal of Fertility and Women's Medicine*, 50(4): 175–9.

Zeitlin, J., Bucourt, M., Rivera, L., Topuz, B. and Papiernik, E. (2004) Preterm birth and maternal country of birth in a French district with a multiethnic population. *BJOG*, 111(8): 849–55.

chapter ten

Occupational health

Andrés A. Agudelo-Suárez,
Elena Ronda-Pérez and
Fernando G. Benavides

Background

The search for jobs and thus for better living conditions is among the principal reasons for migrating to another country. The International Labour Organization estimated that, in 2010, there were 105.4 million economically active migrants worldwide (International Labour Organization 2010). Between 1998 and 2007, the migrant worker population in European OECD (Organisation for Economic Co-operation and Development) countries increased significantly, from 3.5 to almost 6 million workers (OECD 2010). In 2007, the five European countries with the highest proportion of migrant workers as part of their total working population were Belgium (9.5%), Germany (9.4%), Spain (9.0%), Greece (7.5%) and the United Kingdom (7.2%). In countries such as Germany, the proportion of migrant workers has remained relatively stable between 1998 and 2007, whereas in southern European countries such as Spain there has been a sharp increase in this period (Figure 10.1). Although the present economic crisis might dampen the inflow of foreign workers, migration can be expected to resume as the economy improves, since the underlying causes are rooted in long-standing economic and social factors in both countries of origin and destination. In the host countries, falling birth rates and an ageing population will result in continuing demand for new workers, especially for low-qualified jobs, while in countries of origin, emigration is seen as one of few possibilities for improving the prospects of workers and their children.

Given the important role of migrant workers in Europe, research conducted on the occupational health of migrant workers is scarce (Schenker 2010). This might be partly due to the methodological difficulties encountered in such research. The first of these is the definition of migrants (Bhopal 2004; Malmusi et al. 2007). In some studies conducted in countries with a relatively

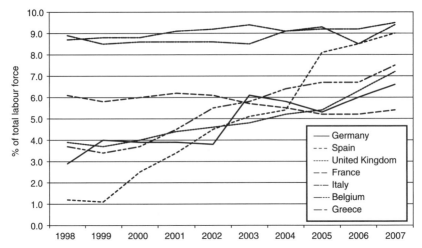

Figure 10.1 Foreign labour force stocks in Europe (% of total labour force), 1998–2007

Source: Authors' compilation, based on OECD (2010)

long tradition of immigration such as the United Kingdom or the Scandinavian countries, ethnicity or "race" have been used as proxies for migrant status (Bhopal 2004). However, migrant status and membership of an ethnic minority group are not necessarily equivalent. In other studies, nationality has been used as a proxy indicator of migrant status. While this information is easily available in some administrative records, there is considerable scope for bias due to classification problems, for example, where nationality has been acquired through marriage (see Chapter 6 on "Monitoring the health of migrants"). A second methodological problem arises from the difficulty of establishing contact with the migrant population, since in many cases individuals are working illegally and fear deportation; even where they have obtained legal status, religious, linguistic and cultural barriers remain. Third, migrants do not form a homogenous population, but vary according to religion, language or country of origin. Fourth, when comparing migrants with the "native" population, there may be a selection bias resulting from the migratory process, as the migrant population tends to comprise individuals in a particularly good state of physical and mental health. The similarity with the "healthy worker effect" (Li and Sung 1999), due to the exclusion of unhealthy workers from employment, has given rise to the term "healthy migrant effect" (Newbold 2005). Finally, migrant workers may work in different jobs than non-migrant workers, making it difficult to compare the two groups (Lee and Wrench 1980). In addition to these methodological problems, research into the relationship between migration, work and health is a politically sensitive subject, for which little funding is forthcoming.

The objective of this chapter is to synthesize and evaluate the available evidence on employment and working conditions and their effects on the health of migrants in Europe, and to identify courses of action that would help to reduce occupational health inequalities between migrant and non-migrant workers.

The employment and working conditions of migrant populations

Migrant workers are important economic agents: in addition to contributing to the wealth of their host countries and making substantial contributions to the social security systems in these countries, they contribute to their countries of origin by sending money to their families. An estimated US$ 250–300 billion is transferred by migrants each year to their countries of origin (World Bank 2008; IOM 2010). The contribution of migrants to social security systems has led, in some places, to the establishment of agreements between different systems, guaranteeing mutual recognition of rights, so that workers can, for example, receive their pension in their country of origin if they so desire. Examples include the multilateral social security agreements in the European Economic Area (EEA), as well as the agreement being promoted by the Ibero-American Social Security Organization between all Latin American countries and Portugal and Spain (Ibero-American Social Security Organization 2009; International Labour Organization 2010).

Yet, despite their significant economic contribution, entry into the labour market is not easy for migrants and they tend to occupy low-qualified, high-risk jobs (Pajares 2008), despite the fact that, in many cases, their educational level and work experience would qualify them to work in much better paid posts and with better contractual conditions (Szczepura et al. 2004; McKay et al. 2006). Table 10.1 shows the occupational differences between migrant and non-migrant workers in Spain. Whereas the non-migrant population occupies a greater proportion of administrative and professional posts, migrants are more frequently employed as domestic workers, builders, waiters, cleaners, and in hotels and catering (Ministry of Work and Immigration & Spanish National Institute of Safety and Hygiene at Work 2008; Spanish National Statistics Institute 2009). Female migrants are especially vulnerable (UNFPA 2007). As a result of workplace segmentation and gender inequalities, most migrants work in occupations which have been called the "3D jobs" – "dirty, demanding and dangerous" (McCauley 2005; Benach et al. 2010).

Some of the main obstacles to labour market entry for migrant workers in Europe include scant opportunities for training and career progression, legal barriers to enforcing employment and social rights, difficulties in having qualifications and experience recognized, limited access to public services, and linguistic difficulties (European Foundation for the Improvement of Living and Working Conditions 2007). Migrants also tend to have low membership of trade unions and professional organizations that can provide support and advice, and a limited capacity for participation in social activities beyond their own communities (García et al. 2009).

Migrants constitute one of the most vulnerable populations in the current economic crisis. Eurostat data reveal that unemployment among migrants has risen sharply and foreign workers, especially those from outside the European

Table 10.1 Distribution of the Spanish and foreign working population by occupation and sex (as %)

Occupation	Males		Females	
	Spanish	Foreign	Spanish	Foreign
Managerial positions in private enterprise or public administration	9.7	4.8	6.5	2.8
Scientific and intellectual specialists and professionals	11.3	3.6	18.4	4.1
Support specialists and professionals	12.6	4.0	14.6	4.3
Employees in administrative posts	5.8	2.7	15.7	6.8
Workers in hotel and catering, personal, security and shop sales services	9.7	11.7	23.2	32.3
Qualified workers in agriculture and fishing	3.5	2.4	1.4	0.3
Qualified artisans and workers in the manufacturing, construction and mining industries, except machine operators	23.7	36.3	2.2	2.1
Machine and factory operators, fitters	14.4	10.8	3.1	2.2
Unqualified workers	8.6	23.5	14.7	45.0
Armed forces	0.8	0.2	0.1	0.0

Source: Compiled by the authors, based on: National Statistics Institute (INE, Spain). *Active Population Survey 2008.*

Union (EU), experience the highest rates of unemployment across the Union (European Commission 2008). Many of these workers survive without unemployment benefits, and some, particularly those who do not fulfil the requirements for legal residence, find themselves obliged to work in the shadow economy (Rial González and Irastorza 2007; European Commission 2010).

Given their vulnerability, employment of migrant workers in precarious conditions has become widespread (Amable et al. 2001; Porthé et al. 2007). These conditions include job insecurity; lack of social benefits; limited capacity for empowerment and exercising rights; poverty; marginalization; and long working hours (Porthé et al. 2010). The degree of precariousness is higher among migrant workers than non-migrant workers, and higher among those migrants who do not hold a residence or work permit (Porthé et al. 2009).

A report on occupational health and safety in Spain showed how migrants were more often exposed to risks in the workplace (Ministry of Work and Immigration & Spanish National Institute of Safety and Hygiene at Work 2008). Migrant workers were more frequently required to adopt painful or tiring postures (9.9% vs 8.2% among non-migrant workers), lift or move heavy weights (8.8% vs 7.2%), use significant force (9% vs 6.4%), and to work with very little space available (6.1% vs 4.7%). Studies from other countries in Europe have identified additional risk factors for occupational diseases, such as monotonous work, lack of clarity in the assignment of tasks and functions, and interpersonal conflict at work (Rial González and Irastorza 2007).

Occupational health in migrant workers

A literature review of articles published between 1990 and 2005 and cited in PubMed (Ahonen et al. 2007) reported that most articles on occupational health in migrant workers came from countries with a long history of migration, such as Australia, Canada and the United States (79.5%), while only 8.3% came from European countries, principally Sweden (Rosmond et al. 1998; Akhavan et al. 2004), Italy (Capacci et al. 2005) and Germany (Elkeles and Seifert 1996). Since 2005, new studies have been published in Spain (Ahonen et al. 2009; García et al. 2009; Agudelo-Suárez et al. 2009b), Italy (Bacciconi et al. 2006; Colao et al. 2006; Marchiori et al. 2008; Patussi et al. 2008) and Finland (Salminen et al. 2009), which have evaluated working conditions and their impact on migrant health, using quantitative and qualitative methodologies. However, it should be borne in mind that much information on this topic is not published in scientific journals, but in institutional reports of varying accessibility and in different languages.

Occupational injuries

Among the effects of working conditions on health, the most evident are injuries resulting from occupational accidents. The working conditions to which migrant workers are exposed, together with their lack of experience of contexts that may be different to those in their country of origin, could explain their higher rates of occupational injuries (Schenker 2008; Schenker 2010). We conducted a basic search in PubMed using the keywords [Occupational injuries OR Injuries AND immigrant OR migrant workers], with a focus on original research published in Europe in 1990–2010 in Spanish and English. Table 10.2 summarizes the nine articles found in this period that reported original research. The majority of these studies found that occupational injury rates were higher among migrants, although one Finnish study of bus drivers found no significant differences in occupational injury rates between Finnish and immigrant workers (Salminen et al. 2009). Several possible explanations for higher rates of occupational injury among migrant workers are given, including difficulties in employment and working conditions; the high incidence of temporary work and rotation between jobs; longer working hours; harsh working conditions; physical and psychological risks; and the fact that many immigrants are in different occupations from those they held in their country of origin (McKay et al. 2006). However, the true extent of these differences might be even greater, as occupational injuries sustained by migrants may be more likely to be unrecorded, especially where workers are not formally employed (Ahonen and Benavides 2006).

Occupational diseases and self-reported health

Some studies carried out among associations that work with migrants suggest that occupational health problems of migrant workers remain largely invisible.

Table 10.2 List of studies on occupational injuries among migrants in the European Union

Author (year)	Country studied	Group studied or comparison	Objective	Results
(Rubiales-Gutiérrez et al. 2010)	Spain	Spanish and workers from low Human Development Index (HDI) countries	To compare the occupational accidents between indigenous and immigrant workers in Spain.	A higher risk of occupational accidents was observed among women from countries with low HDI scores compared to Spaniards (adjusted OR 1.66; 95% CI 1.21–2.28).
(Salminen et al. 2009)	Finland	Finnish and immigrant bus drivers	To examine whether immigrant workers have a higher injury frequency compared to Finnish workers when performing the same tasks under the same working conditions.	Immigrant bus drivers were slightly but not significantly more often involved in occupational injuries than Finnish drivers (13.0% vs 9.8%; $X^2 = 0.72$; df = 1, ns).
(López-Jacob et al. 2008)	Spain	Foreign and Spanish workers	To compare the incidence of both fatal and non-fatal injuries in foreign workers to that of Spanish workers in 2005, by autonomous community and economic activity.	Relative risk for occupational injury in foreign workers in 2005 was elevated for both fatal (1.34; 95% CI 1.11–1.62) and non-fatal injury (1.13; 95% CI 1.13–1.14), although there were important differences by autonomous community and activity sector.
(Benavides et al. 2008)	Spain	Foreign and Spanish workers	To compare the risk of occupational injury by nationality in 2003 and 2004.	There are some contradictory results. The incidence of occupational injuries varied, depending on the definition of a foreigner. In some cases foreign workers reported less risk of occupational injury than Spanish counterparts.
(Patussi et al. 2008)	Italy	Permanent and temporary Italian and immigrant workers	To evaluate the difference in the frequency of occupational injuries between permanent and temporary workers, and between Italian and immigrant workers.	The incidence rate ratio of occupational injury was significantly higher in temporary workers than in permanent workers (IR 2.46; 95% CI 2.02–2.99). Immigrant status appears to be an important risk factor, especially among permanent workers (IR 1.63; 95% CI 1.34–1.98).

Study	Country	Population	Aim	Results
(Marchiori et al. 2008)	Italy	Regular and irregular non-EU workers	The aim of the study was to establish a procedure in order to estimate the rate of occupational accidents in non-EU workers with irregular employment status and/or irregular immigrant status.	Occupational accidents per 1000 irregular non-EU workers in Italy in 2004, at approximately 65 accidents per 1000 irregular non-EU workers, were more than twice as high as those among regular non-EU workers.
(Colao et al. 2006)	Italy	Immigrant and Italian workers	To describe the trend of work accidents in the Local Health Area No. 6 – Fabriano (Marche Region), during the period 2000–2003.	Immigrant workers had a higher risk of accidents at work than Italian workers. Occupational accidents among immigrant workers gradually rose and peaked in 2002. The sectors with high rates of accidents were the mechanical engineering and metallurgic sectors and the construction industry. Accidents occurred mainly among male and female young people (18 to 34 years old). With regard to gender, there was a marked increased prevalence for men (83.3%) over women (16.7%).
(Bacciconi et al. 2006)	Italy	Immigrant women	To describe occupational accidents among foreign women working in two regions of north-eastern Italy.	The most frequent countries of origin of injured workers in Friuli Venezia Giulia (the region bordering Slovenia) were former Yugoslavia (113) and Albania (28). In Veneto, the corresponding regions or countries of origin were Africa (156), Romania (84) and Albania (80).
(Ahonen and Benavides 2006)	Spain	Foreign and Spanish workers	To describe occupational injuries in foreign workers in Spain.	In women and men, and in every age group, foreign workers had an increased risk of non-fatal and fatal occupational injury compared with Spanish workers. The differences were especially notable in foreign women workers and in older workers.

NOTES: CI = confidence interval; d.f. = degrees of freedom; HDI = Human Development Index; IR = incidence rate; n.s. = not significant; OR = odds ratio; X^2 = chi square test.

Source: Authors' compilation

This applies particularly to clandestine workers, but also to those who are formally employed, as companies and insurance companies are sometimes resistant to recognizing injuries of an occupational origin (García et al. 2009). This constitutes a barrier to the establishment of monitoring and surveillance systems on the specific health problems of migrant workers.

In general, it has been reported that migrant workers enjoy better health than non-migrant workers, due to the selection process the former have undergone (the "healthy migrant effect"). However, this advantage deteriorates rapidly as the length of stay in host countries increases, leading to what has been termed the "exhausted migrant" effect (Bollini and Siem 1995; European Foundation for the Improvement of Living and Working Conditions 2007; Rial González and Irastorza 2007).

Self-reported health among migrant workers is worse than among the "native" population, although differences exist according to country of origin, legal status and social, occupational and economic factors. A study in Sweden found that over half of the 60 unemployed migrants included in the study considered their health to be "poor" and reported physical and mental illnesses (unhappiness, fatigue, difficulties in concentrating, cardiovascular disorders, digestive problems, problems related to eyesight and hearing, and migraines) (Akhavan et al. 2004). A similar situation was observed in a study on the unemployed migrant population in Germany, in which subjects reported chronic problems and low levels of satisfaction with their health (Elkeles and Seifert 1996).

The uncertainties involved in the migration process, coupled with poor job and working conditions, often far below the qualifications gained in countries of origin, may be factors that help to explain the high rates of depression, stress, somatic illnesses, anxiety disorders and insomnia found in various studies (Carta et al. 2005; Taloyan et al. 2006; Taloyan et al. 2008). This has been termed the "Ulysses" or "chronic and multiple stress syndrome" (Achotegui 2004), and is characteristic of migrants experiencing adaptation problems in their host country.

Sickness presenteeism

In many European countries working conditions are being restructured, with a reduction in certain social benefits (Benach et al. 2007) that particularly affects migrant workers (Porthé et al. 2007). There also seems to be a trend towards greater controls being exercised in granting these social benefits, which due to discrimination and cultural barriers, also affects the migrant population disproportionally (Agudelo-Suárez et al. 2009a).

One six-month follow-up study conducted in primary health care centres in a Spanish city found that the probability of not attending work due to a health problem was lower among migrants than among non-migrants (Soler-González et al. 2008). In a study in Denmark, it was observed that the risk of absenteeism was lower for migrant workers than for "native" workers, despite the fact that their state of health was worse (Carneiro et al. 2010).

One possible explanation for these findings is "sickness presenteeism", a situation in which workers attend work while ill (Aronsson and Gustafsson

2005). In a study in Spain, migrants showed a higher probability of "sickness presenteeism" than the non-migrant population (with a prevalence of 52% in migrants, compared to 42% in the non-migrant population; OR = 1.40; CI 95% 1.13–1.75), even after adjusting for sociodemographic variables (Agudelo-Suárez et al. 2010). One possible explanation for this finding is that, for the majority of migrants, keeping their job is a very high priority that takes precedence over concerns for their health.

Discrimination in the workplace

For decades, researchers in social epidemiology have been studying the effects of discrimination on the health of vulnerable groups, such as those whose ethnic origin is different from that predominant in the host country (Krieger 1999). Research carried out in Europe has demonstrated that the experience of discrimination of employees in the workplace, together with that experienced outside of work, has an influence on job insecurity and the mental and physical health of migrant workers (Bhui et al. 2005; Jasinskaja-Lahti et al. 2007; Agudelo-Suárez et al. 2009a).

Access to health services

Migrant workers may experience barriers to accessing health services when they need them, due to lack of awareness about entitlements, irregular legal status, fear of deportation or, in some cases, lack of time or administrative difficulties in obtaining access to care (Berra et al. 2004) (see also Chapter 5 on "Migrants' access to health services").

A call for action

In many European countries, the current economic crisis is having an enormous effect on the labour market, with pressures to increase labour market flexibility and reduce social benefits, for example, by delaying the age of retirement (Miguélez and Prieto Rodríguez 2009). One of the groups most vulnerable to these structural changes is the migrant worker population. Furthermore, there are concerns over the effects the economic crisis may have on the health of the population as a whole (Catalano 2009; Dávila Quintana and López-Valcárcel 2009; Stuckler et al. 2009a; Stuckler et al. 2009b).

Based on current evidence, it is reasonable to assume that an increase in temporary, precarious and clandestine work could worsen the health and quality of life of many (migrant and non-migrant) workers. There is an urgent need to put this hypothesis to the test, since, although individual risk may be small, the large number of people affected increases its significance as a public health problem.

However, this requires the availability of better data in order to monitor the effects of employment policies on health. This also applies especially to migrants. Current information systems on the occupational health of migrants in Europe are incomplete and urgently require improvements, including more detailed information in administrative records, which should not only cover nationality, but also country of birth and year of arrival in the host country. Such initiatives, together with the use of qualitative and quantitative surveys and innovative sampling techniques, would help to augment research throughout Europe on this significant public health issue.

Policies to reduce social inequalities in health should incorporate strategies to protect the health of migrant workers (Graham 2004). These policies and interventions will need to be of a multisector nature and be based on coordinated action plans by different departments in public administration, aimed at improving the social, employment and working conditions of migrants.

Protecting the health of migrant workers constitutes one of the most significant challenges for occupational health in Europe. It requires applying the same standards of social security and of health and safety in the workplace to migrants as to non-migrant workers. A crucial first step could be to legalize the presence of undocumented migrant workers in the host country, enabling them to hold a work contract with employers (López-Jacob et al. 2008). Without this, it is impossible for undocumented migrants to insist on their rights or to be protected by the social security system. Recovery from the economic crisis should not be achieved at the expense of this particularly vulnerable group.

Conclusions

Across Europe, the migration of workers from diverse countries and cultures has become a widespread phenomenon that demands action from different sectors of public administration. Migrant workers face numerous problems: they have difficulties entering the workforce and, once they have managed to do so, tend to encounter adverse work conditions in the host country, such as temporary contracts, lack of workers' rights and benefits, and difficulties in legalizing their situation. Furthermore, they lack experience of contexts different to those in their country of origin, and tend to work in occupations that involve a higher risk. As a result, despite experiencing relatively good health on arrival, the health of migrant workers is affected and they suffer higher rates of work-related accidents, a poorer self-reported state of health, and worse indicators of physical, mental and social health. Further research is needed throughout Europe to learn more about the occupational health of migrant workers and to monitor strategies and policies for improving the existing situation and reducing the inequalities experienced by this group of the population.

References

Achotegui, J. (2004) Emigrar en situación extrema. El Síndrome del Inmigrante con estrés crónico y múltiple. Síndrome de Ulises [Emigrating in an extreme situation. The Immigrant's Syndrome with Chronic and Multiple Stress. The Ulysses Syndrome]. *Revista Norte de Salud Mental*, 6(21): 39–53.

Agudelo-Suárez, A.A., Benavides, F.G., Ronda-Pérez, E., et al. (2010) *'Sick but I am working': A Comparison of Presenteeism in Immigrant and Autochthonous Workers in Spain* [Abstract]. 3rd Conference on Migrant and Ethnic Minorities' Health in Europe, 27–29 May 2010, Pecs, Hungary.

Agudelo-Suárez, A., Gil-González, D., Ronda-Pérez, E., et al. (2009a) Discrimination, work and health in immigrant populations in Spain. *Social Science & Medicine*, 68(10): 1866–74.

Agudelo-Suárez, A.A., Ronda-Pérez, E., Gil-González, D., et al. (2009b) Proceso migratorio, condiciones laborales y salud en trabajadores inmigrantes en España (proyecto ITSAL) [The migratory process, working conditions and health in immigrant workers in Spain (the ITSAL project)]. *Gaceta Sanitaria*, 23(Suppl. 1): 115–21.

Ahonen, E.Q. and Benavides, F.G. (2006) Risk of fatal and non-fatal occupational injury in foreign workers in Spain. *Journal of Epidemiology & Community Health*, 60(5): 424–6.

Ahonen, E.Q., Benavides, F.G. and Benach, J. (2007) Immigrant populations, work and health – a systematic literature review. *Scandinavian Journal of Work, Environment & Health*, 33(2): 96–104.

Ahonen, E.Q., Porthé, V., Vazquez, M.L., et al. (2009) A qualitative study about immigrant workers' perceptions of their working conditions in Spain. *Journal of Epidemiology & Community Health*, 63(11): 936–42.

Akhavan, S., Bildt, C.O., Franzen, E.C. and Wamala, S. (2004) Health in relation to unemployment and sick leave among immigrants in Sweden from a gender perspective. *Journal of Immigrant and Minority Health*, 6(3): 103–18.

Amable, M., Benach, J. and González, S. (2001) La precariedad laboral y su repercusión sobre la salud: conceptos y resultados preliminares de un estudio multimétodos [Precarious employment and its health-related impact: concepts and preliminary results of a multi-methods study]. *Archivos de Prevención y Riesgos Laborales*, 4(4): 169–84.

Aronsson, G. and Gustafsson, K. (2005) Sickness presenteeism: prevalence, attendance-pressure factors, and an outline of a model for research. *Journal of Occupational & Environmental Medicine*, 47(9): 958–66.

Bacciconi, M., Patussi, V., Barbina, P., et al. (2006) Gli infortuni sul lavoro tra le donne immigrate nelle regioni del Nord-Est (Veneto e Friuli Venezia Giulia) [Occupational accidents among immigrant women in the Italian North-Eastern regions (Veneto and Friuli Venezia Giulia)]. *Epidemiologia e Prevenzion*, 30(1): 33–9.

Benach, J., Muntaner, C. and Santana, V.; Employment Condition Knowledge Network (EMCONET) (2007) *Employment Conditions and Health Inequalities. Final Report to the WHO Commission on Social Determinants of Health* (http://www.who.int/social_determinants/resources/articles/emconet_who_report.pdf, accessed 20 May 2011).

Benach, J., Muntaner, C., Chung, H. and Benavides, F.G. (2010) Immigration, employment relations, and health: developing a research agenda. *American Journal of Industrial Medicine*, 53(4): 338–43.

Benavides, F.G., Ahonen, E.Q. and Bosch, C. (2008) Riesgo de lesión por accidente laboral en trabajadores extranjeros (España, 2003 y 2004) [Risk of occupational injury in foreign workers in Spain (2003 and 2004)]. *Gaceta Sanitaria*, 22(1): 44–7.

Berra, S., Elorza Ricart, J.M., Bartomeu, N., et al. (2004) Necesidades en salud y utilización de los servicios sanitarios en la población inmigrante en Cataluña. Revisión exhaustiva de la literatura científica [Health needs and health services utilization for the immigrant population in Catalonia. A comprehensive review of the scientific literature]. Barcelona: Agència d'Avaluació de Tecnologia i Recerca Mèdiques.

Bhopal, R. (2004) Glossary of terms relating to ethnicity and race: for reflection and debate. *Journal of Epidemiology & Community Health*, 58(6): 441–5.

Bhui, K., Stansfeld, S., Mckenzie, K., Karlsen, S., Nazroo, J. and Weich, S. (2005) Racial/ethnic discrimination and common mental disorders among workers: findings from the EMPIRIC Study of Ethnic Minority Groups in the United Kingdom. *American Journal of Public Health*, 95(3): 496–501.

Bollini, P. and Siem, H. (1995) No real progress towards equity: health of migrants and ethnic minorities on the eve of the year 2000. *Social Science & Medicine*, 41(6): 819–28.

Capacci, F., Carnevale, F. and Gazzano, N. (2005) The health of foreign workers in Italy. *International Journal of Occupational and Environmental Health*, 11(1): 64–9.

Carneiro, I.G., Ortega, A., Borg, V. and Hogh, A. (2010) Health and sickness absence in Denmark: A study of elderly-care immigrant workers. *Journal of Immigrant and Minority Health*, 12(1): 43–52.

Carta, M.G., Bernal, M., Hardoy, M.C. and Haro-Abad, J.M. (2005) Migration and mental health in Europe (the state of the mental health in Europe working group: appendix 1). *Clinical Practice and Epidemiology in Mental Health*, 1: 13.

Catalano, R. (2009) Health, medical care, and economic crisis. *New England Journal of Medicine*, 360(8): 749–51.

Colao, A.M., Pisciottano, V., Giampaoletti, C. and Cenci, G. (2006) Il fenomeno infortunistico nei lavoratori extracomunitari della zona territoriale n. 6 Fabriano [Occupational accidents among immigrant workers in the Fabriano areas]. *Medicina del Lavoro*, 97(6): 787–98.

Dávila Quintana, C. and López-Valcárcel, B. (2009) Crisis económica y salud [Economic crisis and health]. *Gaceta Sanitaria*, 23(4): 261–5.

Elkeles, T. and Seifert, W. (1996) Immigrants and health: unemployment and health-risks of labour migrants in the Federal Republic of Germany, 1984–1992. *Social Science & Medicine*, 43(7): 1035–47.

European Commission (2008) *Employment in Europe 2008*. Luxembourg: Office for Official Publications of the European Communities (http://www.eurofound.europa.eu/ewco/studies/tn0701038s/, accessed 20 May 2011).

European Commission (2010) *Eurostat: European Statistics* (http://epp.eurostat.ec.europa.eu/portal/page/portal/eurostat/home/, accessed 20 May 2011).

European Foundation for the Improvement of Living and Working Conditions (2007) *Employment and working conditions of migrant workers* (http://www.eurofound.europa.eu/staging/docs/ewco/tn0701038s/tn0701038s.pdf /, accessed 20 May 2011).

García, A.M., López-Jacob, M.J., Agudelo-Suarez, A.A., et al. (2009) Condiciones de trabajo y salud en inmigrantes (Proyecto ITSAL): entrevistas a informantes clave [Occupational health of immigrant workers in Spain (ITSAL Project): key informants survey]. *Gaceta Sanitaria*, 23(2): 91–7.

Graham, H. (2004) Social determinants and their unequal distribution: clarifying policy understandings. *Milbank Quarterly*, 82(1): 101–24.

Ibero-American Social Security Organisation (2009) *Estrategia Iberoamericana de Seguridad y Salud en el Trabajo 2010–2013 [Ibero-American Strategy of Security and Health at Work 2010–2013]*. Madrid: Organización Iberoamericana de Seguridad Social.

International Labour Organization (2010) *International Labour Migration: A Rights-based Approach*. Geneva: International Labour Organization.

IOM (2010) *World Migration Report 2010*. Geneva: International Organization for Migration.

Jasinskaja-Lahti, I., Liebkind, K. and Perhoniemi, R. (2007) Perceived ethnic discrimination at work and well-being of immigrants in Finland: the moderating role of employment status and work-specific group-level control beliefs. *International Journal of Intercultural Relations*, 31(2): 223–42.

Krieger, N. (1999) Embodying inequality: a review of concepts, measures, and methods for studying health consequences of discrimination. *International Journal of Health Services*, 29(2): 295–352.

Lee, G. and Wrench, J. (1980) 'Accident-prone immigrants': an assumption challenged. *Sociology*, 14(4): 551–66.

Li, C.Y. and Sung, F.C. (1999) A review of the healthy worker effect in occupational epidemiology. *Occupational Medicine (London)*, 49(4): 225–9.

López-Jacob, M.J., Ahonen, E., García, A.M., Gil, A. and Benavides, F.G. (2008) Comparación de las lesiones por accidente de trabajo en trabajadores extranjeros y españoles por actividad económica y comunidad autónoma (España, 2005) [Occupational injury in foreign workers by economic activity and autonomous community (Spain 2005)]. *Revista Española de Salud Pública*, 82(2): 179–87.

Malmusi, D., Jansa, J.M. and del Vallado, L. (2007) Recomendaciones para la investigación e información en salud sobre definiciones y variables para el estudio de la población inmigrante de origen extranjero [Recommendations for health research and information on definitions and variables for the study of the foreign-born immigrant population]. *Revista Española de Salud Pública*, 81(4): 399–409.

Marchiori, L., Marangi, G., Mazzoccoli, P., et al. (2008) Una procedura per la stima del tasso di infortunio nei lavoratori extracomunitari irregolar [A procedure for estimating the rate of occupational accidents in non-European-Union workers with irregular immigrant status]. *Medicina del Lavoro*, 99(Suppl. 1): 76–87.

McCauley, L.A. (2005) Immigrant workers in the United States: recent trends, vulnerable populations, and challenges for occupational health. *AAOHN J: Journal of the American Association of Occupational Health Nurses*, 53(7), 313–19.

McKay, S., Craw, M. and Chopra, D. (2006) *Migrant Workers in England and Wales. An Assessment of Migrant Worker Health and Safety Risks*. Norwich: Health and Safety Executive.

Miguélez, F. and Prieto Rodríguez, C. (2009) Transformaciones del empleo, flexibilidad y relaciones laborales en Europa [Transformations of employment, flexibility and industrial relations in Europe]. *Política y Sociedad*, 46(1–2): 275–87.

Ministry of Work and Immigration & Spanish National Institute of Safety and Hygiene at Work (2008) *Informe sobre el estado de la seguridad y la salud laboral en España [Report about Labour Safety and Security in Spain]*. Madrid: National Institute of Safety and Hygiene at Work.

Newbold, K.B. (2005) Self-rated health within the Canadian immigrant population: risk and the healthy immigrant effect. *Social Science & Medicine*, 60(6): 1359–70.

OECD (2010) *OECD Statistics*. Paris: Organisation for Economic Co-operation and Development (http://stats.oecd.org/Index.aspx, accessed 20 May 2011).

Pajares, M. (2008) *Inmigración y mercado de trabajo. Informe 2008 [Immigration and Labour Market. Report 2008]*, Madrid: Ministerio de Trabajo e Inmigración. Observatorio Permanente de la Inmigración.

Patussi, V., Barbina, P., Barbone, F., et al. (2008) Confronto dell'incidenza degli infortuni tra lavoratori tipici, interinali e migrant del Friuli-Venezia Giulia [Comparison of the incidence rate of occupational injuries among permanent, temporary and immigrant workers in Friuli-Venezia Giulia]. *Epidemiologia e Prevenzione*, 32(1): 35–8.

Porthé, V., Ahonen, E., Vázquez, M.L., et al. (2010) Extending a model of precarious employment: a qualitative study of immigrant workers in Spain. *American Journal of Industrial Medicine*, 53(4): 417–24.

Porthé, V., Amable, M. and Benach, J. (2007) La precariedad laboral y la salud de los inmigrantes en España: ¿qué sabemos y qué deberíamos saber? [Precarious employment and immigrant health in Spain: what do we know and what should we know?] *Archivos de Prevención y Riesgos Laborales*, 10(1): 34–9.

Porthé, V., Benavides, F.G., Vázquez, M.L., et al. (2009) La precariedad laboral en inmigrantes en situación irregular en España y su relación con la salud [Precarious employment in undocumented immigrants in Spain and its relationship with health]. *Gaceta Sanitaria*, 23(Suppl. 1), 107–14.

Rial González, E. and Irastorza, X. (eds) (2007) *Literature Study on Migrant Workers*. Bilbao: European Agency for Safety and Health at Work.

Rosmond, R., Lapidus, L. and Bjorntorp, P. (1998) A cross-sectional study of self-reported work conditions and psychiatric health in native Swedes and immigrants. *Occupational Medicine (London)*, 48(5): 309–14.

Rubiales-Gutiérrez, E., Agudelo-Suárez, A.A., López-Jacob, M.J. and Ronda-Pérez, E. (2010) Diferencias en los accidentes laborales en España según país de procedencia del trabajador [Differences in occupational accidents in Spain according to the worker's country of origin]. *Salud Pública de Mexico*, 52(3): 199–206.

Salminen, S., Vartia, M. and GIorgiani, T. (2009) Occupational injuries of immigrant and Finnish bus drivers. *Journal of Safety Research*, 40(3): 203–5.

Schenker, M. (2008) Work-related injuries among immigrants: a growing global health disparity. *Occupational and Environmental Medicine*, 65(11): 717–18.

Schenker, M.B. (2010) A global perspective of migration and occupational health. *American Journal of Industrial Medicine*, 53(4): 329–37.

Soler-González, J., Serna, M.C., Bosch, A., Ruiz, M.C., Huertas, E. and Rue, M. (2008) Sick leave among native and immigrant workers in Spain – a 6-month follow-up study. *Scandinavian Journal of Work, Environment & Health*, 34(6): 438–43.

Spanish National Statistics Institute (2009) *Encuesta de Población Activa [Active Population Survey]* (http://www.ine.es/inebmenu/mnu_mercalab.htm#1, accessed 20 May 2011).

Stuckler, D., Basu, S., Suhrcke, M., Coutts, A. and McKee, M. (2009a) The public health effect of economic crises and alternative policy responses in Europe: an empirical analysis. *Lancet*, 374(9686): 315–23.

Stuckler, D., Basu, S., Suhrcke, M. and McKee, M. (2009b) The health implications of financial crisis: a review of the evidence. *Ulster Medical Journal*, 78(3): 142–5.

Szczepura, A., Gumber, A., Clay, D., et al. (2004) *Review of the Occupational Health and Safety of Britain's Ethnic Minorities*. Norwich: Health and Safety Executive (http://www.hse.gov.uk/research/rrpdf/rr221.pdf, accessed 20 May 2011).

Taloyan, M., Johansson, L.M., Johansson, S.E., Sundquist, J. and Kocturk, T.O. (2006) Poor self-reported health and sleeping difficulties among Kurdish immigrant men in Sweden. *Transcultural Psychiatry*, 43(3): 445–61.

Taloyan, M., Johansson, S.E., Sundquist, J., Kocturk, T.O. and Johansson, L.M. (2008) Psychological distress among Kurdish immigrants in Sweden. *Scandinavian Journal of Public Health*, 36(2): 190–6.

United Nations Population Fund (UNPFA) (2007) *State of the World Population 2006. A Passage to Hope: Women and International Migration*. New York: UNPFA.

World Bank (2008) *Migration and Remittances Factbook*. New York: World Bank.

chapter eleven

Mental health of refugees and asylum-seekers

Jutta Lindert and Guglielmo Schinina

Introduction

Good mental health is crucial for the successful integration of migrants in a new country. However, empirical information on the epidemiology of mental health among migrants remains scarce, posing an obstacle to improving the prevention and treatment of mental disorders among this population group (Lindert et al. 2009). In general, people migrate to improve life chances for themselves or their children and expect gains in well-being. Yet, a large body of literature suggests that migration is a process that involves several stressors, with potentially negative impacts on mental health (Bhugra and Jones 2001).

The European Union (EU)'s Green Paper on mental health (Health & Consumer Protection Directorate-General 2005) and the 2010 World Health Organization–International Organization for Migration report on the health of migrants (WHO-IOM 2010) both recognize migrants as a group particularly at risk of mental disorders in Europe, and one to prioritize in responses. This generalized attribution of vulnerability may however be misleading, as there are many different types of migrants, including refugees and asylum-seekers, foreign students, labour migrants, cyclic or seasonal workers, victims of trafficking, undocumented migrants, and transnational families (IOM 2010).

The evidence is inconclusive and often related to the situation in specific countries, e.g. the Netherlands, Germany or the United Kingdom. Specific groups of migrants, such as refugees who had endured torture (Steel and Chey 2009), victims of trafficking (Zimmerman et al. 2006), or detainees (Cohen 2008) are consistently found to be at higher risk of mental disorders than the general population. However, these rates are often not migration-specific, but instead close to those experienced by similar groups within the non-migrant populations, such as rape victims, victims of political violence, and detainees. Research measuring the ratio of mental disorders in regular migrants against "native" populations in six European countries (France, Belgium, Italy, Spain, the Netherlands and Germany) found that migrants are 2.52 times more likely to develop such disorders than the "native" population (Health & Consumer Protection Directorate-General 2004). However, results show a high degree of variability between countries (ranging from 1.0 to 4.7), highlighting the importance that the receiving systems play in determining those conditions. Moreover, research conducted in the United Kingdom (Cochrane and Ball 1987) and the Netherlands (Selten and Sijben 1994) indicates that the rates of first admission for schizophrenia are higher in several migrant populations than in the "native" population. However, migrants of other nationalities were found to be less prone to mental disorders than the non-migrant population (Carta et al. 2005). Different rates of admission to mental health services can also be due to socioeconomic factors, cultural differences in how mental disorders are perceived, and differences in national legislation (Carta et al. 2005). Several studies have found that the descendants of migrants seem to be at higher risk of mental disorders than their parents or the "native" population (Hjern et al. 2004), confirming the importance of integration.

Given the variety of migrant populations, the mixed evidence, and the diversity of mental health systems in Europe, this chapter reviews the current state of knowledge on mental health of refugees and asylum-seekers only. Refugees and asylum-seekers, together with undocumented migrants, are considered to be particularly at risk, due to past and current predicaments. Research in Switzerland found that irregular migrants were in better mental health than asylum-seekers, who faced the uncertainty of their status (Chimienti and Achermann 2007). The available evidence further suggests that the impact of migration on mental health may differ among permanent and non-permanent labour migrants on the one hand and migrants forcibly uprooted by wars, conflicts or political violence (e.g. refugees and asylum-seekers), or the particularly vulnerable ones, like detainees and victims of trafficking, on the other. Asylum-seekers and refugees are more likely to experience risk factors for mental health, such as exclusion and discrimination (Stillman et al. 2009), and a recent meta-analysis provides evidence that the mental health of labour migrants and refugees is substantially different (Lindert et al. 2008). Refugees and asylum-seekers have often experienced wars, conflicts or political violence that can impact on their mental well-being. Mental health practitioners need to be attuned to such life events in order to best address the needs of this group of the population.

This chapter begins by reviewing the global scope and extent of migration of refugees and asylum-seekers and then explores what is known of their psychopathology, ranging from psychological distress to mental disorder (e.g. depressive disorder and depression, and post-traumatic stress disorder (PTSD)). As robust data on the mental health of refugees and asylum-seekers in the EU are still limited, the chapter draws on literature from both Europe and other parts of the world.

The chapter concludes by drawing lessons on how the mental health sector can meet the mental health needs of refugees and asylum-seekers. The mental health of children of refugees and unaccompanied and separated children falls outside the scope of this chapter, as it would deserve a separate discussion of specific developmental challenges.

Since the early 1980s, there has been a remarkable increase in research on the mental health and psychopathology of refugees and asylum-seekers, in particular in relation to those who have experienced political violence and forced migration. This surge of scientific interest in the mental health impact of political violence began with studies documenting the prevalence of psychiatric disorders among southeast Asian refugees who had fled their homelands in the wake of the Viet Nam war and the Cambodian genocide (Harding and Looney 1977; Kinzie et al. 1986; Felsman et al. 1990). Other conflicts heightened interest in the impact of political violence on psychopathology. These included, among others, conflicts in Latin America (Aron et al. 1991; Bowen et al. 1992), civil wars in Lebanon, Sri Lanka and Sudan (Bryce et al. 1989; Somasundaram 1996; Baron 2002), and "ethnic cleansing" in Bosnia and Herzegovina (Weine et al. 1998).

The terms "refugees" and "asylum-seekers" are legal concepts for people who, in the vast majority of cases, are survivors of political violence. Refugees are individuals who have been forcibly displaced from their home countries, have a well-founded fear of persecution, and are unwilling or unable to return to their home country. Asylum-seekers are individuals who have sought refuge in another country, but whose claim for refugee status has not yet been determined (see Chapter 2 on "Trends in Europe's international migration" and Chapter 3 on "Asylum, residency and citizenship policies and models of migrant incorporation").

The mental health impact of migration for refugees and asylum-seekers is related to the violence they may have experienced in their home country, the conditions under which they flee and travel, and the social and political conditions under which they live in the receiving country. To understand adequately the effects of refugees' experiences on mental health, one would need to compare the mental health of refugees and asylum-seekers to the mental health of those who stayed in their home country, but few such comparative studies are available. There are many additional methodological challenges associated with research into mental health among refugees and asylum-seekers, which will be discussed below.

Life events of refugees and asylum-seekers

Political violence or poor living conditions may affect people at all stages of the refuge process. Prior to fleeing, they may experience torture, witness the disappearance of family members, find themselves close to death, live in poor conditions, and may witness political killings or even massacres. Worse, political violence clusters, so that many refugees and asylum-seekers may have experienced multiple possibly traumatic events. During migration, they may be subject to violence from those trafficking, smuggling or transporting them, or from others exploiting their vulnerability. After arrival, refugees and asylum-seekers may be forced into inadequate living conditions, as a consequence of their initially volatile legal status, often living in detention centres or refugee camps, in overcrowded and unsanitary conditions (Momartin et al. 2006). Yet, despite this catalogue of stressors, controversy about the extent of psychopathology and the mental and psychosocial needs of refugees and asylum-seekers persists (van Ommeren et al. 2005).

Psychopathology among refugees and asylum-seekers

There are two conflicting hypotheses on the relationship between migration and mental health: the hypothesis of acculturation stress ("migration–morbidity hypothesis") and the selection hypothesis ("healthy-immigrant hypothesis"). The first maintains that migration causes distress and predicts greater risks of psychopathology among migrants (Pernice and Brook 1996; Dalgard et al. 2006); the second maintains that it is the healthier, younger and better-educated segments of the population who migrate and that they are at less risk of psychopathology (Alderete et al. 2000; Flores and Brotanek 2005).

The association between migration and the mental health of migrants seems to be even more complicated in the case of refugees and asylum-seekers, as there is wide variability in the rates of the most commonly studied psychiatric conditions and syndromes, such as affective disorders, anxiety and PTSD, and related syndromes of depression, anxiety and post-traumatic stress (de Jong et al. 2001; Fenta et al. 2004). Additionally, some authors have criticized the medicalization of the impact of massive emergencies such as wars or natural disasters, as some emotional reactions to these events could be considered as "normal reactions to abnormal events". On the other hand, evidence is emerging that experience of violence and war may affect the morphology of parts of the brain and the neurobiology of affected individuals (Tynan et al. 2010; Ursano et al. 2010).

Four systematic reviews (Porter and Haslam 2005; Fazel and Silove 2006; Lindert et al. 2009; Steel et al. 2009) and at least four narrative reviews (Karam and Ghosn 2003; Quiroga and Jaranson 2005; Murthy and Lakshminarayana 2006; Johnson and Thompson 2008) have investigated the psychopathology of refugees and asylum-seekers. Fazel et al. (2005) analysed 20 surveys focusing specifically on refugees who had resettled in high-income countries and found that methodological factors, including sample size and type of diagnostic measure used, influenced prevalence rates, as did contextual factors, such as time since resettlement. Porter and Haslam (2005) derived a single measure of psychological distress from the heterogeneous outcome measures used in a subset of 59 surveys that compared a displaced population with a non-displaced control group. Rates of distress were influenced by methodological, ecological and social variables, including restricted economic opportunities, insecure housing and rural residence. Lindert et al. (2008) analysed 36 surveys comparing the prevalence of depression and PTSD among refugees, asylum-seekers and labour migrants, and found that rates differed substantially. However, there remained a lack of clarity on whether the variation in the prevalence of psychopathology persists when differences in methodology and sampling methods are taken into account.

The reviews undertaken so far show clearly, in almost every study that has been done, that refugees and asylum-seekers who reported exposure to political violence prior to migration were more likely to meet criteria for psychopathology (e.g. depression, anxiety, PTSD) than refugees and asylum-seekers who had not been similarly exposed. Violence of all kinds has been shown to be associated with an increase in psychopathology in all countries where studies have been undertaken (Dohrenwend 1998). The effects persist, with increased rates of psychopathology remaining many years after resettlement in the host country (Marshal et al. 2005). However, the long-term effect of living with exposure to violent events needs further elucidation. There seems to be an overall dose–response relationship between political violence and levels of psychopathology, with the worst effects in those who have experienced extremely severe and prolonged political violence, such as those who have survived torture or concentration camps. However, as mentioned above, rates are not dissimilar to those among people affected by the same factors who did not migrate or who sought refuge in a different country. A third model for understanding the mental health of refugees and asylum-seekers, which can be termed the "life-course violence" model, is therefore proposed here.

The life-course violence model and psychopathology of refugees and asylum-seekers

To understand better the effects of political violence on refugees and asylum-seekers, it is useful to distinguish pre-migration, migration and post-migration events. This facilitates identifying and understanding the pathways leading to adverse mental health and psychopathological outcomes, as well as care-seeking behaviour (Table 11.1). The proposed approach builds on concepts of life-course epidemiology and suggests that events that take place during the process of migration may have latent effects, leading to vulnerability to illness being triggered at later stages of refugees' and asylum-seekers' lives, especially when exposed to adverse circumstances following migration (Rutter et al. 2001; Kuh et al. 2004; Pickles et al. 2007). This reflects the consistent finding of the dose–response relationship between the scale of violence experienced before, during and after migration, and the incidence and prevalence of psychopathology.

It is, however, important to recognize the resilience of many people who experience political violence or adverse life events and there has been criticism of what some see as an over-medicalization of the observed responses (Summerfield 1996). Far from all refugees and asylum-seekers have psychologically disabling disorders, but there is a need to be aware of the range of potential psychopathological symptoms and disorders that exist in this population when assessing their needs for mental health and psychosocial care.

Refugees, asylum-seekers and affective disorders and depression

The burden of disease attributable to affective disorders, especially major depressive disorder, in the general population has attracted increased attention as a result of findings by Harvard University and World Bank researchers who undertook surveys of mental health in 17 countries in Africa, Asia, the

Table 11.1 Selected pre-migration, migration and post-migration factors potentially associated with psychopathology

Pre-migration factors	Migration factors	Post-migration factors
Direct violence	**Direct violence**	**Direct violence**
Combat experiences, torture, wartime rape, death or disappearance of friends and family members	Violence during migration (e.g. rape)	E.g. racist attacks, gang violence
Poor living conditions	**Poor living conditions**	**Poor living conditions**
E.g. lack of food and water, poor or no access to health care	E.g. lack of food and water, poor or no access to health care	E.g. in detention centres or refugee camps
Humiliation, exclusion, discrimination	**Humiliation, exclusion, discrimination**	**Humiliation, exclusion, discrimination**
Exclusion from the infrastructure of the home country, loss of persons, possessions, culture	Exclusion from basic services, being vulnerable to abuse	Exclusion from the infrastructure of the host country: living in an unstable and insecure environment that is hostile towards foreigners, discrimination and racism, language and culture barriers, restricted work permits, poor or no access to health care

Source: Authors' compilation

Americas, Europe and the Middle East. They estimated that affective disorders ranked first among the ten leading causes of years lived with disabilities (Kessler et al. 2007). There is rather less research among refugees, but a recent systematic review on the psychopathology of refugees, which compiled evidence on 7000 refugees in seven countries (Australia, Canada, Italy, New Zealand, Norway, the United Kingdom and the United States), identified 14 studies of the prevalence of major depression, which included a total of 3616 adult refugees (Fazel et al. 2005). Somewhat contrary to expectations, the authors reported a 5% prevalence of minor depression, which was similar to the level seen in several western populations (Fazel et al. 2005). Nevertheless, there is some evidence that particular groups may experience greater risk due to particular experiences prior to migration, as has been found among Cambodian refugees (Marshal 2005).

Refugees, asylum-seekers and post-traumatic stress disorder

PTSD is a serious and complex disorder with emotional and psychiatric symptoms and physical consequences. Criterion A of the *Diagnostic and Statistical*

Manual of Mental Disorders IV (Text Revision) (American Psychiatric Association 2000) specifies that, for it to be diagnosed, a person must have "experienced, witnessed, or been confronted with an event that involves actual or threatened death or injury, or a threat to the physical integrity of self or others" (criterion A1) and the person must have a subjective emotional response that involved "intense fear, helplessness, or horror" (criterion A2). PTSD is by far the most common mental health problem diagnosed among refugees and asylum-seekers, as has been documented in numerous studies of populations affected by political violence (LeTouze and Watters 2003). There is consensus that certain PTSD symptoms (nightmares, flashbacks, intrusive images, heightened startle response, sleep disturbances) are found in refugees and asylum-seekers from diverse cultural contexts (de Jong et al. 1999; Sabin et al. 2003; Cardozo et al. 2004; Scholte et al. 2004; Fazel et al. 2005). Current evidence suggests that symptoms of PTSD include certain psycho-physiological correlates that are supposed to be prevalent in all cultural contexts, but there is recognition also that culture may influence the expression of certain symptoms (Summerfield 2003; Kirmayer 2005; Choudhury and Kirmayer 2009; Kirmayer et al. 2010).

Refugees, asylum-seekers and social health

The effects of political violence on the psychopathology of refugees and asylum-seekers are highly relevant to the work of providers of mental and psychosocial care. However, political violence is not only related to the psychopathology of refugees or asylum-seekers at the individual level, but also affects social health, with repercussions for families, communities and social institutions, as has been found in studies of the mental health of other groups affected by violence. At the family level, the adverse impact of political violence on the structure and function of nuclear and extended families has been well documented, for example, with regard to heightened family violence. At the community level, networks of social relations may be shattered, creating profound distrust, animosity and wariness towards social institutions among those affected by political violence. In addition, survivors of political violence have been found to adopt violent solutions to conflict within partnerships (Bryne and Riggs 1996), the community (Jakupcak and Tull 2005), and society at large (Glenn et al. 2002; Bayer et al. 2007).

Help-seeking behaviour of refugees and asylum-seekers

The available evidence indicates that utilization of mental and psychosocial services among refugees and asylum-seekers is low, as reports suggest (e.g. IOM 2010), but studies with representative samples are scarce. The literature attributes the underutilization of mental health services by refugees and asylum-seekers to a multitude of barriers to access. Different researchers have identified four non-exclusive groups of issues, relating to ethnicity, culture, health systems and societal responses, although more empirical research into these different perspectives is needed.

Researchers focusing on ethnicity have identified difficulties with the language of the host country, lack of knowledge about mental health services, failure by those affected to recognize the presence or severity of psychopathology, distrust of mental health services, stigma, and concerns about confidentiality and, in particular, being reported to the authorities. Refugees may also face various contextual and practical difficulties associated with attending health services, such as frequent mobility, difficulties with transport and finance, and a lower priority being placed on obtaining mental health care relative to other basic needs (de Anstiss et al. 2009).

Others have identified "culture" as an important factor in health service utilization (Cauce et al. 2002). Yet, while it is often suggested that cultural differences may be associated with lower use of mental health services, caution should be exercised in making generalizations. Culture is not the only, or even the most central, aspect of identity, as individuals have multiple identities, including age, gender, education and professional background (Nadeau and Measham 2006). Moreover, culture is not uniform, fixed or immutable, and cultural practices are transformed as they engage and interconnect with one another. Nevertheless, low cultural awareness and competence among mental health professionals still features prominently in the literature and is reported not only to inhibit access to services but also seriously to affect the quality of services received. Refugees and asylum-seekers may have understandings of psychopathology that differ from those common in their host countries. In some countries of origin, perceived psychopathology may be attributed to personal weakness, moral transgressions, physical complaints and spiritual causes (Muneghina et al. 2010).

Barriers identified by researchers focusing on the health system include limited access to health professionals from the same country of origin, lack of cultural mediators, high cost of services, lengthy waiting times for specialist counselling services and legal restrictions. Other system-level barriers include service complexity, bureaucracy and fragmentation. Particularly salient to the issue of service utilization is the level of "match" between services offered and those accessing them (Ingleby 2005). "Matching" of offer and needs is possible when the expectations and possibilities of the service providers and the expectations of the help-seeking individuals match. This might not be the case if service providers focus on the individual characteristics of refugees or asylum-seekers, neglecting their wider social and cultural environment and migration history.

From a societal perspective, researchers have identified restricted access to services for refugees and asylum-seekers, as well as detention practices, as possible causes of low utilization rates and higher rates of psychopathology (Silove et al. 2000).

The literature frequently identifies a mismatch between the emphasis on individual psychopathology and mental health symptoms and the actual health concerns of refugees and asylum-seekers. It is known that refugees and asylum-seekers are likely to perceive mental and psychosocial services to be most relevant when they target their immediate priorities, such as concerns about poverty, isolation and other stressors in their host countries. Such concerns underscore the importance of mental and psychosocial health interventions that transcend a narrow focus on psychopathology and include social health issues. It can be particularly helpful to identify resources locally available within communities that can promote healing and adaptation.

Conclusions

Refugees and asylum-seekers may remain at increased risk of psychopathology for many years, due to the life events many of them experience prior to having to flee, during their often prolonged travel and then after arrival. Strengthening mental health services for refugees and asylum-seekers requires attention from policy-makers, service planners, researchers and mental health professionals to match services more appropriately to needs.

However, there are still many gaps in our knowledge and more research is needed on the aetiology and effective responses to the psychopathology and mental disorders associated with political violence. Specifically, we need to learn more about the mental health problems and psychosocial stressors that refugees and asylum-seekers identify as most salient to their problems, as well as the impact that other forms of violence (e.g. the structural violence of poverty, institutionalized racism, gender-based discrimination, and the acute violence of spouse and child abuse) may have on mental health in the context of political violence and forced migration. There is also a need to understand how healthy and impaired psychosocial functioning are defined locally in countries of origin and how these definitions vary by factors such as age, gender, ethnicity and marital status. The help-seeking behaviour of refugees and asylum-seekers in the area of mental health is another neglected area of theory and research. This is one of the reasons for the apparent lack of effectiveness of mental health and psychosocial interventions (Tol et al. 2010). Other important areas for future research include explanatory models of psychopathology among refugees, preferred strategies for recovery (including through the use of informal networks), barriers to accessing mental health services, and experience of and satisfaction with services. There seems to be sufficient evidence to suggest that a focus on individual psychopathology that fails to address the wider social environment will not fully meet the needs of refugees and asylum-seekers (Vinck et al. 2007).

References

Alderete, E., Vega, W.A., Kolody, B., et al. (2000) Lifetime prevalence of and risk factors for psychiatric disorders among Mexican migrant farmworkers in California. *American Journal of Public Health*, 90(4): 608–14.

American Psychiatric Association (2000) *Diagnostic and Statistical Manual of Psychiatric Disorders-DSM-IV-TR*, 4th edn. Washington, DC: American Psychiatric Association.

Aron, A., Corne, S., Fursland, A. and Zelwer, B. (1991) The gender-specific terror of El Salvador and Guatemala: PTSD in Central American refugee women. *Women's Studies International Forum*, 14(1–2): 37–47.

Baron, N. (ed.) (2002) Community based psychosocial and mental health services for southern Sudanese refugees in long term exile in Uganda. In: de Jong, J. (ed.) *Trauma, War, and Violence: Public Mental Health in Socio-cultural Context*. New York: Kluwer Academic.

Bayer, C.P., Klasen, F. and Adam H. (2007) Association of trauma and PTSD symptoms with openness to reconciliation and feelings of revenge among former Ugandan and Congolese child soldiers. *JAMA*, 298(5): 555–9.

Bhugra, D. and Jones, P. (2001) Migration and mental illness. *Advances in Psychiatric Treatment*, 7: 216–33.

Bowen, D.J., Carscadden, L., Beighle, K. and Fleming, I. (1992) Post-traumatic stress disorder among Salvadoran women: empirical evidence and description of treatment. *Women & Therapy*, 13(3): 267–80.

Bryce, J.W., Walker, N., Ghorayeb, F. and Kanj, M. (1989) Life experiences, response styles and mental health among mothers and children in Beirut, Lebanon. *Social Science & Medicine*, 28(7): 685–95.

Bryne, C.A. and Riggs, D.S. (1996) The cycle of trauma: relationship aggression in male Vietnam veterans with symptoms of posttraumatic stress disorder. *Violence and Victims*, 11(3): 213–25.

Cardozo, B.L., Bilukha, O.O., Crawford, C.A., et al. (2004) Mental health, social functioning, and disability in postwar Afghanistan. *JAMA*, 292(5): 575–84.

Carta, M., Bernal, M., Hardoy, M.C., Haro-Abad, J.M.; Report on the Mental Health in Europe Working Group (2005) Migration and mental health in Europe. *Clinical Practice and Epidemiology in Mental Health*, 1: 1–16.

Cauce, A.M., Domenech-Rodriguez, M., Paradise, M., et al. (2002). Cultural and contextual influences in mental health help seeking: a focus on ethnic minority youth. *Journal of Consulting and Clinical Psychology*, 70(1): 44–55.

Chimienti, M. and Achermann, C. (2007) Coping strategies of vulnerable migrants: the case of asylum seekers and undocumented migrants in Switzerland.

Choudhury, S. and Kirmayer, L.J. (2009) Cultural neuroscience and psychopathology: prospects for cultural psychiatry. *Progress in Brain Research*, 178: 263–83.

Cochrane, R. and Bal, S.S. (1987) Migration and schizophrenia: an examination of five hypotheses. *Social Psychiatry*, 22(4): 181–91.

Cohen, J. (2008) Safe in our hands? A study of suicide and self-harm in asylum seekers. *Journal of Forensic and Legal Medicine*, 15(4): 235–44.

Dalgard, O.S., Thapa, S.B., Hauff, E., et al. (2006) Immigration, lack of control and psychological distress: findings from the Oslo Health Study. *Scandinavian Journal of Psychology*, 47(6): 551–8.

de Anstiss, H., Ziaian, T., Procter, N., et al. (2009) Help-seeking for mental health problems in young refugees: a review of the literature with implications for policy, practice, and research. *Transcultural Psychiatry*, 46(4): 584–607.

de Jong, J.T., Komproe, I.H., Van Ommeren, M., et al. (2001) Lifetime events and posttraumatic stress disorder in 4 postconflict settings. *JAMA*, 286(5): 555–62.

de Jong, K., Ford, N. and Kleber, R. (1999) Mental health care for refugees from Kosovo: the experience of Medecins Sans Frontières. *Lancet*, 353(9164): 1616–17.

Dohrenwend, B. (ed.) (1998) *Adversity, Stress and Psychopathology*. Oxford: Oxford University Press.

Fazel, M. and Silove, D. (2006) Detention of refugees. *BMJ*, 332(7536): 251–2.

Fazel, M., Wheeler, J. and Danesh, J. (2005) Prevalence of serious mental disorder in 7000 refugees resettled in western countries: a systematic review. *Lancet*, 365(9467): 1309–14.

Felsman, J.K., Leong, F.T., Johnson, M.C. and Felsman, I.C. (1990) Estimates of psychological distress among Vietnamese refugees: adolescents, unaccompanied minors and young adults. *Social Science & Medicine*, 31(11): 1251–6.

Fenta, H., Hyman, I. and Noh, S. (2004) Determinants of depression among Ethiopian immigrants and refugees in Toronto. *Journal of Nervous and Mental Disease*, 192(5): 363–72.

Flores, G. and Brotanek, J. (2005) The healthy immigrant effect: a greater understanding might help us improve the health of all children. *Archives of Pediatrics & Adolescent Medicine*, 159(3): 295–7.

Glenn, D.M., Beckham, J.C., Feldman, M.E., et al. (2002). Violence and hostility among families of Vietnam veterans with combat-related posttraumatic stress disorder. *Violence and Victims*, 17(4): 473–89.

Harding, R.K. and Looney, J.G. (1977) Problems of Southeast Asian children in a refugee camp. *American Journal of Psychiatry*, 134(4): 407–11.

Health & Consumer Protection Directorate-General (2004) *The State of Mental Health in Europe*. Luxembourg: European Commission.

Health & Consumer Protection Directorate-General (2005) *Green Paper: Improving the mental health of the population: Towards a strategy on mental health for the European Union*. Luxembourg: European Commission.

Hjern, A., Wicks, S. and Dalman, C. (2004) Social adversity contributes to high morbidity in psychoses in immigrants – a national cohort study in two generations of Swedish residents. *Psychological Medicine*, 34(6): 1025–33.

ILO (2000) *Mental Health in the Workplace*. Geneva: International Labour Office.

Ingleby, D. (ed.) (2005) *Forced Migration and Mental Health: Rethinking the Care of Refugees and Displaced Persons*. New York: Springer (International and Cultural Psychology Series).

IOM, WHO, CDC (2005) *International Dialogue on Migration No. 6 – Health and migration: bridging the gap*. Geneva: International Organization for Migration.

IOM (2010) *World Migration Report 2010*. Geneva: International Organization for Migration.

Jakupcak, M. and Tull, M.T. (2005) Effects of trauma exposure on anger, aggression, and violence in a nonclinical sample of men. *Violence and Victims*, 20(5): 589–98.

Johnson, H. and Thompson, A. (2008) The development and maintenance of post-traumatic stress disorder (PTSD) in civilian adult survivors of war trauma and torture: a review. *Clinical Psychology Review*, 28(1): 36–47.

Karam, E. and Ghosn, M.B. (2003) Psychosocial consequences of war among civilian populations. *Current Opinion in Psychiatry*, 16(4): 413–19.

Kessler, R.C., Angermeyer, M., Anthony, J.C., et al. (2007) Lifetime prevalence and age-of-onset distributions of mental disorders in the World Health Organization's World Mental Health Survey Initiative. *World Psychiatry*, 6(3): 168–76.

Kinzie, J.D., Sack, W., Angell, R., Manson, S. and Rath, B. (1986) The psychiatric effects of massive trauma on Cambodian children: I. The children. *Journal of the American Academy of Child Psychiatry*, 25(3): 370–6.

Kirmayer, L.J. (2005) Culture, context and experience in psychiatric diagnosis. *Psychopathology*, 38(4): 192–6.

Kirmayer, L.J., Narasiah, L., Munoz, M., et al. (2010) Common mental health problems in immigrants and refugees: general approach in primary care. *Canadian Medical Association Journal* [Epub ahead of print].

Kuh, D., Ben-Shlomo, Y. and Susser, E. (eds) (2004) *A Life Course Approach to Chronic Disease Epidemiology*. Oxford: Oxford University Press.

LeTouze, D. and Watters, C. (2003) Good practices in mental health and social care provision for refugees and asylum seekers. Report on the United Kingdom. In: Watters, C. and Ingleby, D. *Final Report on Good Practices in Mental Health and Social Care Provision for Refugees and Asylum Seekers*. Brussels: European Commission (European Refugee Fund).

Lindert, J., Brahler, E., et al. (2008) Depressivität, Angst und posttraumatische Belastungsstörung bei Arbeitsmigranten, Asylbewerbern und Flüchtlingen

Systematische Übersichtsarbeit zu Originalstudien [Depression, anxiety and posttraumatic stress disorders in labour migrants, asylum seekers and refugees. A systematic overview]. *Psychotherapie, Psychosomatik, Medizinische Psychologie*, 58(3–4): 109–22.

Lindert, J., Ehrenstein, O.S., Priebe, S., Mielck, A. and Brähler, E. (2009) Depression and anxiety in labor migrants and refugees – a systematic review and meta-analysis. *Social Science & Medicine*, 69(2): 246–57.

Marshal, G.N., Schell, T.L., Elliott, M.N., Berthold, S.M. and Chun, C.A. (2005) Mental health of Cambodian refugees after resettlement in the United States. *JAMA*, 294(5): 571–9.

Momartin, S., Steel, Z., Coello, M., et al. (2006). A comparison of the mental health of refugees with temporary versus permanent protection visas. *Medical Journal of Australia*, 185(7): 357–61.

Muneghina, O., Papadopoulos, R., et al. (2010) *Enhancing Vulnerable Asylum Seekers Protection in Europe*. Transnational Report. IOM-EU-Defense for Children-University of Essex (www.evasp.eu, accessed 20 May 2011).

Murthy, R.S. and Lakshminarayana, R. (2006) Mental health consequences of war: a brief review of research findings. *World Psychiatry*, 5(1): 25–30.

Nadeau, L. and Measham, T. (2006) Caring for migrant and refugee children: challenges associated with mental health care in pediatrics. *Journal of Developmental & Behavioral Pediatrics*, 27(2): 145–54.

Pernice, R. and Brook, J. (1996) Refugees' and immigrants' mental health: association of demographic and post-immigration factors. *Journal of Social Psychology*, 136(4): 511–19.

Pickles, A., Maughan, B. and Wadsworth, M. (eds) (2007) *Epidemiological Methods in Life Course Research*. Oxford: Oxford University Press (Lifecourse Approach to Adult Health Series).

Porter, M. and Haslam, N. (2005) Predisplacement and postdisplacement factors associated with mental health of refugees and internally displaced persons: a meta-analysis. *JAMA*, 294(5): 602–12.

Quiroga, J. and Jaranson, J.M. (2005) Politically-motivated torture and its survivors: a desk study review of the literature. *Torture*, 15(2–3): 1–112.

Rutter, M., Pickles, A., Murray, R. and Eaves, L. (2001) Testing hypotheses on specific environmental causal effects on behavior. *Psychological Bulletin*, 127(3): 291–324.

Sabin, M., Lopes Cardozo, B., Nackerud, L., Kaiser, R. and Varese, L. (2003) Factors associated with poor mental health among Guatemalan refugees living in Mexico 20 years after civil conflicts. *JAMA*, 290(5): 635–42.

Scholte, W.F., Olff, M., Ventevogel, M.D., et al. (2004) Mental health symptoms following war and repression in eastern Afghanistan. *JAMA*, 292(5): 585–93.

Selten, J.P. and Sijben, N. (1994) First admission rates for schizophrenia in immigrants to the Netherlands. The Dutch National Register. *Social Psychiatry and Psychiatric Epidemiology*, 29(2): 71–7.

Silove, D., Steel, Z. and Watters, C. (2000) Policies of deterrence and the mental health of asylum seekers. *JAMA* 284(5): 604–11.

Somasundaram, D.J. (1996) Post-traumatic responses to aerial bombing. *Social Science & Medicine*, 42(11): 1465–71.

Steel, Z., Chey, T., Silove, D., et al. (2009) Association of torture and other potentially traumatic events with mental health outcomes among populations exposed to mass conflict and displacement: a systematic review and meta-analysis. *JAMA*, 302(5): 537–49.

Stillman, S., McKenzie, D. and Gibson, J. (2009) Migration and mental health: evidence from a natural experiment. *Journal of Health Economics*, 28: 677–87.

Summerfield, D. (1996) *The Impact of War and Atrocity on Civilian Populations: Basic Principles for NGO Interventions and a Critique of Psychosocial Trauma Projects*. Network Paper 14. London: Overseas Development Institute.

Summerfield, D. (2003) Mental health of refugees. *British Journal of Psychiatry*, 183: 459–60; author reply 460.

Tol, W., Kohrt, B.A., Jordans, M.J.D., et al. (2010) Political violence and mental health: a multi-disciplinary review of the literature on Nepal. *Social Science & Medicine*, 70(1): 35–44.

Tynan R.J., Naicker, S., Hinwood, M., et al. (2010) Chronic stress alters the density and morphology of microglia in a subset of stress-responsive brain regions. *Brain, Behavior, and Immunity*, 24(7): 1058–68.

Ursano, R.J., Goldenberg, M., Zhang, L., et al. (2010) Posttraumatic stress disorder and traumatic stress: from bench to bedside, from war to disaster. *Annals of the New York Academy of Science*, 1208: 72–81.

van Ommeren, M., Saxena, S. and Saraceno, B. (2005) Mental and social health during and after acute emergencies: emerging consensus? *Bulletin of the World Health Organization*, 83(1): 71–5.

Vinck, P., Pham, P.N., Stover, E., et al. (2007) Exposure to war crimes and implications for peace building in northern Uganda. *JAMA*, 298(5): 543–54.

Weine, S.M., Vojvoda, D., Becker, D.F., et al. (1998) PTSD symptoms in Bosnian refugees 1 year after resettlement in the United States. *American Journal of Psychiatry*, 155(4): 562–4.

World Health Organization (2005) *Promoting Mental Health: Concepts, Emerging Evidence, Practice*. Summary Report. Geneva: World Health Organization.

WHO–IOM (2010) *Health of Migrants – The Way Forward*. Madrid: World Health Organization and International Organization for Migration.

Zimmerman, C., Hossain, M., Yun, K., et al. (2006) *Stolen Smiles: A summary report on the physical and psychological health consequences of women and adolescents trafficked in Europe*. London: London School of Hygiene & Tropical Medicine.

Section VI

Policy response

twelve

Migrant health policies in Europe

Philipa Mladovsky

Introduction

Studies from across the European Union (EU) demonstrate considerable, but varied, health inequalities between migrants and non-migrants (Mladovsky 2007). While certain types of migrants, such as asylum-seekers and undocumented migrants, face restrictions in their statutory rights to health care, most EU countries grant full equality of treatment to "third-country nationals" (non-EU citizens) who have achieved long-term residence status, putting them on an equal standing to residents from other EU countries (see Chapter 3 on "Asylum, residency and citizenship policies and models of migrant incorporation"). However, there is a growing recognition that migrants face specific obstacles in accessing health services that go beyond legal restrictions, such as lack of information, cultural and linguistic barriers, and socioeconomic deprivation. A succession of policies and initiatives have been initiated by the EU to improve migrants' access to health care in these respects (Peiro and Benedict 2009). In addition, a small but growing number of EU countries have also started developing national policies. This chapter provides an overview of migrant health policies and programmes in 11 European countries.

Analysing migrant health policies

The country information presented in this chapter is based on several sources. The first is a survey conducted in 2008 among health policy experts from 19 European countries (including one non-EU country): Austria, Belgium, Bulgaria, Czech Republic, Denmark, England, Estonia, Finland, France, Germany, Ireland, Italy, Lithuania, the Netherlands, Romania, Slovenia, Spain, Sweden and Turkey.

Further information on six additional countries (Greece, Hungary, Norway, Poland, Portugal and Switzerland) was obtained from MIGHEALTHNET country reports and country wikis (see: http://mighealth.net) and Chimienti (2009). Information on policies regarding asylum-seekers was obtained from some key publications (Nørredam et al. 2006; Huber et al. 2008; Vazquez et al. 2010), while information on undocumented migrants was retrieved from *Health care in NowHereland* country reports (see: http://www.nowhereland.info).

The results suggest that in most European countries migrants' health and access to health services are not addressed by specific policies. Only eleven of the 25 countries for which information was available have established specific national policies aimed at improving migrant health that go beyond statutory or legal entitlements: Austria, England, France, Germany, Ireland, Italy, the Netherlands, Portugal, Spain, Sweden and Switzerland. This chapter provides information on migrant health policies in these eleven countries along four dimensions: population groups targeted, health issues addressed, whether providers or patients are the focus of interventions, and whether policies are being implemented.

Population groups targeted

Migrant health policies can either focus on migrants in general or on specific migrant groups, such as asylum-seekers or undocumented migrants. However, policies may also be directed at broader population groups that include migrants, such as "ethnic minorities" or "socioeconomically disadvantaged groups".

Policies targeting migrants in general

In England, Ireland and the Netherlands, migrant policies are integrated into broader policies that also encompass ethnic minorities. In England, migrant health policy is largely subsumed under policies concerned with "race" and "black and minority ethnic" (BME) groups. This is reflected, for example, in Sir Donald Acheson's *Independent Inquiry into Inequalities in Health* (Acheson 1998) and the Department of Health *Race Equality Scheme 2005–2008* (Department of Health 2005). This categorization does not consider country of birth and therefore does not distinguish between different migrants and their descendants. As a result, the specific health needs of newly arrived migrants might be overlooked (Jayaweera 2010). A sign that the limitations of this approach have been recognized is the launch in 2010 of a "Migrant Health Guide" by the Health Protection Agency of the United Kingdom (http://www.hpa.org.uk/MigrantHealthGuide/).

Ireland's first National Intercultural Health Strategy covering 2007–2012 was published by its Health Service Executive in February 2008. In addition to migrants (including asylum-seekers, refugees and undocumented migrants), it covers travellers, other ethnic minorities and children of migrants born in Ireland. Policy recommendations of the strategy focus on anti-discrimination and "interculturalism" in the provision of health services to users from diverse cultures and ethnicities.

In the Netherlands, the government addresses health inequalities of both migrants and ethnic minorities under the broad conceptual umbrella of "cultural difference". In 1997, the Dutch Scientific Foundation established a working party on "culture and health" to stimulate research and care innovations in this area and, in 2000, the Council for Public Health and Health Care published two reports highlighting the health needs of migrants and ethnic minorities and their problems in accessing services (RVZ 2000a; RVZ 2000b). In response to these developments, the Minister of Health established a project group in 2001, which developed a strategy for "interculturalising" health care. However, this group resigned in 2003 when the new Minister of Health announced that he saw no role for the government in this area.

In Austria, France, Germany, Italy, Portugal, Spain, Sweden and Switzerland, the focus of health policy and programme development is more narrowly on migrants. In Austria, a working group of experts was created by the Ministry of Health with the aim of analysing migrant health issues. The working group produced a report on intercultural competence in the health sector (Bundesministerium für Gesundheit und Frauen 2005) that focuses on migrants and asylum-seekers, but does not consider undocumented migrants.

In Germany, a working committee on migration and public health was founded in 1997 (Berens et al. 2009) and produced a handbook on best practice models in the area of "Health and Integration" (Beauftragte der Bundesregierung für Migration 2007). However, specific national policy recommendations were not made until the National Integration Plan was issued in July 2007 (German Federal Government 2007). The plan lists a number of areas for action to improve integration. While the focus is not principally on health, the plan asks state governments (*Länderregierungen*) to set up projects to reduce barriers to access that would lead to an "intercultural opening" of the health system, including the creation of migrant-specific services and tailored information on health issues. However, the health of asylum-seekers and undocumented migrants is not specifically addressed in the plan. Further developments in the area of migrant health are described at a dedicated website of the federal government (http://www.bundesregierung.de/Webs/Breg/DE/Bundesregierung/ BeauftragtefuerIntegration/ThemenNeu/GesellschaftlicheIntegration/ Gesundheit/gesundheit__soziales.html).

In Italy, the Ministry of Health established a "national reference centre for health and immigration and the fight of diseases due to poverty" (*Centro di riferimento nazionale per la promozione della salute delle popolazioni migranti e il contrasto alle malattie della poverta*) at the Scientific Research Institute (*Istituto San Gallicano*) in Rome (Morrone 2006).

In Sweden, in 2004, government agencies dealing with health and social affairs, education, employment, integration and immigration services agreed on a common policy document, the *"Nationell samsyn kring hälsa och första tiden i Sverige"* (National agreement on health and the first years in Sweden), which aims to coordinate services in a way that promotes the health of migrants (asylum-seekers and others) during their first 2–5 years in Sweden

(Integrationsverket 2004). Migrants also have a right to interpreters guaranteed by law.

In Portugal, the Health Office of the National Centre for the Support of Immigrants was established in 2004. It disseminates information on the rights of migrants to health care and aims to improve access of migrants (both regular and irregular) to health services. During Portugal's Presidency of the EU in 2007, the issue of international migration was a health policy priority. The country's "Plan for the Integration of Immigrants 2007–2009" addressed a number of obstacles in migrants' access to the Portuguese national health service and aimed to improve the quality of services (Fonseca et al. 2009).

In Spain, a first Immigrant Social Integration Plan was adopted in 1994 as a framework of reference for the national government and a proposal for action at the regional level. In 2001, the Global Programme for Regularization and Coordination of Foreigners and Immigration was adopted. In 2005, relations between employers and irregular foreign workers (who were not authorized to reside and work in Spain) were regularized. In February 2007, the Secretary of State on Emigration and Immigration (at the Ministry of Labour and Social Affairs) approved the Strategic Plan on Citizenship and Integration 2007–10. The health-related goals were to guarantee migrants the right to health protection, better identify their social and sanitary needs, and to train health professionals. In addition, by 2008, 15 of the country's 17 autonomous communities (the exceptions being Asturias and Galicia) had developed regional immigration plans with more detailed health policies for migrants than in the regional health plans. Examples of regional plans or guidelines that include health objectives are:

- In Catalonia, the objectives of the Citizenship and Immigration Plan 2005–08 included ensuring better access to health care for migrants. The Catalan Immigration Master Plan for Health that was published in 2006 specified a number of health-related objectives for migrants.
- The regional Department of Health of Aragon has drawn up a document entitled "Immigration and Health" which gives guidance to health professionals providing care to migrants.
- The Immigration Plan of the Basque Country for 2007–09 identifies the provision of health care to migrants as one of the priorities for action.
- The Madrid Health Plan for 2006–10 dedicates a special chapter to improving the health status of migrants.
- The Valencia Immigration Plan for 2004–07 includes six sub-plans related to different areas of migrant health.
- The Andalusian Health Department has developed a "Guide to health care provision for immigrants". As part of the second Integral Immigration Plan of Andalusia, the department also published a document entitled *Providing Health Care to Immigrants.*

In Switzerland, the "Migration and Public Health Strategy 2002–2006" envisaged that policy initiatives on the topics of migration and health and awareness-raising measures would be taken in all health institutions in what is a highly decentralized health system. A small unit at the Federal Office of Public Health is charged with encouraging measures within this programme.

In 2006–07, the programme was evaluated and a new strategy formulated for 2008–13 which aims to continue and consolidate the measures from the first phase (Chimienti 2009).

In France, since the introduction of the Code of Admission and Residence of Foreign Persons and the right to asylum in 2006, each foreign person wishing to reside in the country must sign an accommodation and integration contract with the state. Part of this contract is the requirement to attend a "medical visit", which is compulsory for all foreigners residing in France for more than three months.

Many of the countries discussed in this section have developed migrant health policies as part of wider integration policies. Some of them (for example, Italy, Portugal and Spain) started to experience large-scale immigration more recently than England and the Netherlands, so their focus on newly arrived migrants is understandable. However, policies targeting the second and third generation will soon become relevant. By contrast, other countries such as France, Germany and Austria already have large numbers of descendants of migrants in their population and access to health care for these groups is likely to benefit from increased policy attention.

Policies targeting specific types of migrants

Although asylum-seekers and undocumented migrants tend to be at particularly high risk of health problems (Ingleby 2004; Björngren-Cuadra and Cattacin 2010), they are often confronted with barriers to accessing health care. Policies targeting asylum-seekers and undocumented migrants in Europe vary in the scope of care covered (e.g. whether they cover emergency services at all), the depth of financial protection (in terms of higher user charges or exemptions), the quality of care provided, levels of access to health care among different types of asylum-seekers (such as those whose claims have failed, are in detention, or are appealing a decision), and types of health care providers (the main health system or separate services provided in reception centres for asylum-seekers or by non-governmental organizations (NGOs)).

Asylum-seekers

The Council of the European Union has outlined minimum standards for the reception of asylum-seekers, which include emergency care, essential treatment of illness, and necessary medical or other assistance to applicants who have special needs (Council of the EU 2003). A comparative study of the 25 EU member states before 2004 (except Portugal) found legal restrictions in access to health care for asylum-seekers in 2004 in Austria, Denmark, Estonia, Finland, Germany, Hungary, Luxembourg, Malta, Spain and Sweden (Nørredam et al. 2006). In all of these countries, except Austria, legal restrictions were due to the fact that asylum-seekers were only entitled to emergency care. In Austria, asylum-seekers were only entitled to emergency care once they were released from reception centres. In Germany, Luxembourg, Spain and Malta, asylum-seekers' access to care changed over time. In Germany, asylum-seekers received full access to care 36 months after arrival. In Luxembourg, asylum-seekers were granted access to care comparable to citizens after 3 months of stay, and in Spain as soon as they had registered at a town council. Malta did not describe the nature of the change in status (Nørredam et al. 2006). In all countries studied, except Cyprus, Latvia and Luxembourg, some kind of access to specialized treatment was provided for tortured and traumatized asylum-seekers.

The study also covered medical screening practices and found that, in 2004, medical screening of newly arrived asylum-seekers existed in all the countries studied, except Greece, where it was only offered to asylum-seekers who applied for a work permit. In the Nordic countries (Denmark, Finland and Sweden), medical screening for diseases was systematically offered to all new asylum-seekers, whereas in other countries, such as Austria, France, Spain and Britain, it was only carried out in so-called "induction" or "reception" centres, so that newly arrived asylum-seekers who did not enter these centres did not have systematic access to medical screening. In all countries, medical screening was financed by the state authorities, which also provided the screening services, except in Denmark where they were provided by the Danish Red Cross (Nørredam et al. 2006).

Huber et al. (2008) provide more detailed policy information on access of asylum-seekers to health care in Finland, Germany, Greece, the Netherlands, Poland, Spain and the United Kingdom (Table 12.1). Further research is needed on access of asylum-seekers to health care in other European countries.

Table 12.1 Coverage regulations for asylum-seekers, selected EU countries

Finland	Free services are provided through designated reception centres; for urgent treatment, the municipal health system can also be used.
Germany	Access is limited to acute care, maternity care and pain relief.
Greece	Free services are only provided to those with a health card.
Netherlands	Health and long-term care are free, with coverage similar to standard benefit packages. However, there is no free choice of physicians and dental care for adults is restricted to acute treatment or pain relief.
Poland	Free services are provided, first at the reception centre and then upon referral. Transportation costs are also refunded.
Spain	Free services are provided in reception centres and the general health system.
United Kingdom	Free services are provided to accepted refugees, those given leave to remain, asylum-seekers, those waiting for a decision, appealing against a decision or detained in detention centres.
	Failed asylum-seekers have no right to treatment in the National Health Service (NHS), except for emergency services, sexually transmitted diseases (except HIV/AIDS), communicable diseases, family planning, compulsory psychiatric care and emergency care. There is a user fee for secondary care not considered "immediately necessary".

Source: adapted from Huber (2008)

Undocumented migrants

Undocumented migrants include visa or permit "overstayers", rejected asylum-seekers and individuals who have entered a country illegally. The "Health Care in NowHereland" project has classified EU27 countries into three groups, according to the rights of undocumented migrants to health care (Björngren-Cuadra and Cattacin 2010):

- EU countries in which undocumented migrants have no rights to free emergency health care: Bulgaria, Czech Republic, Finland, Ireland, Latvia, Luxembourg, Malta, Romania and Sweden.
- Countries in which undocumented migrants have "minimum rights| to health care": Austria, Belgium, Cyprus, Denmark, Estonia, Germany, Greece, Hungary, Lithuania, Poland, Slovakia, Slovenia and the United Kingdom. In most of these countries undocumented migrants have the right to access emergency care free of charge, but are required to pay for primary and secondary care.
- Countries in which undocumented migrants have the right to receive health services for no fee or a moderate fee: France, Italy, the Netherlands, Spain and Portugal.

This illustrates the wide diversity of rights to health care granted to undocumented migrants across the EU. The "Health Care in NowHereland" project points out that in countries with no or minimum entitlement to health services, providers are confronted with a dilemma: if they provide care, they may act against national regulations, but if they do not provide care, they may violate basic human rights and their own moral obligations (Björngren-Cuadra and Cattacin 2010). Various mechanisms have been developed as approaches to dealing with this dilemma. The two approaches identified by Karl-Trummer et al. (2010: 15) are "functional ignorance", where the legal status of somebody who needs health care is not asked for or is not monitored, and "partial acceptance", where, for example, specific sub-groups of migrants without permission to stay may have the right to certain limited hospital and outpatient treatment in the case of sickness or accidents, as well as to preventive treatments. More evidence is needed on how entitlements to health services are realized in practice, as well as on which health services are provided to undocumented migrants without legal entitlements.

Health issues addressed

Migrant health policies in the eleven countries covered in this chapter diverge considerably in the types of health issues addressed. Broadly speaking, in England, Spain and the Netherlands, there has been a strong focus on improving mental health care for migrants and ethnic minorities. For example, in the Netherlands in 2000, a four-year action plan for intercultural mental health was approved, to be supervised by the coordinating agency for mental health services. In the same year, an "intercultural mental health centre of expertise" called MIKADO was set up, with financing guaranteed until 2007 (Ingleby et al. 2005). In England, the action plan on "Delivering racial equality in mental health care" was published in 2005. Apart from mental health, considerable attention is paid in England to chronic physical illness, which may be related to the fact that there is a relatively high proportion of older migrants. In Austria, the 2005 *"Interkulturelle Kompetenz im Gesundheitswesen"* report focuses on mental health, in addition to gynaecology, obstetrics and paediatrics.

By contrast, in Italy there is no specific mention of migrant mental health in the national health plans. Instead, the focus is on sexual and reproductive health care and communicable disease (Vazquez et al. 2010). The 2001–03 plan, for example, set a target of a 10% reduction in elective abortion rates among migrant women. Similarly, in Germany, specific health-related issues in the National Integration Plan are covered mainly under the chapter on strategies for improving the situation of women and girls and fostering gender equity (German Federal Government 2007).

In Spain, regional plans focus on different health issues, as can be illustrated by the following examples:

- The Catalan Immigration Master Plan for Health sets targets for infant and maternal mortality, HIV infection, sexually transmitted diseases, tuberculosis and cancer.
- The Madrid Health Plan addresses preventive care, family planning for migrant women, promotion of healthy lifestyles among migrant children and adolescents (for example, through physical activity), improving school outcomes, and reducing the time migrant children spend alone.
- The Andalusian Integral Immigration Plan addresses services for children and women, diseases with high prevalence rates among migrants (for example, tuberculosis, hepatitis, HIV and dengue fever), long-term care, and specific risks such as prostitution, violence against women, and genital mutilation.
- Aragon's guide on Immigration and Health addresses pathologies related to adaptation problems, prevention and health promotion, immunization, paediatric services, the inclusion of migrant children in already existing programmes, recognizing potential risks of violence or harmful practices (including female genital mutilation), and referrals to social services.
- The Basque plan focuses on prevention and early detection of infectious diseases and immunization.
- The Valencian plan addresses health prevention and promotion activities, academic research, and nurse-led activities aimed at specific groups of migrants (e.g. women or older people) or organized under specific topics (e.g. nutrition or reproductive health).

In Switzerland, the "Migration and Public Health Strategy 2002–2006" grew out of a national HIV/AIDS prevention strategy which had been developed in the 1990s. HIV/AIDS remained a priority in the 2002–06 strategy, but the topics covered were broadened to include sexuality, pregnancy, birth and neonatal care under the national coordination centre for reproductive health; occupational safety and workplace health promotion; substance abuse through a migrant-specific outpatient project and a national feasibility study of the "Migration and dependency" pilot project; and therapy for traumatized asylum-seekers (Chimienti 2009).

In France, the afore-mentioned "medical visit" includes: a general clinical examination; radiographic examination of the lungs; and verification of vaccination status. Some people may also be screened for diabetes and be offered screening for other diseases. The following conditions may preclude the issuance of the final medical certificate: certain diseases covered by the World Health Organization (WHO) International Health Regulations (diseases which have a serious public health impact); active pulmonary tuberculosis if the person refuses treatment; and mental disorders requiring treatment, endangering others or likely to endanger public order if the examinee refuses treatment.

Ireland's National Intercultural Health Strategy covers a wide range of health issues, including specific care and support needs of ethnic minority women, mental health services for minority ethnic groups, care needs of children and families, as well as older people of diverse ethnicities and cultures, and improvements in disability, sexual health, alcohol, addiction and screening services.

This overview illustrates how health issues addressed differ across the eleven countries covered in this chapter. Ideally, these differences should reflect different health needs of migrants and deficiencies in existing health service structures, but this does not always seem to be the case. Specifically, given generally lower immunization rates among migrants (see Chapter 8 on "Communicable diseases"), preventive services do not seem to receive sufficient attention. The increasing importance of older migrants and the resulting need to develop culturally appropriate long-term care is another area that seems to have been ignored in most countries.

Targeting patients or providers

Migrants face many barriers to accessing health services (see Chapter 13 on "Differences in language, religious beliefs and culture: the need for culturally responsive health services" and Chapter 5 on "Migrants' access to health services"). In order to overcome these barriers, governments will need to decide on the appropriate balance between targeting patients (demand) and providers (supply).

On the demand side, migrants may benefit from better information on health services and entitlements, as well as from education programmes to improve health literacy (Netto et al. 2010). On the supply side, migrants often require extra interventions to ensure access. This typically involves improving the cultural competence of providers. Recently, emphasis has been placed on the development of the "whole organization approach", in which cultural competence is no longer regarded as a property of individuals but of organizations. In the United States, for example, the Department of Health (OMH 2000) redefined "cultural competence" as "culturally and linguistically appropriate services (CLAS)". "Good practices" in culturally competent health care include the training of staff, diversification of the workforce, use of "cultural mediators", and adaptation of protocols, procedures and treatment methods (Fernandes and Pereira Miguel 2009) (see Chapter 14 on "Good practice in emergency care" and Chapter 15 on "Good practice in health service provision for migrants").

Across the eleven countries covered, there is a mix of policies, programmes and projects at all levels of the health system to improve both the supply of and demand for health care for migrants. Some examples are provided here. On the supply side, the English Department of Health has set specific goals under the Delivering Racial Equality initiative which commits primary care trusts (local health authorities) to provide race equality training in their mental health services and to appoint race equality leads and community development workers. The project "Pacesetters, Race for Health" was established in 2003 to enable primary care trusts to make health services fairer for black and minority ethnic communities.

In France, the "medical visit" includes information on how to access the health system, as well as on the major diseases that may affect migrants. If a need for treatment is identified, the patient is referred and a copy of the medical certificate is forwarded to the doctor, with the permission of the patient.

In Italy, efforts have been made to improve the health information system covering migrants registered with the National Health Service (*Servizio Sanitario Nazionale*), as well as registration rates of foreigners with a residence permit. In 2007, the Minister of Health established the "Commission for the Health of Migrants". The Commission aims, among other things, to monitor the quality and equity of health services provided to both regular and irregular migrants.

In the Netherlands, supply-side interventions include migrant health promoters who give patients information in their own language and mediate between care providers and migrants. Their activities are coordinated by the Netherlands Institute for Health Promotion and Disease Prevention.

In Austria, the focus is on improving the intercultural competence of health services provided by hospitals and general practitioners, for example, through interpreter services and the training of physicians and nurses. The Migrant-Friendly Hospitals project (see Chapter 13 on "Differences in language, religious beliefs and culture: the need for culturally responsive health services") was designed and coordinated by an Austrian research institute, but has found limited resonance among hospitals in Austria.

In Ireland, the National Intercultural Health Strategy aims to improve:

- training for culturally competent, antiracist and non-discriminatory services;
- referrals of ethnic minority service users to secondary and tertiary care;
- the management of conditions disproportionately affecting ethnic minority communities;
- working with the NGO sector in the design and delivery of services;
- using cultural mediators at the community level;
- guidelines on providing translated material;
- interpretation and a national interpretation service;
- data and research, including the rollout of an ethnic identifier and the development of a database on ethnic minority health;
- conducting health impact assessments;
- organizational and human resource development through a "whole organizational approach" to support interculturalism.

The Portuguese "Plan for the Integration of Immigrants 2007–2009" introduced measures which included training, education and communication programmes to inform health professionals of the legal rights of migrants, plus the promotion of partnerships to improve the quality of services provided and facilitate change in organizational culture. Furthermore, the High Commission for Immigration and Intercultural Dialogue established a telephone interpretation service for migrants for use by public and private health care providers (Fonseca et al. 2009).

In Spain, activities differ across autonomous communities.

- The Catalan Immigration Master Plan for Health's objectives include the development of better data collection systems on migrant health and health care utilization, adapting the health system to the reality of immigration (for example, through training), better preparedness for specific health problems migrants may have (e.g. "imported diseases"), and reorganization and coordination of the network of International Health Units providing care to migrants.
- The Madrid Health Plan envisages measures to improve access to health services by migrants.
- Andalusia's "Guide to health care provision for immigrants" focuses on protocols for migrants' first contact with the health system, recommendations for nursing professionals, with particular attention to providing long-term care for migrants, and a central role for intercultural mediation.
- The guide on "Immigration and Health" in Aragon focuses on interventions by health professionals, including guidelines for general practitioners on paying attention to cultural differences.
- The Basque plan includes the objective of training health professionals.
- The Valencian plan envisages the provision of free interpretation services, training programmes for health professionals, and the development of clinical protocols.

In Switzerland, the "Migration and Public Health Strategy" envisages the provision of training programmes for officially recognized professional interpreters and the promotion of basic, advanced and continuous education in migration-specific matters for health professionals. It also aims to remove barriers to access through "Migrant-Friendly Hospitals", coordination services (the "Integration and Health" service in east Switzerland), and the use of interpreters and cultural mediators (Chimienti 2009).

Other types of intervention aim to modify demand for health care among migrants by influencing their care-seeking behaviour. In Ireland, the intercultural strategy aims to adapt information for service users, and use peer-led approaches, as well as the participation of ethnic minority communities in the rollout of the primary care strategy process. In Italy, the 2001–03 plan stated that local health offices (*Azienda Sanitaria Locale*) should promote information campaigns for migrants, while the 2006–08 plan aimed to promote education programmes in cooperation with volunteer and non-profit organizations. The Swedish "National agreement on health and the first years" also aims to improve the provision of information to migrants on the right to health care. In Germany, the National Integration Plan proposes projects in kindergarten and primary schools that link German language support with health-related education. The Federal Ministry of Health (via the Federal Centre for Health Education, the *Bundeszentrale für gesundheitliche Aufklärung*), the German Cancer Society and a few other country-wide initiatives also provide telephone services or leaflets in migrant languages, although the general use of interpreters by health care providers has not yet been established (Berens et al. 2009). The Portuguese "Plan for the Integration of Immigrants 2007–2009" provides for training, education and communication programmes to improve information among migrants on available health services and to encourage the use of the national health service. All the regional plans in Spain promote the improvement of information for migrants on health services. The Swiss strategy aims to provide health information materials to migrants by distributing and updating the "Health Guide Switzerland".

To summarize, in all eleven countries, there is a mix of interventions targeting patients and providers in order to improve migrants' access to health services. A notable weakness of most demand-side policies and programmes (with the exception of Ireland) is that they do not seem to aim at increased participation and empowerment of migrants, but are instead limited to providing basic information on available services.

Implementation

The development and implementation of migrant health policies is a potentially challenging task for governments, considering the highly contested and political nature of any public policy related to immigration in many European countries. Implementation is affected by a number of factors, including the administrative set-up of the country and its health system, demographic patterns of immigration, election cycles, data availability, collaboration with other sectors and budgetary restraints due to the current economic crisis.

In England, the Race Relations Amendment Act (2000) imposes on all public bodies the legal obligation to outlaw racial discrimination and promote equal opportunities. However, a review of 300 primary care trusts found that compliance has been patchy and that a significant minority of primary care trusts did not appear to have made public their race equality schemes (Thorlby and Curry 2007). A review of "Delivering Race Equality" was published (Wilson 2009), but it is mainly an overview of activities undertaken and does not provide an in-depth analysis of problems of implementation. In Germany, the federal state governments (*Länderregierungen*) rather than the national government are tasked with implementation of the goals of the National Integration Plan. Implementation of the proposed projects is therefore likely to vary across federal states, although regular monitoring of implementation is planned. In Spain, implementation is also decentralized to the regional level, resulting in a wide heterogeneity of plans, programmes and implementation strategies. Implementation of the Swiss strategy takes place in cooperation with federal agencies and organizations and is coordinated by an inter-institutional group at the federal level (Chimienti 2009).

Apart from uneven implementation across regions and geographical areas, another challenge of implementation is sustainability. While the Netherlands stands out in Europe for its long-standing and systematic attention to migrant health, these initiatives might be in danger of stagnating. The "Culture and Health" programme and the Action Plan both ended in 2004, and the government which came to power in 2002 distanced itself from the policy of interculturalization announced by the previous Minister of Health in 2000, instead placing the onus on migrants to adapt to Dutch society (Ingleby et al. 2005). In 2005, the then Minister of Health, Welfare and Sport found that no additional government policies on migrant health were needed, although the Secretary of the State of Health noted in 2006 that, at least with respect to older immigrants, new programmes might be needed to improve care (Clemence Ross-van Dorp, Secretary of the State of Health, 9 October 2006). However, since 2002, migrant health policy in the Netherlands has been almost entirely regressive, with the exception of a reform increasing access to health care for undocumented migrants in some respects, which came into force in 2009 (Björngren-Cuadra 2010).

The Austrian report on "Intercultural Competence in the Health Sector" provided no details on implementation. In Ireland, the implementation of the intercultural strategy is planned to take place mainly through existing health service structures, with a central role for consultation with and participation of ethnic minority groups. The establishment of a National Advisory Body is planned to guide the implementation of the intercultural strategy. This representative, multisectoral body is envisaged to link with national, regional and local organizations and groups, and to report to the Social Inclusion Directorate and the Health Services Executive. In Portugal, the multidisciplinary group "Health & Migrants" was established to support the implementation of the "Plan for the Integration of Immigrants" under the coordination of the General Directorate of Health. The High Commissariat for Immigration and Intercultural Dialogue reports annually on the implementation of the plan, but has found it difficult to establish whether some goals have been achieved, due to a lack of statistical information (Fonseca et al. 2009). This lack of information on the implementation of migrant health policies is a challenge in most of the countries covered in this chapter, which makes it very difficult to assess the success of many of the policy initiatives discussed above.

Discussion

As the preceding sections have shown, each country has taken a different approach, with some producing detailed policies and others, such as Germany, providing only a few objectives as part of a wider integration plan. All eleven countries have developed a minimum set of policies with regard to asylum-seekers, mostly in terms of establishing legal provisions and screening. However, there is a need for more detailed information on specific policy initiatives, programmes and practices.

Across the eleven countries there seems to be a tendency to focus policy either on newly arrived migrants or on more established ethnic minorities. However, high immigration countries may need to focus on both of these groups given their divergent health and health care problems (Jayaweera 2010; Vazquez et al. 2010). The Netherlands and Ireland, with their focus on "intercultural health care", are perhaps the countries with the most balanced approach in this regard.

Another issue is whether specific diseases affecting migrants should be prioritized. For example, sexual and reproductive health seems to take priority in Italy and Germany, whereas mental health has been a particular focus in England and the Netherlands. More research is needed to understand whether such differences in policy accurately reflect real differences in need among migrants across these countries. It is, for example, conceivable that migrants in Italy have as much need for targeted mental health care services as those in England and the Netherlands, which would present an opportunity for knowledge transfer from one context to another. As mentioned above, there may also be gaps in the provision of preventive and long-term care for migrants in all of the eleven countries.

All the countries adopt a mix of interventions targeting both patients and providers. However, there may be more scope for promoting the participation of migrants in developing health care that is responsive to their needs.

The wide differences observed across and sometimes even within countries, in the different dimensions of migrant health policies, suggest that there are considerable opportunities for learning and policy dialogue across contexts. However, it is also important to recognize that countries have varying traditions in social welfare, so there can be no "one size fits all" approach to migrant health policies. It has, for example, been argued that welfare systems based on a "communitarian" approach to diversity (for example, in the United Kingdom and the Netherlands) are relatively well-adapted to incorporating migrant health policies, while such policies challenge the logic of systems based on a "republican" approach, such as in Austria, France, Germany and Sweden (Cattacin et al. 2006). Indeed, this might help explain why a country with a relatively long history of immigration such as France focuses narrowly on newly arrived migrants and has not developed intercultural or ethnic minority health policies. Further research is needed to understand how migrant health policies can be developed in various types of social welfare systems.

Conclusions

The findings presented here may assist countries to learn from each others' experiences and to design more appropriate migrant health policies. However, the analysis of migrant health policies is still in its infancy. There is a need to further refine the analytical framework, evaluate the effectiveness of policies, and better understand how migrant health policies can be developed in countries with varying political and social welfare systems.

There is also a clear need for better monitoring and evaluation. Even where migrant health policies have been elaborated at the national level, due to a lack of data and information it is often unclear to what extent they have been implemented. Furthermore, little information is available on policies relating to asylum-seekers.

Finally, there is the challenge of sustaining momentum, in particular in the current context of economic crisis and budgetary constraints. As illustrated by the Netherlands, migrant health policies are situated in the politically sensitive and contested policy area of immigration and may thus fall victim to anti-immigration sentiments.

Acknowledgements

This chapter is an adaptation and extension of Mladovsky (2009). The survey on which this chapter is based was collected within the project "Health Status and Living Conditions" (VC/2004/0465), funded by the European Commission, DG Employment and Social Affairs, and implemented by the European Observatory on the Social Situation.

The following experts contributed to this chapter by providing country reports: Austria – Sascha Müller and Iris Saliterer (Wiener Gebietskrankenkasse, Abteilung Gesundheitspolitik und Prävention); Germany – Stefanie Ettelt (London School of Hygiene & Tropical Medicine) and Marcial Velasco (Berlin University of Technology); Ireland – Helen McAvoy (Institute of Public Health, Belfast); Italy – Margherita Giannoni-Mazzi (University of Perugia) and Zahara Ismail; Netherlands – Jeanine Suurmond and Karien Stronks (Department of Social Medicine, Academic Medical Centre, University of Amsterdam); Spain – Alexandrina Stoyanova (University of Barcelona); Sweden – Anna Melke (Göteborg University and Vårdal Institute). The author is very grateful to David Ingleby for his input into earlier drafts of this chapter.

References

Acheson, D. (1998) *Independent Inquiry into Inequalities in Health.* Report. London: The Stationery Office.

Beauftragte der Bundesregierung für Migration, Flüchtlinge und Integration (2007) *Gesundheit und Integration. Ein Handbuch für Modelle guter Praxis* (http://www.bundesregierung.de/Content/DE/Publikation/IB/Anlagen/2007-08-31-gesundheit-und-integration,property=publicationFile.pdf, accessed 20 May 2011).

Berens, E., Spallek, J., Razum, O. (2009) *Summary of State of the Art Report: Germany.* MIGHEALTHNET (http://mighealth.net/management/images/4/4c/Germany_summary_SOAR_EN.doc, accessed 1 June 2011).

Björngren-Cuadra, C.B. (2010) *Policies on Health Care for Undocumented Migrants in the EU27. Country Report: The Netherlands.* Malmö: Malmö University.

Björngren-Cuadra, C. and Cattacin, S. (2010) *Policies on Health Care for Undocumented Migrants in the EU27: Towards a Comparative Framework. Summary Report.* Malmö: Health Care in NowHereland, Malmö University.

Bundesministerium für Gesundheit und Frauen (2005) *Interkulturelle Kompetenz im Gesundheitswesen* (http://www.bmg.gv.at/cms/site/attachments/6/5/0/CH0772/CMS1126253889077/bericht_interkulturelle_kompetenz_im_gesundheitswesen.pdf, accessed 20 May 2011).

Cattacin, S., Chimienti, M. and Björngren-Cuadra, C. (2006) *Difference Sensitivity in the Field of Migration and Health: National Policies Compared.* Research Report. Geneva: Department of Sociology, University of Geneva.

Chimienti, M. (2009) Migration and health: national policies compared. In: Fernandes, A. and Pereira Miguel, J. (eds) *Health and Migration in the European Union: Better*

Health for All in an Inclusive Society. Lisbon: Instituto Nacional de Saúde Doutor Ricardo Jorge (http://www.insa.pt/sites/INSA/Portugues/Publicacoes/Outros/Documents/ Epidemiologia/HealthMigrationEU2.pdf, accessed 1 June 2011).

Chimienti, M. (2009) *State of the Art Report: Switzerland.* MIGHEALTHNET (http:// mighealth.net/ch/images/1/11/Soar.doc, accessed 1 June 2011).

Clémence Ross-van Dorp, Secretary of the State on Health, Well-being and Sport (9 October 2006) *Spreektekst voor de staatssecretaris van Volksgezondheid, Welzijn en Sport, Clémence Ross-van Dorp, bij de bijeenkomst Interculturalisatie in de Ouderenzorg op 9 Oktober 2006 in Rotterdam [Text of the speech of the Secretary of State on Health, Well-being and Sport, Clémence Ross-van Dorp, at the meeting on interculturalization of the care for the elderly, on 9 October 2006 in Rotterdam]* (http://www.informelezorg.info/eiz/ docs/pdf/toespraakrossintercultuuralisatie.pdf, accessed 1 June 2011).

Council of the EU (2003) *Council Directive 2003/9/EC of 27 January 2003 laying down minimum standards for the reception of asylum seekers.* Brussels: Council of the European Union: L 31/18.

Department of Health (2005) *Race Equality Scheme 2005–2008.* London: Department of Health.

Fernandes, A. and Pereira Miguel, J. (eds) (2009) *Health and Migration in the European Union: Better Health for All in an Inclusive Society.* Lisbon: Instituto Nacional de Saúde Doutor Ricardo Jorge (http://www.insa.pt/sites/INSA/Portugues/Publicacoes/Outros/ Documents/Epidemiologia/HealthMigrationEU2.pdf, accessed 1 June 2011).

Fonseca, M.L., Silva, S., Esteves, A. and McGarrigle, J. (2009) *Portuguese State of the Art Report.* MIGHEALTHNET (http://mighealth.net/pt/images/0/00/Mighealthnet_SOAR_ eng.pdf, accessed 1 June 2011).

German Federal Government (2007) *National Integration Plan* (http://www. bundesregierung.de/nsc_true/Content/DE/Archiv16/Artikel/2007/07/Anlage/2007-07-12-nationaler-integrationsplan-kurzfassung,property=publicationFile.pdf/2007-07-12-nationaler-integrationsplan-kurzfassung, accessed 1 June 2011).

Huber, M., Stanciole, A., Wahlbeck, K., et al. (2008) *Quality in and Equality of Access to Healthcare Services.* Brussels: European Commission (http://www.euro.centre.org/ data/1237457784_41597.pdf, accessed 1 June 2011).

Ingleby, D., Chimienti, M., Hatziprokopiou, P., Ormond, M. and De Freitas, C. (2005) The role of health in integration. In: Fonseca, L. and Malheiros, J. (eds) *Social Integration and Mobility: Education, Housing and Health.* Lisbon: Centro de Estudos Geográficos: 101–37.

Ingleby, D. (ed.) (2004) *Forced Migration and Mental Health: Rethinking the Care of Refugees and Displaced Persons.* New York: Springer.

Integrationsverket (2004) *Nationell samsyn kring hälsa och första tiden i Sverige [National agreement on health and the first years in Sweden.]* Norrköping: Integrationsverket [Swedish Integration Board].

Jayaweera, H. (2010) *Health and Access to Health Care of Migrants in the UK.* London: Race Equality Foundation.

Karl-Trummer, U., Novak-Zezula, S. and Metzler, B. (2010) Access to health care for undocumented migrants in the EU: a first landscape of NowHereland. *Eurohealth,* 16(1): 13–16.

Mladovsky, P. (2007) *Migration and Health in the EU.* Brussels: European Commission.

Mladovsky, P. (2009) A framework for analysing migrant health policies in Europe. *Health Policy* 93(1): 55–63.

Morrone, A. (2006) Salute e immigrazione: un Centro di riferimento Nazionale Immigrati e Assistenza Sanitaria [Health and immigration: a national reference centre on immigrants and health care]. *Monitor,* 5(18): 63–6.

Netto, G., Bhopal, R., Lederle, N., et al. (2010) How can health promotion interventions be adapted for minority ethnic communities? Five principles for guiding the development of behavioural interventions. *Health Promotion International*, 25(2): 248–57.

Nørredam, M., Mygind, A. and Krasnik, A. (2006) Access to health care for asylum seekers in the European Union – a comparative study of country policies. *European Journal of Public Health*, 16(3): 286–90.

OMH (2000) *National Standards on Culturally and Linguistically Appropriate Services (CLAS) in Health Care*. Excerpted from the Federal Register, 22 December 2000, 65(247): 80865–80879. Washington, DC: Office of Minority Health, Department of Health And Human Services (http://minorityhealth.hhs.gov/templates/browse.aspx?lvl=2&lvlID=15, accessed 20 May 2011).

Peiro, M.-J. and Benedict, R. (2009) *Migration Health: Better Health for All in Europe*. Brussels: International Organization for Migration.

RVZ (2000a) *Allochtone Cliënten en Geestelijke Gezondheidszorg [Migrant and Ethnic Minority Clients and Mental Health Care]*. Zoetermeer: Raad voor de Volksgezondheid en Zorg [Council for Public Health and Healthcare].

RVZ (2000b) *Interculturalisatie van de Gezondheidszorg [Interculturalization of Health Care]*. Zoetermeer: Raad voor de Volksgezondheid en Zorg [Council for Public Health and Healthcare].

Thorlby, R. and Curry, N. (2007) *PCTs and Race Equality Schemes*. London: King's Fund.

Vazquez, M-L., Terraza-Nunez, R., Vargas, I., Rodriquez, D. and Lizana, T. (2010) Health policies for migrant populations in three European countries: England; Italy and Spain. *Health Policy* [Epub ahead of print].

Wilson, M. (2009) *Delivering Race Equality in Mental Health Care: A Review*. London: Mental Health Division, Department of Health.

chapter thirteen

Differences in language, religious beliefs and culture: the need for culturally responsive health services

Sophie Durieux-Paillard

Introduction

In 2004, the "Amsterdam Declaration towards Migrant-Friendly Hospitals in an ethno-culturally diverse Europe" responded to one of the major challenges facing European health professionals, recognizing that "migration, ethno-cultural diversity, health and health care are closely interlinked in many ways" (Amsterdam Declaration 2004: 1). The declaration was followed by the resolution on the "Health of Migrants" by the World Health Assembly in 2008 (World Health Assembly 2008). A combination of globalization, European integration and international migration means that the intermixture of nationalities and cultures is a daily reality, with an estimated 214 million migrants worldwide and 72.6 million migrants in the WHO European region in 2010 (IOM 2010).

International conventions, such as the International Covenant on Economic, Social and Cultural Rights (UNHCHR 1976), which has been ratified by all EU member states, establish that access to health care is a basic human right for everyone (see Chapter 4 on "The right to health of migrants in Europe"). Health systems therefore have a particular responsibility to meet the diverse needs that come with a multiethnic society. Health service providers have to realize that culture and diversity affect clinical practice (Kleinman et al. 1978; Kleinman 1983; Betancourt et al. 2003; Lee 2010), and that they must also enhance their ability to provide "culturally responsive health care". However, doing so poses new challenges for health professionals, managers, and those responsible for monitoring quality (Amsterdam Declaration 2004). Investing in a generation of European health workers more aware and open to different cultures and diversity was also one of the recommendations of the EU Level consultation on "Migration Health – Better Health for All in Europe" (Peiro and Benedict 2009).

The term "culture" has many meanings, which makes defining "culturally responsive health care" challenging. This chapter follows the broad definition given by Mezzich et al. (2009: 384):

> Culture has been defined as a set of meanings, behavioral norms, values and practices used by members of a particular society, as they construct their unique view of the world. As such, culture deeply informs *every aspect of life and health.*

This implies that "culture" embraces not only ethnicity and religion but also socioeconomic factors, including levels of education, housing conditions, and access to information. Yet, much of the medical literature takes a narrower view. Research in the United States (Todd 2000; Williams 2003), has focused mainly on "racial and ethnic disparities", leaving out socioeconomic dimensions of cultural concerns. Other authors, like Marmot and Syme (1976), studying coronary heart disease among Japanese migrants in the United States, and, later, among migrants from a number of countries living in the United Kingdom, found that links between social environment and health may be more important than the country of origin. Appadurai (1996) argues that traditional cultural identities cross national boundaries, partly through the advent of modern mass media. At the same time, it can be argued that there are more "cultural" differences between a business executive and a homeless person sharing the same country of origin, than between two colleagues from different countries with the same profession and level of education.

The social determinants of health can be defined as: "the circumstances, in which people are born, grow up, live, work and age, and the systems put in place to deal with illness" (WHO 2010). These circumstances are in turn shaped by wider economic, social and political forces (WHO 2010). However, there is also extensive evidence of the importance of ethnic, religious and linguistic factors, interacting with socioeconomic factors. Examples include language barriers, but also lack of appropriate information and resources for migrants. In times of economic crisis and in the face of rising nationalism in a number of European countries, enlarging the cultural dimension of migrant health to include their economic and social context is an option to avoid what could be called "ghetto medicine". This chapter therefore argues that the concept of "migrant-friendly services" should be considered within a broader perspective that includes other forms of vulnerability. The emphasis then shifts to the wider question of whether health systems have competence in managing diversity.

Overcoming language barriers

Delivering adequate and appropriate health care to migrant patients thus raises wider questions about medical culture and values and how to improve medical care for all patients, *inter alia* by enhancing the communication skills of health professionals and their diagnostic sensitivity (Partida 2007; Lee 2010). It has become generally accepted that clinical practice should be patient-centred and, in most medical schools, communication skills are now an important part of the curriculum. However, when doctors encounter patients from different ethnic backgrounds, cultural differences are often assumed.

Language barriers are one of the main obstacles in medical consultations involving migrant patients (Terraza-Núñez et al. 2010; see also Chapter 15 on "Good practice in health service provision for migrants"). Bischoff et al. (2003) use the term "allophone", derived from linguistics, to describe patients whose first language is not the one spoken in the country they live in. In the EU, there are 23 official languages, 60 regional languages and around 175 languages spoken by migrants (Euranet 2010). Several studies have found that language barriers linked to medical encounters with allophone patients are associated with greater use of diagnostic investigations, lower uptake of preventive services (such as breast examinations), lower adherence to self-monitoring of blood glucose, and lower patient satisfaction (Bischoff et al. 2003). Other studies have shown that training health professionals in working with qualified interpreters when communicating with migrant patients improves quality of care and patient satisfaction (Harmsen et al. 2005; Leanza et al. 2010).

Given the language barrier encountered in interactions with migrants, some countries, such as Sweden and the Netherlands, organized "community interpreting" systems at the beginning of the 1980s, especially in the social and health sectors (Sauvetre 2002). In Sweden, the right to interpreters has been established by law. In southern and central Europe, interpreting services, where available, are often offered by "cultural mediators" (Loutan 1999). However, some European health systems still fail to systematically recognize that language barriers contribute to poor quality of care. This contrasts with the situation in the United States, where interpreter services are more widely available, at a moderate cost of an estimated US$ 279 per non-English speaking patient per year in 2004 (Jacobs 2004). In some European countries, interpreter services have started to become more widely available. In 2011, the Swiss Federal Office of Public Health, for example, set up a telephone interpreter service, accessible to health professionals in private or public practice, and subsidized by the federal government.

Apart from an absence of national health policies on interpreting services, there seem to be other reasons why health professionals do not use interpreters, as identified in several studies from outside Europe. In Australia, for example, although the Royal Australian College of General Practitioners recommends the use of professional interpreters (Bird 2010; Philips 2010), two-thirds of general practitioners (GPs) have reported in a survey in 2006 never to use the "Doctors Priority Line", which provides the world's largest free telephone interpreter service for doctors, available also to those in private practice (Atkin 2008). The availability of the service is not the reason for the low uptake, as the provider can connect to an interpreter by phone within 3 minutes and free onsite interpreters can be booked in advance. Yet, 82% of interviewed Australian GPs in the 2006 survey did not see the need to use any professional interpreters in their practice, and reported that they instead use patients' family members or friends as interpreters when needed (Atkin 2008).

Other studies find that health professionals can sometimes be reluctant to use trained interpreters because of negative feelings associated with the "trialogue" setting, such as loss of control and fear of being excluded from the conversation (Leanza et al. 2010). Two approaches could be considered to overcome these attitudes: legislating medical interpreting and training health professionals, so that using a third person during medical consultations becomes a new routine. Passing legislation is a long-term procedure which requires political will and convincing economic arguments to finance the running costs of interpreting services. Although it seems intuitively plausible that it would be cost-effective, this is difficult to demonstrate because of the multiplicity of factors involved in the process. However, recent studies (Jacobs 2004; Muela Ribera et al. 2008) illustrate how language barriers can increase medical costs, for example, from the higher risk of medical errors and disease complications. Other studies (Bischoff 2003; Flores 2005; Leanza 2010) have demonstrated that the use of professional interpreters, in addition to improving the satisfaction of both patients and health professionals, increases the use of preventive care, improves the reporting of symptoms and decreases misunderstandings.

The effectiveness of training health professionals in the use of interpreters has also been documented by several studies that have underlined the benefits of turning to trained interpreters rather than family members (Flores 2005; Thornton et al. 2009). The main way of ensuring that this training takes place is to include it in medical curricula and in continuing education (Karliner 2004). The training of interpreters is another critical issue. Transmission of medical information to patients and communicating the patient's reactions to health professionals are challenging; yet, many community interpreters have not received any formal training in these skills (Angelelli 2004; Ertl, 2010). In addition to training health workers and interpreters, the provision of culturally responsive health services depends on broader organizational development (see Chapter 15 on "Good practice in health service provision for migrants").

Another way to deal with language barriers is to promote diversity among health professionals through the enrolment of staff with diverse linguistic and cultural competences. Countries like Australia, Canada and the United States have developed this approach in the framework of affirmative action programmes, promoting the registration of students from migrant communities in medical and nursing schools (Lakhan 2003; Fox 2005).

Overcoming stereotypes

Although addressing language barriers is crucial, the concept of cultural competence in medicine goes much further. Patients and health professionals may share the same language but misunderstand each other because of cultural differences. Practising medicine, particularly family medicine, in a multicultural society benefits from the use of approaches and tools originating from many scientific disciplines, including cultural anthropology. The use of concepts such as cultural patterns and shared experiences, as developed by Kirmayer et al. (2003) and Mezzich et al. (2009) can enrich the clinical relationship between health professional and patient and help to understand patients' expectations, as well as culturally patterned interpretations of morbidity.

When post-war migration to western Europe resulted in the settlement of large migrant communities in some countries, such as Turks in Germany, north Africans in France, and Pakistanis in the United Kingdom, doctors were confronted with new medical complaints and created new diagnoses. The *"syndrome méditerranéen"* in France (also called *"syndrome transalpin"* in Switzerland (Durieux-Paillard and Loutan 2005)), describing the "excessive" complaints of migrant patients from southern Europe (e.g. women during delivery, or men complaining of back pain in emergency rooms), is a good example of this cultural classification of diseases. Nowadays, we know that the construction of these diagnoses was scientifically unfounded. However, they illustrate how western health professionals can become perplexed when interacting with patients of different origin, leading to attempts to "culturalize" diagnoses where biomedicine fails to provide obvious answers to differences in the expression of symptoms.

In today's multicultural Europe, with patients coming from very diverse backgrounds, it could appear difficult to practice "culturally competent medicine". Being aware of one's own culture, and specifically of one's medical culture, is a major first step (Fox 2005). In hospitals, services like "cultural consultations" (Kirmayer et al. 2003) may help clinicians to deal with cultural misunderstandings, but such services are not available everywhere. Other authors offer "tips" to become more culturally competent, such as Dosani (2001), whose recommendations are to:

• elicit patients' language, culture and ethnic group;
• be aware of cultural stereotypes;
• avoid using patients' families as interpreters;
• familiarize oneself with culturally specific expressions of distress;
• maintain confidentiality;
• avoid religious and social taboos;
• use same-sex chaperones;
• remember potential prescribing pitfalls;
• allow culturally specific rituals, for example, after death;
• not make assumptions.

Such "tips" can be useful, but some are ambiguous, such as the concept of "social taboos" which can be based on cultural stereotypes.

Even if the *"syndrome méditerranéen"* is a diagnosis of the past, cultural stereotypes are long-lasting and still influence medical practice (Geiger 1996, 2001). For example, Todd et al. (2000) found that the risk of receiving no analgesic while being in an emergency ward in Atlanta, United States for a long-bone fracture was 66% greater for black than for white patients. A study analysing the prescriptions of opioid analgesics in emergency wards in the United States several years later concluded that differences in opioid prescribing by race and ethnicity had not diminished (Pletcher et al. 2008). Astonishingly, these differences also existed for children attending emergency wards. The odds ratio for children under the age of 12 receiving an opioid during a pain-related visit to emergency wards (adjusted for a wide range of factors including pain and severity) was 0.66 (95% confidence interval (CI) 0.62–0.70) for black,

0.67 (95% CI 0.63–0.72) for Hispanic and 0.79 (95% CI 0.67–0.93) for Asian children (Pletcher et al. 2008). This illustrates how clinical decision-making may be affected by health professionals projecting cultural stereotypes onto individual patients. Although there are no comparable data from emergency wards of European hospitals, where ethnicity or migration status are not usually recorded (Simon 2007), these findings emphasize the importance of becoming aware of the influence of cultural stereotypes on medical practice, as a first step to overcoming them (see Chapter 15 on "Good practice in health service provision for migrants").

Religious considerations: a medical concern?

Religious beliefs of migrant patients are sometimes considered by health professionals in Europe to be a critical issue, particularly where health professionals may have to deal with patients who disagree with medical recommendations for religious reasons (Curlin et al. 2005). An example is the management of people with chronic disease who are fasting during Ramadan. For Muslim migrants living in non-Muslim countries, fasting during Ramadan can be a way of identifying with their cultural group, and it is therefore an important practice, even for people with chronic diseases such as diabetes. Recognizing this, there are a number of publications offering guidance for health professionals and patients (Sheikh et al. 2007). Fasting is the choice of the patient and religion is a private affair; it is unlikely that patients will tackle the subject with health professionals, especially if they do not share the same religion. However, one can argue that it is the responsibility of health professionals to anticipate the fasting period. This applies particularly when Ramadan falls in the summer months and the time period between dawn and sunset (when participating Muslims refrain from eating and drinking) can extend to more than 18 hours.

In many cultures, traditional medicine is linked to religious practices, and it is therefore not uncommon for migrants in western countries to turn to biomedicine and traditional medicine at the same time (Sloan et al. 1999). Most of the time, the interaction between these two practices has no negative consequences (McCord et al. 2004). However, taking the opportunity to discuss this issue with patients might help to improve the relationship between patients and health professionals while increasing the understanding of health workers of traditional practices (Curlin et al. 2005). For example, while a western point of view might at first suggest that the efficacy of traditional medicine relies on a placebo effect, a more careful analysis might show that good traditional healers can also act as family therapists or as mediators between different cultures.

The interaction of religion and gender is particularly sensitive in the western medical context. In several European countries, the clinical encounter between male doctors and Muslim women has become a highly politicized question in recent years. It is interesting to note how health professionals in Arab countries deal with this issue. In a study of a public hospital in the United Arab Emirates, McLean et al. (2010) interviewed 218 female patients. Only 16% of them answered that they would agree for a male medical student to be present at a gynaecological consultation (compared to 87% agreeing for female medical students to be present), and only 69% said they would agree to a male medical student participating in a consultation involving examination of the face. The authors concluded that it will be very difficult to overcome these religious and cultural beliefs (McLean et al. 2010).

In most European countries, patients in primary care services can choose whether they want to be seen by a male or female physician. However, in hospitals, especially emergency departments and maternity wards, the issue may be more difficult. Most of the time, an open-minded attitude of medical staff can resolve the situation if it is not possible to reschedule the consultation. Some of the gestures with which health professionals can demonstrate goodwill and cultural know-how include allowing a same-sex chaperone to participate in the consultation if the patient so wishes, explaining through an interpreter or cultural mediator what will be done during the examination, agreeing that the patient only partially undresses, and discussing the medical procedures with patients and their families before and after the consultation.

Female genital mutilation (FGM) is another issue that illustrates challenges in providing culturally responsive care. It is estimated that, globally, 100–140 million women have been victims of some form of FGM and that every year 3 million girls are at risk of being submitted to this practice (Kaplan-Marcusán et al. 2010). Primary health care professionals, paediatricians and gynaecologists in host countries can be instrumental in dealing with and preventing FGM and should be trained appropriately (Kaplan-Marcusán et al. 2009). This will allow them to tackle the subject with their patients during routine consultations, to identify the different types of FGM, to evaluate consequences for health, and to offer adequate support for women with FGM, as well as to their relatives. However, so far, FGM is not routinely included in the curricula of most medical schools in Europe.

Conclusions

In their interactions with migrant patients, health professionals need to be aware and prepared to address differences in language, religious beliefs, culture and origin (Gijon Sanchez et al. 2009). Many so-called "ethnic misunderstandings" are linked to poor linguistic comprehension. Where patients and health professionals do not share a common language, the use of trained interpreters is therefore an essential prerequisite for bridging cultural differences.

It is, however, important to avoid making assumptions based on "ethnic" considerations without discussing them with the patient. A common problem facing medical practitioners when dealing with migrant patients is how to achieve a balance that avoids going too far in cultural interpretations (for example, when confronted with an apparent aggressive attitude of a male patient towards a female doctor) and also avoids a reluctance to take up sensitive subjects (for example, alcohol use or sexuality) altogether, for fear of causing "cultural offence". Indeed, the application of cultural generalities based on language, religion, country of origin, and cultural or socioeconomic grouping of patients can easily degenerate into stereotyping (Fiore 2008). It is necessary to reiterate that stereotypical perceptions of patterns of illness among migrants and ethnic minorities are rarely scientifically based.

Whether they attend to migrants or other patients, self-awareness of health professionals of their preconceptions, as well as knowing the history and circumstances of patients is fundamental to providing adequate prevention, diagnosis and treatment. This could be summarized as adopting a humble and culturally open-minded approach. Concurrently, health service providers need to have an understanding of the determinants of migrant health and have the capacity to advise migrant patients on their entitlements to health services (Gijon Sanchez et al. 2009). Cultural competence needs to be part of the overall skills, knowledge and attitudes of health professionals and they need to be adequately trained in order to be able to provide appropriate care to diverse patients.

References

Amsterdam Declaration (2004) *The Migrant-friendly Hospitals Project, 2004* (http://www.mfh-eu.net/public/home.htm, accessed 20 May 2011).
Angelelli, C.A. (2004) *Medical Interpreting and the Cross-cultural Communication*. Cambridge: Cambridge University Press.
Appadurai, A. (1996) *Modernity at Large: Cultural Dimensions of Globalization. Public World, Volume 1*. Minneapolis: University of Minnesota Press.
Atkin, N. (2008) Getting the message across – professional interpreters in general practice. *Australian Family Physician*, 37(3): 174–6.
Betancourt, J.R., Green, A.R., Carillo, J.E. and Ananeh-Firempong, O., 2nd. (2003) Defining cultural competence: a practical framework for addressing racial/ethnic disparities in health and health care. *Public Health Reports*, 118(4): 293–302.
Bird, S. (2010) Failure to use an interpreter. *Australian Family Physician*, 39(4): 241–2.
Bischoff, A., Perneger, T.V., Bovier, P.A., Loutan, L. and Stalder, H. (2003). Improving communication between physicians and patients who speak a foreign language. *British Journal of General Practice*, 53(4920): 541–6.
Curlin, F.A., Roach, C.J., Gowara-Baht, R., et al. (2005) When patients choose faith over medicine: physician perspectives on religiously related conflict in the medical encounter. *Archives of Internal Medicine*, 165(1): 88–91.
Dosani, S. (2001) How to practise medicine in a multicultural society. *Student BMJ*, 9: 357–98.
Durieux-Paillard, S. and Loutan, L. (2005) Diversité culturelle et stéréotypes, la pratique médicale est aussi concernée. *Revue Medicale de la Suisse Romande*, 1(34): 2208–13.
Ertl, A. and Pöllabauer, S. (2010) Training (medical) interpreters – the key to good practice. MedInt: a joint European training perspective. *Journal of Specialised Translation*, 14: 165–93.
Euranet (2010) *Préserver la diversité linguistique de l'union européenne* (http://www.euranet.eu/fre/Dossiers/Dialogue-interculturel/Preserver-la-diversite-linguistique-de-l-Union-europeenne, accessed 1 June 2011).
Fiore, R.N. (2008) Ethics, culture and clinical practice. *Northeast Florida Medicine Journal Supplement,* January: 33–6.
Flores, G. (2005) The impact of medical interpreter services on the quality of health care: a systematic review. *Medical Care Research and Review*, 62(3): 255–99.
Fox, R.C. (2005) Cultural competence and the culture of medicine. *New England Journal of Medicine*, 353(13): 1316–19.

Geiger, H.J. (1996) Race and health care – an American dilemma? *New England Journal of Medicine*, 335(11): 815–16.

Geiger, H.J. (2001) Racial stereotyping and medicine: the need for cultural competence. *Canadian Medical Association Journal*, 164(12): 1699–700.

Gijon Sanchez, M.T., Pinzon Pulido, S., Kolehmainen Aitken, R.L., et al. (2009) *Developing a Public Health Workforce to Address Migrant Health Needs in Europe*. Background Paper. Brussels: International Organization for Migration.

Harmsen, H., Bernsen, R., Meeuwesen, L., et al. (2005) The effect of educational intervention on intercultural communication: results of a randomised controlled trial. *British Journal of General Practice*, 55(514): 343–50.

IOM (2010) *World Migration Report 2010. The future of migration: Building capacities for change*. Geneva: International Organization for Migration.

Jacobs, E.A., Shepard, D.S., Suaya, J.A. and Stone, E.L. (2004) Overcoming language barriers in health care: costs and benefits of interpreter services. *Am J Public Health*, 94(5): 866–9.

Kaplan-Marcusán, A., Torán-Monserrat, P., Moreno-Navarro, J., Castany Fàbregas, M.J. and Muñoz-Ortiz, L. (2009) Perception of primary health professionals about female genital mutilation: from healthcare to intercultural competence. *BMC Health Services Research*, 9: 11.

Kaplan-Marcusán, A., del Rio, N.F., Moreno-Navarro, N., et al. (2010) Female genital mutilation: perceptions of healthcare professionals and the perspective of the migrant families. *BMC Public Health*, 10: 193.

Karliner, L.S., Pérez-Stable, E.J. and Gildengorin, G. 2004. The language divide. The importance of training in the use of interpreters for outpatient practice. *Journal of General Internal Medicine*, 19(2): 175–83.

Kirmayer, L.J., Groleau, D., Guzder, J., et al. (2003) Cultural consultation: a model of mental health service for multicultural societies. *Canadian Journal of Psychiatry*, 48(3): 145–53.

Kleinman, A., Eisenberg, L. and Good, B. (1978) Culture, illness, and care: clinical lessons from anthropologic and cross-cultural research. *Annals of Internal Medicine*, 88(2): 251–8.

Kleinman, A. (1983) The cultural meaning and social issues of illness. *Journal of Family Practice*, 16(3): 539–45.

Lakhan, S.E. (2003) Diversification of U.S. medical schools via affirmative action implementation. *BMC Medical Education* 2003, 3: 6 (doi:10.1186/1472-6920-3-6).

Leanza, Y., Boivin, I. and Rosenberg, E. (2010) Interruptions and resistance: a comparison of medical consultations with family and trained interpreters. *Social Science & Medicine*, 70(12): 1888–95.

Lee, R. (2010) Culture and diversity. *Australian Family Physician*, 39(4): 181.

Loutan, L. (1999) The importance of interpreters to insure quality of care for migrants. *Sozial und Präventivmedizin*, 44(6): 245–7.

Marmot, M. and Syme, S.L. (1976) Acculturation and coronary heart disease in Japanese-Americans. *American Journal of Epidemiology*, 104(3): 225–47.

Marmot, M. (2005) Social determinants of health inequalities. *Lancet*, 365(9464): 1099–104.

McCord, G., Gilchrist, V.J., Grossman, S.D., et al. (2004) Discussing spirituality with patients: a rational and ethical approach. *Annals of Family Medicine*, 2(4): 356–61.

McLean, M., Al Ahbabi, S., Al Ameri, M., Al Mansoori, M., Al Yahyaei, F. and Bernsen, R. (2010) Muslim women and medical students in the clinical encounter. *Medical Education*, 44: 306–15.

Mezzich, J.E., Caracci, G., Fabrega, H. Jr, and Kirmayer, L.J. (2009) Cultural formulation guidelines. *Transcultural Psychiatry*, 46(3): 383–405.

Muela Ribera, J., Hausmann-Muela, S., Peeters Grietens, K. and Toomer, E. (2008) *Is the use of interpreters in medical consultation justified? A critical review of literature*. Partners for Applied Social Sciences (PASS) International (http://pass-international.org/site/index.php?option=com_content&task=view&id=45&Itemid=59, accessed 1 June 2011).

Partida, Y. (2007) Addressing language barriers: building response capacity for a changing nation. *Journal of General Internal Medicine*, 22(Suppl. 2): 347–9.

Peiro, M.-J. and Benedict, R. (2009) *Migration Health: Better Health for All in Europe*. Brussels: International Organization for Migration.

Philips, C. (2010) Using interpreters – a guide for GPs. *Australian Family Physician*, 39(4): 188–95.

Pletcher, M.J., Kertesz, S.G., Kohn, M.A. and Gonzales, R. (2008) Trends in opioid prescribing by race/ethnicity for patients seeking care in US emergency departments. *JAMA*, 299(1): 70–8.

Sauvetre, M. (2002) L'interprète en milieu social en Europe. *Ecarts d'identité*, 99: 48–53 (http://www.revues-plurielles.org/_uploads/pdf/6_99_9.pdf, accessed 1 June 2011).

Sheikh, A. and Wallia, S. (2007) Ramadan fasting and diabetes *BMJ*, 335(7620): 613–14.

Simon, P. (2007) *'Ethnic' Statistics and Data Protection in the Council of Europe Countries*. Study Report of the European Commission against Racism and Intolerance. Strasbourg: Council of Europe.

Sloan, R.P., Bagiella, E. and Powell, T. (1999) Religion, spirituality and medicine. *Lancet*, 353(9153): 664–7.

Terraza-Núñez, R., Vázquez, M.L., Vargas, I. and Lizana, T. (2010) Health professional perceptions regarding healthcare provision to immigrants in Catalonia. *International Journal of Public Health*, 9 Dec 2010 [Epub ahead of print].

Thornton, J.D., Pham, K., Engelberg, R.A., Jackson, J.C. and Curtis, J.R. (2009) Families with limited English proficiency receive less information and support in interpreted intensive care unit family conferences. *Critical Care Medicine*, 37(1): 89–95.

Todd, K.H., Deaton, C., d'Amado, A.P. and Goe, L. (2000) Ethnicity and analgesic practices. *Annals of Emergency Medicine*, 35(1): 11–16.

UNHCHR, Office of the United Nations High Commissioner for Human Rights (1976) *International Covenant on Economic, Social and Cultural Rights* (http://www2.ohchr.org/english/law/cescr.htm, accessed 1 June 2011).

WHO (2010) *Social Determinants of Health: Key Concepts* (http://www.who.int/social_determinants/thecommission/finalreport/key_concepts/en/, accessed 1 June 2011).

WHO Regional Office for Europe (2010) *How Health Systems can Address Health Inequities Linked to Migration and Ethnicity*. Copenhagen: WHO Regional Office for Europe.

Williams, D.R., Neighbors, H.W. and Jackson, J.S. (2003) Racial/ethnic discrimination and health: findings from communities studies. *American Journal of Public Health*, 93(2): 200–8.

World Health Assembly (2008) *Health of Migrants, Resolution* 61.17. Geneva: World Health Organization.

chapter fourteen

Good practice in emergency care: views from practitioners

Stefan Priebe, Marija Bogic, Róza Ádány,
Neele V. Bjerre, Marie Dauvrin,
Walter Devillé, Sónia Dias,
Andrea Gaddini, Tim Greacen,
Ulrike Kluge, Elisabeth Ioannidis,
Natasja K. Jensen, Rosa Puigpinós i Riera,
Joaquim J.F. Soares,
Mindaugas Stankunas,
Christa Straßmayr, Kristian Wahlbeck,
Marta Welbel and Rosemarie McCabe
for the EUGATE study group

Introduction

Health services across Europe are faced with the increasing challenge of delivering accessible, appropriate and effective care for migrants. Some service providers already have a long tradition of delivering health care to migrants, particularly in large cities such as London and Paris. Elsewhere, as in central and eastern Europe, immigration on a substantial scale is a much more recent phenomenon and health services have only recently begun to see significant numbers of migrants as patients. Available evidence on how services across Europe treat migrants, what problems health workers regard as most important and what solutions have been found has mainly been anecdotal, with no systematic research basis.

Accident and emergency (A&E) departments are the first point of contact with organized health care for many migrants in Europe. They are usually attached to general hospitals and, while there are variations in the way they are organized and operate in different countries, they have many common features: they provide acute care in emergency situations, dealing with problems affecting all body systems. Often, they are the entry point for further treatment, not only in other departments of the hospital they are attached to, but also in other in- and outpatient services in the local health system.

Care provided in these settings often involves a rapid response. Clinicians need to obtain information about the patient's condition (frequently including additional information from family members or friends of the patient), establish a positive rapport with the patient, and make a decision about the most appropriate subsequent management, all within a short period of time. Care in this setting typically involves multidisciplinary team work with different health professionals (and sometimes also administrative staff) communicating with the patient, but none of them necessarily aiming to establish a longer-term relationship, as is the case in many other health care settings. Many patients only stay in the health facility for a few hours. The workload in these facilities typically fluctuates. At peak times there can be great pressure on staff to deliver care to a large number of patients with very different needs, and the atmosphere may be perceived as stressful.

A&E departments are the only services in the health system that are accessible to all types of migrants in most EU member states, including undocumented migrants who – depending on the precise legislation in the given host country – may have limited or no entitlement to receive medical treatment beyond emergency care. Exceptions are Sweden, where undocumented migrants do not have access to any health care free of charge, and Germany, where the obligation to denounce undocumented migrants used to override the entitlement to free-of-charge emergency care (HUMA network 2009), although this obligation was abolished in 2009.

Given this situation, it might be expected that migrants would be over-represented in such facilities. Yet the evidence is contradictory, with higher utilization levels compared to non-migrants in some places, and equal or lower levels in others (Nørredam et al. 2004; Hargreaves et al. 2006; Nørredam et al. 2009). Regardless of the actual situation, it is reasonable to assume that migrants may pose additional challenges for health workers, making it more difficult to provide high-quality care.

So, what constitutes good practice in providing acute health care to migrants in A&E departments? What do those who work in A&E departments across Europe see as their greatest problems, what do they regard as the strengths of their service and in what respects do they think the care for migrants using their services might be improved? Drawing on findings of the EUGATE ("Best Practice in Health Services for Immigrants in Europe") study, funded by the European Commission, this chapter describes the views of practitioners who were interviewed in A&E departments in 16 European countries. While problems of access to care and of care delivery can overlap, the focus of the study was on delivery rather than access.

Methods

In each participating country we identified three A&E departments operating in areas with relatively high levels of migrants. The areas selected, and the countries they are in, are shown in Table 14.1. We conducted face-to-face interviews with one practitioner in each service, resulting in a total of 48 in-depth interviews.

The interview schedule was developed in English and piloted in each country. The final version was translated into the languages of the participating countries. The data presented here are based on two components of the interview: a) open questions on general experiences; and b) mostly open

Table 14.1 Selected A&E departments in each country

Country	Cities	Selected areas
Austria	Vienna	2nd district – Leopoldstadt 16th district – Ottakring 20th district – Brigittenau
Belgium	Brussels	Brussels City Saint Josse Schaerbeek
Denmark	Copenhagen	Bispebjerg Hospital Glostrup Hospital Hvidovre Hospital
Finland	Oravais Pietarsaari Vaasa	Oravais Pietarsaari Vaasa
France	Paris	Bichat Lariboisiere La Roseraie
Germany	Berlin	Kreuzberg Tiergarten Wedding
Greece	Athens	Thrakomakedones Voula
Hungary	Budapest	VI district – Terézváros VII district –Erzsébetváros XX district – Pesterzsébet
Italy	Rome	I district VIII district XX district
Lithuania	Kaunas	Downtown of Kaunas Silainiai district Zaliakalnis
Netherlands	Amsterdam The Hague Utrecht	Amsterdam The Hague Utrecht

Continued overleaf

Table 14.1 *Continued*

Country	Cities	Selected areas
Poland	Warsaw	Mokotov Praga Południe Srodmiescie
Portugal	Lisbon	Amadora Lisboa Loures
Spain	Barcelona	Ciutat Vella Eixample Nou Barris
Sweden	Stockholm	Central Stockholm Southeast Stockholm Southwest Stockholm
United Kingdom	London	Hackney Newham Tower Hamlets

questions on how practitioners would deal with patients as represented in three case vignettes. The questions and vignettes are presented in Table 14.2. For the general questions, a consistent understanding of the term migrant was required. We defined migrants as persons who were born outside the country of current residence, arrived in the host country within the last five years and, in recognition of the very specific issues relating to children and elderly people, those between 18 and 65 years of age. In line with EU directives, five groups of migrants were considered: regular migrants (e.g. labour migrants), irregular (illegal, undocumented) migrants, asylum-seekers, refugees and victims of trafficking. In the vignettes, the characteristics of migrants were specified in more detail. The origin of the migrant described in the vignette was chosen as somewhere contributing a high proportion of all migrants in the country of the interviewee, but otherwise the vignettes were identical. This adaptation was made to ensure that the scenario would be seen as realistic by the interviewee.

Interviews were recorded, transcribed verbatim and subjected to content analysis (Hsieh and Shannon 2005). In a stepwise analysis, lists of emerging codes were generated based on a line-by-line analysis of the initial interviews (Miles and Huberman 1994). Codes and the associated text were then translated into English. These data were used to develop a codebook, which was then reviewed and agreed among all collaborators. The agreed codebook was then used to code the interviews. In the second step of data analysis, the translated codes were sorted into categories based on how different codes were related and linked. The emergent categories were then used to form meaningful themes (Patton 2002). Final verification by the collaborating institutions ensured that the emergent categories and themes accurately presented the data. In a final step, simple descriptive counts of themes, categories and codes were used to provide a summary of the data set (Morgan 1993). Based on all 48 interviews with practitioners in A&E departments (three in each country) common

Table 14.2 Questions and case vignettes used in the interviews

General experiences	1. In your experience, what are the specific problems for you in the care of an immigrant patient in your service that you would not have in the care of a patient with a similar condition from the indigenous population?
	2. In your experience, what are the specific problems faced by an immigrant patient coming into your service that are different from those faced by a patient with a similar condition coming from the indigenous population (e.g. communication)?
	3. In your experience, what are the strengths of your service in the care of immigrants?
	4. What would improve the care for immigrants in your service?
	5. EUGATE aims to create a repertoire of best practice models for immigrant care in Europe. Please indicate three services in your field of work (other than your service) that you would recommend as models of best practice in care provision for immigrants in your city. For each of these services, please give one or two reasons why you recommend them.
Case vignettes	<u>Illegal immigrant</u> The patient arrived in the host country as an illegal immigrant about 1 year ago. He is 25 years of age and of *[insert a country]* origin. He does not speak any language that the A&E staff understand and presents with an intense lower abdominal pain.
	<u>Refugee</u> The female patient is 19 years of age and arrived from *[insert a country]* 10 months ago. She has refugee status and speaks only *[insert language of origin]* and a few words of English. She is in her fifth month of pregnancy and has a serious complication (pre-eclampsia). She is reluctant to be examined by a male doctor.
	<u>Labour immigrant</u> The male patient is 35 years of age and arrived from *[insert a country]* 2 years ago. He has a regular residence permit. He was brought to A&E by the police because of his aggressive behaviour following heavy drinking. He suffered external head injuries in a fight. He is fully conscious and accessible for examination.
Case vignette questions	Questions asked for all three case vignettes:
	1. What are the differences, if any, in the treatment for this patient compared to a patient with a similar condition from the indigenous population?
	2. What are the specific problems this patient would encounter that are different from those of a patient with a similar condition from the indigenous population, and how would they be overcome?
	3. What are the specific further pathways and treatment options, if any, for this patient that are different from those of a patient with a similar condition from the indigenous population?
	Vignette-specific questions
	1. Would you inform the police and/or other authorities? (illegal immigrant)
	2. Would it be arranged for a female doctor to examine her? (refugee)

themes were then described. In the analysis, the responses of the interviewees to all questions, including the case vignettes, were considered and eight main themes identified. The majority of these were similar across all countries, and the findings presented here focus on consistent aspects rather than differences. The themes are linked, but each focuses on a distinct aspect of care.

Results

Language

Language was raised as a crucial issue in all interviews, with most practitioners identifying communication problems as a result of language barriers as the main problem in delivering appropriate care to migrants, who were often unable to provide relevant information. Clinicians struggled to establish a diagnosis and felt compelled to arrange additional examinations and diagnostic tests, often absorbing more staff time and resources. Communication problems also led to misunderstandings between staff and patients. As a consequence, patients sometimes felt badly treated, resulting in a strained relationship between staff and patient. Sometimes this led to verbal aggression or even physical violence. The availability of good interpreters was identified as an obvious solution. Most practitioners used professional interpreting services, but some also reported using bilingual staff or the patient's family and friends for interpreting.

While the language barrier was regarded by practitioners as the most important issue they faced, many interviewees felt that health services dealt with this very well. In fact, 40% of interviewees stated that the provision of services in different languages was one of the main strengths in their delivery of health care to migrants, with many regarding their interpreting services as easily accessible and of good quality. At the same time, involving a third party in the consultation was seen as a potential barrier to good communication with the patient and the establishment of a positive relationship.

Several interviewees did, however, express concerns regarding the use of professional interpreters. Professional interpreting services do not always provide excellent quality, but quality tends to be even poorer when family members or friends step in to interpret. Thus, poor interpretation was seen as a significant hindrance to appropriate communication. Some also described difficulties in mobilizing interpreting services quickly. In A&E departments, immediate and easy access is essential, as the nature of the medical problem does not allow for complicated or time-consuming booking procedures. An additional problem is that professional interpreters may come from the same migrant community as the patient, which often comprises a relatively small group in which many of the migrants know each other. In such cases, patients can be reluctant to reveal confidential information. Finally, consultations and examinations take more time when conducted with an interpreter, an issue that relates to the general need for more time and resources when dealing with migrant patients (see section below on time and organizational resources).

"Cultural" factors

All interviewees identified "cultural" factors as an important issue. These comprise both general ones, not specifically related to the patient's health problem, as well as health-related ones that directly affect the management of the patient's condition and its treatment. Since these are closely linked, they are combined into a single theme.

Interviewees accepted the importance of understanding the patient's cultural and religious norms and values, such as dietary needs, dress code and attitude to nudity. In some cultures, family links are stronger than the norm in most European countries, and interviewees reported how this can be an advantage if recognized and addressed early and actively in the patient's attendance.

Differences in understanding gender roles (e.g. male patients may have less confidence in female doctors because of the role of females in their own culture) may act as a barrier to good care. This was raised particularly in response to a vignette describing a refugee woman (see Table 14.2). Most practitioners stated that they would arrange for a female clinician to examine the patient if one was available at the time. However, other interviewees stated that in an emergency situation the priority was delivering effective care rather than accommodating the patient's cultural preferences.

Among issues specifically related to the health problem, the majority of interviewees identified cultural differences in the understanding of illness or its treatment. Different medical paradigms can act as barriers in reaching appropriate diagnoses and may affect treatment choice and adherence. Treatment may not be adhered to if it clashes with the patient's cultural norms and values, and some migrants prefer traditional healers to the western-style medicine provided in A&E departments.

Patients may also have culturally determined understandings of their own health and the problem they are presenting with that differ from those in western medicine. Some interviewees reported that certain migrants, especially those with the least education, often lacked the basic biological knowledge needed to have an appropriate understanding of their disease process.

Despite all these difficulties, about half of the interviewees reported that their department provided culturally responsive services and saw this as being a particular strength of the service they offered. Several interviewees emphasized that their service had specific expertise in delivering care to migrants, although this is likely to be related to the fact that we interviewed practitioners in A&E departments operating in areas with high levels of immigration. Some services were said to be particularly responsive to patients' cultural needs and customs, while for others the promotion of cultural awareness through staff training and education was reported as a strength.

The existence of multicultural staff was also perceived as a strength. In addition to facilitating consultation with a clinician from the same culture, it supports the wider acquisition of an understanding of different cultures. In most services, the adaptation of care to the cultural needs of their patients was perceived as a strength. At the same time, interviewees underlined the importance of good medical care independent of cultural issues. They stressed that patients should be seen by specialists with expertise in the presenting health problem rather than by health professionals with a specific focus on the health of migrants.

About a third of interviewees felt that further improvements in the provision of culturally sensitive care were needed in their service. Suggestions for improvements included the promotion of cultural awareness through staff training or education (including training in culturally specific and tropical diseases), more multicultural staff, and improved responsiveness or adaptation of care to patients' cultural or religious norms and values (e.g. by having staff of both genders available all the time).

Treatment expectations and understanding of the health system

Many migrants come from countries with very different health systems and may therefore not understand how the health system in their host country operates. Lack of awareness of the role and availability of services can lead to no or inappropriate service use. About two-thirds of interviewees felt that migrants tend to overuse emergency services.

There may be substantial differences in the expectations of migrant patients and staff as a result of cultural factors or insufficient understanding of the health system in the host country. This was particularly seen to be a problem among older patients, while younger migrants were perceived as adapting faster and having treatment expectations more in line with those of the non-migrant population. As a typical example of differing treatment expectations, it was reported that some migrants relied heavily on medication, even if it was viewed as inappropriate by clinicians. Differing treatment expectations can complicate the communication between patients and clinicians, lead to misunderstandings about further procedures and result in patients being dissatisfied with the care provided.

The provision of educational programmes for migrants, and of information on health and the health system of the host country in the patient's language and a culturally appropriate style, was reported as a strength of the service they provided by approximately 20% of interviewees. A further third of interviewees felt that such programmes and material would be useful to improve care in their services.

Access to health services and service use

Another problem mentioned in almost all interviews was access to health services and their utilization by migrants. Due to an often limited understanding of the health system (see previous section), migrants were reported as using different pathways to access services. This resulted in inappropriate service use, including more frequent use of emergency services, but also in delaying health care utilization until the problem was very severe and emergency care was required, which earlier intervention would have avoided. A tendency by some migrants (especially irregular ones) to seek care with private practices first was noted, attributed to a wish to avoid any questions about their legal or residential status, or to obtain traditional medicine. Once they have accessed care, some migrants may have restricted (or no) free treatment options available, due to their legal or insurance status. This was viewed as a key problem for undocumented migrants but varied for other types of migrants, depending on their legal and insurance status.

Despite these restrictions, some interviewees noted that they provide treatment anyway and, if necessary, look for funding elsewhere, e.g. by using special hospital funds, approaching non-governmental organizations (NGOs) or social services. Where this is not possible, some clinicians try to use their own resources, such as samples of free medicine, prescribing medication in their own name and accessing specialists through their personal contacts. Sometimes, undocumented migrants use other people's identification or health insurance document to access emergency services. The provision of equal treatment to all patients and the additional efforts of clinicians to achieve this were seen as the main strengths in some services and suggested as areas for improvement in others.

Staff–patient relationships

Poor staff–patient relationships can be especially problematic with migrant patients. Several interviewees reported negative attitudes and hostile behaviour by staff towards migrants, potentially impairing empathy and invoking discrimination. Once perceived as "difficult", migrant patients can be referred from one service to another. Some services also reported negative attitudes and hostile behaviour of migrant patients towards staff, sometimes associated with aggression and a lack of respect. Approximately 20% of interviewees thought that the presence of non-discriminatory, helpful and friendly staff was one of the strengths of their service in providing health care for migrants.

Time and organizational resources

On a practical level, care for migrant patients was thought to require more time and resources. Compared to non-migrant patients with the same medical problem, the consultations may take longer due to the language barrier and more administrative steps may be required when admitting the patient. This was reported as a substantial problem in emergency services, which interviewees felt were already understaffed and overstretched. The strain on resources was frequently reported in response to the vignette describing an undocumented migrant (see Table 14.2). Only 15% of health professionals reported that their service had good human and technical resources, including an administration that could help with bureaucratic problems and staff that would generally devote more time and effort when caring for migrants. About a further 20% felt that care for migrants in their services would improve if there were dedicated programmes for especially frequent diseases among migrant groups, more staff specialized in mental health care, more time for consultations, and generally more staff and resources.

Migration stressors and post-migration status

Migrant patients may have experienced stressors linked to the process of migration and to their status following migration (see Chapter 11 on "Mental health of refugees and asylum-seekers"). A majority of interviewees mentioned such factors as being relevant to the provision of health care in emergency situations. They included the uncertainties and difficulties involved in migration, low socioeconomic status in the host country, problems with acquiring residency status and poor mental health as a result of the various stressors faced by migrants. Migrant patients were reported as being more likely than non-migrant patients to present with socioeconomic and legal problems, and to be involved in illicit drug use, sex work or crime. They were also reported to have generally poorer health than non-migrants, which interviewees attributed to unhealthy lifestyles or poor personal hygiene and, for some groups, a greater risk of certain diseases, especially tropical infections, tuberculosis and HIV.

When asked whether they would report an undocumented migrant to the police, most stated that the duty of health professionals was not to check the legal status of the patients but to treat them and 90% stated that they would not inform the police or would do so only under certain circumstances (if patients were a danger to themselves or others, if they were suspected to be involved in a crime, or if this was requested by the authorities). However, the remaining 10% reported that they would inform the police.

Because of the high prevalence and severity of social problems faced by migrant patients, some interviewees reported a close collaboration with social services to be an important component of good health care. However, only two interviewees described such a collaboration as a current strength of their service. Others felt a need for improvement in this type of collaboration, particularly for undocumented migrants.

Difficulties in accessing records on medical history

Interviewees cited difficulty in obtaining medical records for patients. The records of many migrants were assumed to be held in their country of origin and were generally not accessible in their new host country. Even where records were available (for example, when the patient or a family member brought them along), staff in the A&E department sometimes struggled to use them if they were written in a foreign language.

Discussion

An important limitation of the findings presented here is that they are based on the perceptions of a comparatively small number (48) of health workers from a number of different countries and that their statements cannot be taken at face value. However, we believe that they provide insights into challenges and opportunites for the provision of A&E services to migrants in Europe.

While the adaptation of services to patients' cultural preferences was perceived by most health professionals to be an example of best practice, others stressed the importance of not making stereotypical assumptions about the needs of migrant patients. The prevailing view was that every patient should be entitled to the best medical care available and that culturally sensitive care was required to achieve this in A&E departments, but there was no support for separate and specific care for migrants. There was, however, some concern that certain aspects of culturally specific care could impede the successful integration of migrants and worsen their social isolation.

In many countries of the EU, migrants whose status is irregular or who have no insurance have only limited entitlements to medical care. Our findings suggest that practitioners are aware of the ethical problems this may pose, i.e. that their ethical responsibility for the welfare of the patient can clash with official policies or even legislation. Most practitioners stated that they would not report irregular migrants to the police. Instead, they sought and often found ways to provide care for all patients, frequently without proper funding. Professional values and ethical principles appeared to overrule official policies, at least to some extent, and some may argue that this is a virtue of the health professionals interviewed.

Although the reported themes reflect various problems in delivering good care to migrants as perceived by providers, most interviewees stated that the actual care provided for the labour migrant described in one of the case vignettes (Table 14.2) and the further pathways for that patient would not differ from the care provided to a non-migrant patient with the same medical problem. This seems to be an encouraging sign that these emergency services have integrated care for migrants into their practice, developing a "normality" in dealing with, and not necessarily providing poorer quality care for, this population group.

The identified themes are consistent with other reports in the literature. Several studies have shown that health workers experience language difficulties in dealing with migrant populations and that there is a need for professional interpreters (Flores et al. 2002; Flores 2005; Hultsjo and Hjelm 2005), as a lack of skilled interpreters can result in poor communication and misunderstandings, medical errors, poorer treatment adherence and treatment satisfaction, increased use of emergency services and less efficient resource utilization (Manson 1988; Waxman and Levitt 2000; Flores et al. 2002; Flores 2005; Bagchi et al. 2010).

Differences in cultural norms and in explanatory models of illness and treatment between the patient and the health worker have been found to complicate cross-cultural consultations in emergency care (Flores et al. 2002; Scheppers et al. 2006). Further reports emphasized the importance of individual care, i.e. care that goes beyond cultural issues. Wachtler et al. (2006) reported that primary care health workers view consultations as a meeting between individuals, where cultural differences are only one of the factors affecting health worker–patient communication.

Migrants may also have a different understanding and expectations of health care based on their experience of health care in their country of origin (Ivanov and Buck 2002; O'Donnell et al. 2008), which has been found to lead to inappropriate use of health services (Scheppers et al. 2006; Nørredam et al. 2007) and treatment dissatisfaction (Reiff et al. 1999).

Obstacles in accessing health care by migrants have been frequently reported in the literature (Scheppers et al. 2006; Nørredam et al. 2007), in particular for undocumented migrants (PICUM 2007). Likewise, it has been reported that health workers are often torn between conflicting legal requirements and professional ethics regarding the delivery of care to undocumented migrants (PICUM 2007).

In terms of staff–patient relationships, the quality of relationships has been found to be potentially poorer when there are differences in "race", ethnicity and language between health workers and patients. In a systematic review, Ferguson and Candib (2002) found consistent evidence that "race", ethnicity and language have a substantial influence on the quality of the health worker–patient relationship. Patients from ethnic minorities, especially those who did not speak the same language as the physician, were less likely to engender an empathic response from physicians, establish rapport, receive sufficient information, or be encouraged to participate in medical decision-making.

Studies confirm that the service workload is higher with large numbers of migrant patients due to communication difficulties, different demands and a higher frequency of service use (Hargreaves et al. 2006).

Conclusions

Our study obtained and analysed the experiences and views of selected practitioners in emergency services. It did not assess what actually happens in these services, nor were other important stakeholders, most notably the migrant patients concerned, interviewed. The barriers patients had to overcome in order to reach emergency services and how access can be improved were also not addressed in this study.

The results suggest several implications for policies to improve the quality of health care for migrants who utilize emergency services. The most important components of good practice in emergency services to emerge from our study are good quality and easily accessible professional interpreting services, and treatment delivered by staff sensitive to diversity that accommodates patient preference where possible. This may be helped by the presence of staff from different ethnic origins, the promotion of cultural awareness through education and training, education programmes and translated materials for migrants on health issues, and information for migrants on the health system of the host country. Close collaboration between health and social care services was perceived as facilitating appropriate care for patients with substantial social problems. Finally, information and guidelines for practitioners about what care undocumented migrants are entitled to receive was considered helpful in efforts to arrange care for these patients. None of these components alone can guarantee good quality emergency services, and policies may have to address comprehensively several or all of them in order to achieve the best possible practice for migrants. In many emergency services, some or all of the identified components are already part of daily practice, but there seems to be substantial scope for further improvements.

References

Bagchi, A.D., Dale, S., Verbitsky-Savitz, N., et al. (2010) Examining effectiveness of medical interpreters in emergency departments for Spanish-speaking patients with limited English proficiency: results of a randomized controlled trial. *Annals of Emergency Medicine*, Aug 3 [Epub ahead of print].

Ferguson, W.J. and Candib, L.M. (2002) Culture, language and the doctor–patient relationship. *Family Medicine*, 34(5): 353–61.

Flores, G. (2005) The impact of medical interpreter services on the quality of health care: a systematic review. *Medical Care Research and Review*, 62(3): 255–99.

Flores, G., Rabke, J., Pine, W. and Sabarwhal, A. (2002) The importance of cultural and linguistic issues in the emergency care of children. *Pediatric Emergency Care*, 18(4): 271–84.

Hargreaves, S., Friedland, J.S., Gothard, P., et al. (2006) Impact on and use of health services by international migrants: questionnaire survey of inner city London A&E attenders. *BMC Health Services Research*, 6: 153.

Hsieh, H.F. and Shannon, S.E. (2005) Three approaches to qualitative content analysis. *Qualitative Health Research*, 15(9): 1277–88.

Hultsjo, S. and Hjelm, K. (2005) Immigrants in emergency care: Swedish health care staff's experiences. *International Nursing Review*, 52(4): 276–85.

HUMA network (2009) *Law and Practice: Access to health care for undocumented migrants and asylum seekers in ten EU countries.* Health for Undocumented Migrants and Asylum seekers (HUMA) network (http://www.huma-network.org/Publications-Resources/Our-publications/Law-and-practice.-Access-to-health-care-for-undocumented-migrants-and-asylum-seekers-in-10-EU-countries, accessed 1 June 2011).

Ivanov, L.L. and Buck, K. (2002) Health care utilization patterns of Russian-speaking immigrant women across age groups. *Journal of Immigrant Health*, 4(1): 17–27.

Manson, A. (1988) Language concordance as a determinant of patient compliance and emergency room use in patients with asthma. *Medical Care*, 26(12): 1119–28.

Miles, M.B. and Huberman, A.M. (1994) *Qualitative Data Analysis* (2nd edn). Thousand Oaks, CA: Sage.

Morgan, D.L. (1993) *Successful Focus Groups: Advancing the State of the Art.* Newbury Park, CA: Sage.

Nørredam, M., Nielsen, S.S. and Krasnik, A. (2009) Migrants' utilization of somatic healthcare services in Europe – a systematic review. *European Journal of Public Health*. 29 Dec 2009 [Epub ahead of print].

Nørredam, M., Mygind, A., Nielsen, A.S., Bagger, J. and Krasnik, A. (2007) Motivation and relevance of emergency room visits among immigrants and patients of Danish origin. *European Journal of Public Health*, 17(5): 497–502.

Nørredam, M., Krasnik, A., Moller Sorensen, T., Keiding, N., Joost Michaelsen, J. and Sonne Nielsen, A. (2004) Emergency room utilization in Copenhagen: a comparison of immigrant groups and Danish-born residents. *Scandinavian Journal of Public Health*. 32(1): 53–9.

O'Donnell, C.A., Higgins, M., Chauhan, R. and Mullen, K. (2008) Asylum seekers' expectations of and trust in general practice: a qualitative study. *British Journal of General Practice*, 58(557): e1–11.

Patton, M.Q. (2002) *Qualitative Research and Evaluation Methods* (3rd edn). Thousand Oaks, CA: Sage.

PICUM (2007) *Access to Health Care for Undocumented Migrants in Europe.* Brussels: Platform for International Cooperation on Undomented Migrants (http://picum.org/picum.org/uploads/file_/Access_to_Health_Care_for_Undocumented_Migrants.pdf, accessed 6 June 2011).

Reiff, M., Zakut, H. and Weingarten, M.A. (1999) Illness and treatment perceptions of Ethiopian immigrants and their doctors in Israel. *American Journal of Public Health,* 89(12): 1814–18.

Scheppers, E., van Dongen, E., Dekker, J., Geertzen, J. and Dekker, J. (2006) Potential barriers to the use of health services among ethnic minorities: a review. *Family Practice*, 23(3): 325–48.

Wachtler, C., Brorsson, A. and Troein, M. (2006) Meeting and treating cultural difference in primary care: a qualitative interview study. *Family Practice*, 23(1): 111–15.

Waxman, M.A. and Levitt, M.A. (2000) Are diagnostic testing rates higher in non-English-speaking versus English-speaking patients in the emergence department? *Annals of Emergency Medicine*, 3(5): 456–61.

chapter fifteen

Good practice in health service provision for migrants

David Ingleby

Introduction

This chapter reviews the ways in which health services may need to be adapted to meet the needs of migrants and their descendants. Health services have the same task in relation to migrants as they have for the rest of the population, i.e. to provide them with accessible and high-quality care (preventive, curative and palliative), as well as health promotion and education. Before reviewing the different measures or "good practices" that have been proposed to this end, this chapter will briefly consider how concern about this issue has arisen. Ideas on this topic do not form a single, unified body of knowledge; different ideas have arisen in different times and places, and to assess them it is necessary to take account of the context in which they were formulated. A more detailed account of policy differences in European Union (EU) member states is given in Chapter 12 on "Migrant health policies in Europe".

Where and when has concern about adapting services arisen?

The realization that inequities exist in the field of migrant health, including the provision of health services, is fairly recent. Health was one of the issues raised by the Civil Rights Movement in the United States during the 1960s and 1970s (Dittmer 2009), when the focus was on ethnicity or "race", rather than migration. Later, concern began to be voiced in the traditional "countries of immigration" (Australia, Canada, New Zealand and the United States) about the health problems of migrants and the necessity of adapting health services to their needs. With regard to service provision, the two main issues singled out for attention were language barriers and cultural differences. This is reflected in the terminology: the government of the United States supported the development of standards for "culturally and linguistically appropriate services" (the CLAS standards, OMH 2000), while in Australia concern focused on "culturally and linguistically diverse" (CALD) groups.

In Europe, such concern arose a little later. Levels of migration to Europe during the second half of the twentieth century were lower than to the traditional countries of immigration, although some European countries have recently caught up with, and sometimes even overtaken, those countries. As might be expected, the level of interest in migrant health has largely followed the growth of migration itself, which can be roughly divided into three main phases.

The first phase of post-war economic expansion took place in northwest Europe (Austria, Belgium, Denmark, France, Germany, Luxembourg, the Netherlands, Sweden, Switzerland and the United Kingdom) from the 1950s to the 1970s and was accompanied by substantial levels of immigration. Gradually, concern began to be voiced about the health problems of migrant workers and the fact that many were not receiving adequate health care. The first European conference on migrant health was held in the Netherlands in 1983 under the auspices of the World Health Organization (WHO) and the Dutch government (see Colledge et al. 1986).

During the 1980s and 1990s, the economies of southern European countries began to expand and immigrants to these countries started to outnumber emigrants. In this phase, the response to the health needs of migrants was often quicker; Italy, Portugal and Spain made rapid efforts to improve health services for this segment of the population.

Around the turn of the twentieth century, eastern Europe, Finland, Iceland, Ireland and Norway experienced a rise in immigration, although in eastern Europe emigration – especially to other EU countries – also remained high. The economic crisis that began in 2007 brought a sudden end to the boom years and many migrants returned to their country of origin. While it is still unclear what the final effect of the economic crisis will be on migrant populations in Europe, the negative attitudes towards migrants that have been strengthened by the crisis are unlikely to make efforts to improve their health easier.

The particular health problems that have been emphasized in different countries reflect, to some extent, the characteristics of the respective migrant populations. In northwest Europe, where the first wave of post-war migrants is already swelling the ranks of the elderly, attention is paid to the care of older migrants and to chronic and non-communicable diseases, such as diabetes, cardiovascular disease and cancer. By contrast, countries where migration is a new phenomenon show more concern with issues such as contagious disease, sexual and reproductive health, and health in the workplace. Where a sizeable proportion of the migrant population consists of asylum-seekers and refugees (as in the Netherlands, Scandinavia and the United Kingdom), extra attention is paid to mental health problems caused by exposure to traumatic pre-flight experiences and stressful asylum procedures (Ingleby 2005).

Nevertheless, it would be an oversimplification to assume that a country's interest in migrant health is purely determined by the number and characteristics of the migrants it harbours. Political and ideological factors are also involved. Where pluralist or multicultural policies have been adopted (as in the Netherlands, Portugal, Spain, Sweden and the United Kingdom), the idea of accommodating the health needs of newcomers has been more readily accepted. Elsewhere (as in Austria, France and Germany), more emphasis has been placed on the need for migrants themselves to adapt. Political attitudes, of course, are constantly changing and, since 2003, an increasingly assimilationist approach has been adopted in the Netherlands (Ingleby 2006), while Germany has begun to show more openness to the idea of adapting health services to the needs of migrants (Berens et al. 2008).

Furthermore, there are regional or local differences within many countries. Regional governments may have their own health policies, and in the big cities and industrial areas – where more migrants tend to be found – more efforts are usually made to adapt health services to the needs of migrants. Initiatives do not only originate from national, regional or municipal authorities ("top-down"), but also from service providers, professional organizations, employers, non-governmental organizations (NGOs) and migrant organizations ("bottom-up").

As migrants tend to constitute only a small proportion of national populations and often do not have the right to vote, their interests tend to be poorly represented in national politics. For this reason, their cause is often taken up by international organizations and intergovernmental bodies. Since 2000, the United Nations, WHO, the International Organization for Migration (IOM), the EU and the Council of Europe have all launched new initiatives on migrant health (Peiro and Benedict 2010). Nevertheless, the impact of these initiatives at the national level remains slight, because the ability of international bodies to mandate changes is limited. An exception is the EU, which can mandate changes in all member states, but health systems and policies still fall to a large degree into the remit of national governments (see Chapter 4 on the "The right to health of migrants in Europe").

The following section will discuss the kinds of measures that have been put forward to improve the matching of health services to migrant users. It is important to bear in mind, however, that the ultimate goal of health equity for these groups cannot be achieved by improving health services alone. It is also necessary to tackle the underlying social determinants of ill health using the multisectoral approach characterized by the Council of the European Union (Council of the EU 2010) as "equity and health in all policies" (see also WHO Regional Office for Europe 2010 and Chapter 1 on "Migration and health in the European Union: an introduction").

The importance of inclusive research policies

The task of monitoring health problems and identifying risk factors is not only carried out by health service providers, but also by public health agencies, municipal or government departments, research institutes, NGOs and universities. Close contact between service providers and these bodies is important, because those providing care can play a crucial role in monitoring disparities in health and health care. Clinical research on the effects of migrant status or ethnicity is hampered when service providers are not willing to classify patients according to these variables. Service providers also need to be well-informed about problems that research has identified among particular groups.

The exclusion of minority groups from high-quality health care is closely linked to their exclusion from research. The title of an influential book on the history of psychological research in the United States, *"Even the Rat Was White"* (Guthrie 1976), could just as well apply to mainstream medical research. In the United States, extensive measures were introduced towards the end of the twentieth century mandating the inclusion of ethnic minorities in both medical and psychological research. Regrettably, Europe lags behind in this respect.

The collection of data on the health of migrants faces several serious obstacles (Ingleby 2009). One is the lack of consensus about the categories that should be used, another is the additional burden placed on staff. Yet another obstacle in some countries is the political sensitivity of ethnic coding and the concern, rooted in Europe's twentieth-century history, about possible misuse of such data. Some regard this concern as outdated, but there is no shortage of politicians in Europe whose success is due to their ability to mobilize hostility towards migrants or ethnic minorities (UN News Centre 2010). This does not make it easier for researchers to persuade health workers that there can be no harm in recording the national origins of their patients (see Chapter 6 on "Monitoring the health of migrants").

Adapting service delivery to the needs of migrants

The provision of equitable health services involves making sure that access to services and their quality do not differ between groups. Although access and quality are distinct concepts, there is a great deal of overlap in the factors influencing them. Moreover, access is influenced by quality, because lack of confidence in the quality of services will deter people from accessing them. This chapter argues that equity cannot be reached simply by giving all groups access to the same care. Indeed, giving the same care to people whose needs are different is a form of inequity (see Chapter 13 on "Differences in language, religious beliefs and culture: the need for culturally responsive health services").

Ensuring entitlement to use the health system

The notion of "equity of access" is a very complex one (Oliver and Mossialos 2004). Discrepancies come to light when particular services are not utilized to the extent that data on patterns of health problems suggest they should be, or when there is a tendency for care to be sought only when problems have reached an advanced stage (see Chapter 5 on "Migrants' access to health services"). The most fundamental element of access is entitlement to use the health system. In practice, this usually means entitlement to participate in the scheme of health care coverage that has been adopted in the country in question. People who can afford to pay the full costs themselves can almost always access health services.

Most European countries have either a tax-based or a statutory insurance-based system of coverage for health expenses, or a mixture of both. However, not everyone is entitled to join these systems, and entitlements for migrants vary from country to country. Particular barriers may exist for unemployed and undocumented migrants. There are wide differences in the willingness of countries to provide any health care at all for the latter group; ironically, some economically weaker countries, such as Italy, Portugal and Spain, offer better coverage for undocumented migrants than more wealthy ones, such as Germany, Sweden and the United Kingdom (Björngren-Cuadra and Cattacin 2010). For all people on low incomes (which includes many migrants), the out-of-pocket payments (informal as well as formal) that are routinely demanded may be difficult to meet.

The rules governing entitlement to care are not usually laid down by service providers, but by governments or insurance companies. However, service providers have to implement these rules, and they may sometimes sidestep them by giving help to people who are not really entitled to it, or, conversely, by denying help to those who are. They may do this deliberately or through ignorance or inability to understand the rules. Finally, entitlement to health care may depend on satisfying administrative criteria (such as registration of one's place of residence or proof of one's income), which are either hard to fulfil or involve complicated bureaucratic procedures. Good practice in this area entails not just having equitable policies in place, but implementing them in such a way that they achieve what they are supposed to achieve. Common shortcomings of implementation of the provision of health care to undocumented migrants (see MdM 2007; PICUM 2007; HUMA 2009) are:

- inadequate dissemination of information to both migrants and health workers about what the policies are;
- inconsistencies in the application of rules defining the range of eligible treatments and the criteria for inability to pay, so that the fear of incurring crippling debts may deter migrants from seeking treatment;
- uncertainty about the risk for the migrant of being denounced to the authorities; even if the latter risk is objectively speaking non-existent, a formidable barrier can exist if the migrant has no way of knowing for sure that this is the case.

Health promotion, health education and "health literacy"

Another determinant of access, which is largely outside the control of service providers but crucial to their good functioning, is the availability of information for patients about health and the health system. To be able to benefit from their entitlements, people need to know what these are and how to make use of them. Unfortunately, knowledge and skills of this kind (often subsumed under the concept of "health literacy") are unequally distributed throughout the population. Socially excluded and less well-educated groups, in particular, may be handicapped by lower health literacy (Kutner et al. 2006). To improve health literacy among the general population, many initiatives are undertaken by public health agencies, service providers and NGOs (including representatives of health professions and the pharmaceutical industry). However, these initiatives are generally targeted at the majority population and may not reach, or have much impact on, migrants (Simich 2009).

This is a serious shortcoming, because health inequalities among these groups often appear to be linked to inadequate knowledge about health problems and the services that can prevent or treat them. A targeted, outreaching approach to improving health literacy for migrants is urgently needed, particularly in the case of sexual and reproductive health, diet-related illnesses, cancers and mental illnesses, and healthy living in general. There are opportunities for educating newly arrived migrants about these matters in the context of integration programmes, but these opportunities are rarely taken. One possible reason is the difficulty of getting different ministries to cooperate with each other.

It is important to realize that the concept of "health literacy" contains concealed normative aspects. Often, what is regarded as ignorance would be more accurately described as a discrepancy between the health knowledge and skills that people have and those that are assumed by health workers. We will return to this theme below under the heading of "cultural barriers".

Making health services easily reachable

If people are entitled to use health services and they possess the knowledge and skills necessary for doing so, the next question is: how easily can they reach them? This concerns issues such as the geographical location of services, the availability of transport and the services' capacity to cope with demand. General practitioners may be unable to accept new patients because their list is full; they may also use their discretion to accept or reject new patients in a discriminatory way. In addition, the tendency towards concentrating specialized facilities in a small number of widely separated health centres can create problems of access for many people, not just migrants and minorities. However, many of the latter will be dependent on public transport and may live in neighbourhoods that are located far from such centres. If users cannot come to the services, an obvious answer is to bring the services to the users, e.g. by using mobile clinics as is done in Portugal (Fonseca et al. 2009).

Other issues concern waiting lists and opening hours. The capacity of service providers is not always distributed equitably. Opening hours are a crucial factor for those who may not be able to afford to take time off work to get treatment or who may not be able to get permission to do so. This seems to be one of the reasons why many migrants utilize accident and emergency services (see Chapter 14 on "Good practice in emergency care: views from practitioners"). However convenient such services may seem to migrant users, they cannot provide a substitute for the timely prevention and treatment of illness in primary care facilities.

A further problem of access stems from the increasing fragmentation of disciplines and specialties within the health system. Because different tasks tend to be carried out by different people, it may be necessary to make multiple appointments, sometimes at different locations, in order to get attention for the same problem. "One-stop" services for migrants are one way of mitigating this (e.g. the Migrant Helpline in London). A related issue is the poor integration of health and social care services in many countries. Many migrants have a need for several different kinds of help, but may be daunted by the task of negotiating two or more separate access procedures.

Finally, services that are not concerned with treatment, but with prevention, screening, health education and health promotion must also make allowance for the circumstances in which migrants live, as well as for cultural and language differences. Health promotion activities carried out by "ethnic health educators" in migrants' languages are a particularly effective form of intervention that has been practised in the Netherlands since the 1980s (Voorham 2003; Singels 2009), although the Dutch government has recently stopped subsidizing health education that is not in the Dutch language.

Addressing language barriers

One of the greatest problems undermining both the accessibility of health services for migrants and their quality is the existence of language barriers. The Institute for Healthcare Advancement (IHA 2003) estimated that US$ 73 billion were wasted annually in the United States as a result of communication problems in health care, many of which originate in language differences. Contributing to this wastage are faulty diagnoses, lack of compliance with therapies, lower patient safety and lower treatment satisfaction on both sides.

A level of language proficiency enabling a patient to get by in everyday interactions may be quite inadequate in health service encounters, which require clear communication about non-everyday matters and may be accompanied by considerable stress. Language proficiency has become a politically sensitive topic, especially in countries where migrants are accused of not making enough effort to integrate. However, to make health care inaccessible as a means of motivating migrants to learn the national language would be a bizarre approach to integration policy and unlikely to produce positive effects. Where language barriers jeopardize high-quality health care, measures should be taken to reduce them.

What means have been proposed for doing this? Where written materials are involved (such as forms, information brochures and health promotion or education materials), the obvious solution is to translate them. The use of pictures and diagrams can also facilitate understanding. Multilingual materials are often already made available by major health agencies dealing with diverse populations across Europe. Where there are only a few large language communities, this presents few problems. However, the ever-increasing diversity of migrant populations sets limits to the possibility of providing translations for everybody. Eversley et al. (2010) found that 233 different languages were spoken by London's schoolchildren. Clearly, health authorities cannot be expected to provide information in this number of languages. Fortunately, this is not necessary, since many migrant users of health services in London have a good command of English.

Concerning interactions in health care, a variety of methods have been proposed for overcoming language barriers:

- **Professional face-to-face interpretation** is the most accurate method, but it has many drawbacks. It requires organization in advance and may introduce delays with urgent procedures. Sometimes the patient may resent the presence of a third party in the consulting room, fearing that intimate details may not be kept confidential (especially when the interpreter is from their own community). Health professionals will require special training in order to be able to work effectively with interpreters. Last but not least, this method is costly.
- **Professional interpretation by telephone** can solve many of the logistical problems discussed above, as centralized services can offer interpretation at very short notice, for example, to ambulance personnel. However, interpreters find this work harder because they lack important visual cues, although technological advances make it increasingly possible to add a visual dimension. Because the interpreter does not have to be physically present, costs can be reduced considerably.
- **Informal face-to-face interpretation** is perhaps the most widely used method, and at the same time the most widely criticized (Flores 2005). Reliance on family members (in particular children) destroys the confidentiality of the encounter and may be emotionally challenging for those involved. Sometimes a member of staff in the health care setting may be called in to provide interpretation (e.g. a doctor, nurse, receptionist, cleaner or cook). However, this may not be as economical as it sounds, because they are not able to carry out their own work while they are interpreting. The main objection to any kind of informal interpreter though is that they may simply lack the necessary skills to avoid potentially dangerous misunderstandings; they are unlikely to have the specialized vocabulary or skills required to ensure that their interpretation will help rather than hinder the medical encounter.
- **Bilingual professionals** with a command of the migrant or minority patient's language present many advantages over the above-mentioned methods. However, their proficiency in the migrant's language needs to be quite high, and the range of languages catered for can only be slightly increased by this method. Here again, if one is dealing with large minority groups such as Spanish-speakers in the United States or Russian-speakers in Latvia or Estonia, this may not be a serious drawback.
- **"Cultural mediators"** are health workers who not only provide linguistic interpretation but also mediate actively between health professionals and service users. They are concerned with overcoming not only language barriers but cultural and social ones as well. The minorities concerned must be fairly large, but this method has many advantages and the role of "cultural mediators" may be varied and extensive, involving trying to help caregivers and users understand each other's point of view and offering advice on ways to solve problems. Some may even operate independently of medical professionals and function as a kind of "gatekeeper". European countries where cultural mediation seems to be a favoured approach include Belgium, France, Ireland, Italy, the Netherlands, Spain and the United Kingdom.

Both in the traditional countries of immigration and in European countries responding to the challenge of diversity, debates among health professionals over the pros and cons of these different approaches to overcoming language barriers are in full swing. An issue that is increasingly coming to the fore is how these services should be paid for. Some countries provide government subsidies for interpretation services and translation, while others require service providers to pay, many of which place the responsibility squarely on the shoulders of the patient. There are large variations between countries in the degree to which patients are accorded legal rights to interpretation and translation services. In Britain, the "race equality obligation" can be interpreted as requiring service providers to provide language assistance in order to avoid "institutional discrimination", while in the Netherlands, a law from 1995 obliges all health care providers to communicate with patients "in [a] language they can understand". In Sweden, there is also a legal requirement to provide interpreting services. However, in neither country do these legal instruments seem to be used to enforce the provision of better interpreter services, and in most European countries such legislation does not exist.

What is often overlooked, however, is the cost of not providing these services. Although litigation over medical errors in Europe seldom involves the astronomical sums seen in the United States, the human and financial cost of mistakes, misunderstandings and ineffective health care delivery may be substantial. There is still a long way to go in developing a rational, evidence-based approach to overcoming language barriers in European health systems. Many issues also need to be resolved concerning the training and licensing of interpreters. Clear leadership from national governments on all these issues is necessary if language barriers are to be tackled effectively.

Addressing cultural barriers

For decades it has been almost an axiom that matching health services to the needs of migrant users involves bridging "cultural gaps". Terms such as "cultural sensitivity" and "cultural competence" have come to be used as synonyms for good practice. Ironically, cultural anthropologists have been among the fiercest critics of the way in which "culture" has come to dominate the discourse on health, migration and ethnicity (Kleinman and Benson 2006). Partly as a result of this criticism, the concept of culture assumed by writers on health services has changed considerably over time.

Early work tended to view culture as a sort of mental baggage that migrants bring with them from their country of origin. The labels on the baggage (e.g. Nairobi, Fez, Santiago) were assumed to tell us what we could expect to find inside. Culture in this sense was an exotic attribute, the possession of which set the migrant apart from "us". Cultural sensitivity was a matter of adapting care to the presumed contents of the baggage. Starting from this assumption, textbooks were produced which informed health workers what to expect from people originating from different parts of the globe.

Gradually, however, it became clear that not all people with the same country of origin had the same ideas and attitudes regarding health. Regional, religious, generational and socioeconomic differences often led to greater variation within groups than between them. Moreover, these ideas and attitudes were neither homogenous nor static. According to Geertz (1973), this heterogeneity was an intrinsic property of culture itself. Migrants, in particular, typically live "between two cultures". Lastly, it was not only the "other" who possessed a culture, "we" had one too – many different ones, in fact. In this way, the textbook approach to understanding cultures came to be regarded as a source of stereotypes, which, far from reducing the gap between health workers and users, might actually increase it.

Coincidentally or not, the reaction against textbook approaches occurred at the same time as an increase in the number of different sender countries. The only way to avoid an uncontrollable growth in the number of chapters required in textbooks was to create absurdly broad categories like "Asian" or "African".

Towards the end of the twentieth century, new approaches came to the fore, responding to the realization that culture was not a fixed attribute (Carpenter-Song et al. 2007). The starting-point of these approaches was not knowledge about other people's cultures, but awareness of one's own. Only by first exploring one's own preconceptions and values could one learn to recognize and accept those of others. The only way to find out about patients' "cultural baggage" was to get to know them better and to discuss it with them. This approach shows a great deal of overlap with the concept of "patient-centred care" (Saha et al. 2009). However, such ideas were unwelcome to many health service managers, because instead of being able to take a ready-made care package off the shelf, the caregiver was now expected to invest time in developing personal rapport with the patient. Between the "static" and the "dynamic" views of culture a pragmatic middle way has to be found. Migrant cultures are undoubtedly more complex than the "textbook" approach suggests; nevertheless, migrants are likely to appreciate a health worker who knows and respects their traditions and shows an informed interest in their country of origin. In addition, although a huge variety of cultural and ethnic groups can be found across Europe, large migrant communities tend to gravitate to specific locations, making it possible for service providers to focus on the needs of particular groups without necessarily pigeon-holing them into rigid stereotypes.

There are other respects in which the current concept of "cultural competence" differs from the textbook approach of its predecessors. First, it involves not just knowledge, but also skills and attitudes. It cannot be learned from a book, but has to be practised and be based on a commitment to valuing and respecting diversity. Second, the concept has been broadened to encompass organizations, in addition to individual caregivers. This shift was already apparent in the use of the phrase "culturally and linguistically appropriate services" (OMH 2000) by the government of the United States. "Cultural competence" must reside in all aspects of an organization's activities and be anchored in an explicit "commitment to diversity". Systematic training and education, not only of health workers, but also of policy-makers, managers and researchers, is required to bring about these changes.

Other insights have stretched the concept of "culture" to its limits and, some would say, beyond. The Council of Europe's recommendations on health services in a multicultural society (Council of Europe 2006) adopt a broad definition of culture that recognises cultural subcategories based on shared attributes (such as gender) or shared life experiences (such as education, occupation, socio-economic status, trauma, homelessness, being without ID papers).

However, it could be argued that instead of treating traumatized or undocumented migrants as "cultural groups", it would be more logical to replace "culture" by a broader term, such as "social context". Moreover, when migrants arriving in a new country have inappropriate expectations of the health system because they assume it resembles the system in their country of origin, it is hardly appropriate to label their expectations as "culturally determined".

Some researchers (e.g. Renschler and Cattacin 2007) propose that "sensitivity to diversity" would be a more comprehensive aim for health services than "cultural competence". Moreover, this aim is not just relevant to the care of migrants, but refers to all forms of diversity. Such a shift would fit in with the tendency in some countries to subsume ethnic and cultural differences under broader policies relating to diversity that also encompass gender, age, religion, disability, sexuality and socioeconomic position (for example, the UK equality legislation into which race equality legislation has been incorporated). Such proposals are often resisted by advocates of better care for migrants, however, on the grounds that the specific concerns of migrants would easily get submerged under other issues.

Applications of "cultural competence"

What sorts of barriers is "cultural competence" required to break down? In the first place, it can facilitate interactions between people with widely differing frames of reference and aim to avoid misunderstandings and affronts, whether intentional or unintentional. In this sense, there is nothing specifically medical about it. Perhaps the most fundamental component concerns attitudes, i.e. the need to overcome deep-rooted prejudices and resistance to diversity.

A more specific application to health-care situations concerns the different beliefs and attitudes people may have concerning health. Health workers and users of health services may differ widely in their understandings of health and illness in general, as well as the nature, manifestations, causes, effects and social meanings of particular illnesses. The influential concept of "explanatory models" (Kleinman et al. 1978) was intended to draw attention to these divergences. The task of interpreters is not simply to translate words, but to get across the meanings they convey. In this sense, language barriers nearly always involve cultural barriers too. Treatment adherence is likely to be lower when the caregiver and the patient are not "on the same wavelength" regarding the nature of the problem and the best way to solve it.

Expectations concerning appropriate behaviour for doctors and patients may also vary. To what extent is the patient supposed to take responsibility for their condition? Should doctors always tell the truth about the prognosis? How many family members is it reasonable to bring on a hospital visit, and how long should they be allowed to stay?

Adapting services to users with different beliefs and expectations does not necessarily mean that services should abandon their own commitments, but it does mean showing respect for other people's standpoints instead of just dismissing them as a sign of backwardness or ignorance. For example, stigmas attached to mental illness are not necessarily irrational; they may simply reflect the fact that migrants are used to health services that provide psychiatric help only for the most extreme and acute problems. As Netto et al. (2010) argue, targeted health promotion interventions for migrants cannot be effective if they do not take account of the different ways in which people perceive and experience health problems.

So far this chapter has discussed "cultural competence" as an ingredient that has to be added to the routine activities of health workers, not in terms of new methods that may need to be developed. However, to match services to the differing needs of users and make services "diversity-proof", it may be necessary not only to change the way existing methods are applied, but also to develop new methods of diagnosis and treatment. It is perhaps in the mental health field that new methods have most often been explored. Instruments for psychiatric diagnosis such as the Diagnostic and Statistical Manual (DSM) are of unknown cross-cultural validity. In an effort to remedy this weakness, some mental health workers carry out a "cultural interview" to supplement such diagnoses (Mezzich and Caracchi 2008). Methods of treating mental illness that have been developed in a western context may not be the most effective way of helping people from different cultural backgrounds (Moodley and Stewart 2010). Even in the field of physical medicine, there is a cautious willingness among some mainstream providers to accept that traditional treatment methods may be effective for migrant patients – and even, to a certain extent, for western patients too (Institute of Medicine 2005).

Implementing change

Separate versus integrated services

A perennial issue in dealing with the special needs of particular groups is whether provisions should be separate or integrated into mainstream services (Healy et al. 2004). The dilemmas here are familiar from the history of women's health care. Separate facilities permit concentration of expertise and can reduce barriers between staff and patients. However, they may be less easy to reach and may not be able to offer a full range of services.

In the case of migrants, separate service provision has often arisen in response to the failure of mainstream providers to take account of their needs. Specialized centres have played a pioneering role in developing appropriate methods of care, but where migrants are widely dispersed in the community, the only way to ensure wide coverage is to adapt all services to diversity. The greater the diversity of the local community, the more impetus there will be to implement change in mainstream services. However, systematic changes have proved extremely hard to implement in Europe, even in the rare cases where governments have taken measures to embed them in policy.

Sustainability of changes

Characteristic of the history of this topic is the large number of initiatives that spring up (often instigated by a charismatic individual or a dynamic group), flourish for a while, then die out because of lack of structural support. Many "good practices" have been developed and become extinct in this way. For example, the Dutch government provided substantial funding between 1986 and 1991 for a project to stimulate the development of "culturally competent" mental health services, but failed to incorporate this aim into national policy, so that in 2000 the Council for Public Health and Healthcare (RVZ 2000) reported serious inadequacies in services for migrants and ethnic minorities. As Padilla et al. (2009: 107) put it, "good practices are not enough"; they must be embedded in policy.

In connection with this, the important role of NGOs deserves mention. These carry out the essential task of providing services for groups left out in the cold by mainstream providers, as well as advocating for the interests of these groups (Padilla et al. 2009). They often enjoy excellent contact with their beneficiaries and may be able to offer highly accessible services. However, their role is an ambiguous one. The long-term interest of the groups they serve would almost always be better served by improving provisions in the mainstream, which leaves NGOs in the awkward position of campaigning for their own abolition. An ideal system would be one that combined the strengths of NGOs with the resources, sustainability and accountability of the public health system.

User involvement

The need to involve users in decisions about their care has become something of a mantra in health policy discourse, but this ideal has proved extraordinarily difficult to realize with regard to health care for migrants. Getting well-educated middle-class members of the dominant cultural group to join in client councils and patient platforms is hard enough, but ensuring participation from socially excluded groups is even harder. Nevertheless, the involvement of local communities seems to be extremely important for reducing barriers between health services and their (migrant) users (García-Ramirez and Hatzidimitriadou 2009).

Conclusions

In this chapter we have examined the demands that the increasing diversity of users places on health service providers. We have considered the entitlements of migrants, issues surrounding the accessibility of services, language barriers, "cultural barriers" and the need to critically examine the appropriateness of diagnostic tools and treatment methods. We have seen that in order to match services to the differing needs of users and make services "diversity-proof", it may be necessary not only to change the way existing methods are applied, but also to develop new methods of diagnosis and treatment. Changes should be integrated in the mainstream of health services, embedded in policy and supported by communities.

In an ideal world, inequities in health and health care would come to light automatically as a result of monitoring. Researchers would then investigate the causal mechanisms underlying the inequities, and, on the basis of their findings, proposals would be made for innovations ("good practices") to put matters right. Finally, the success of these innovations would be evaluated in pilot studies, and, after the necessary adaptations, they would be implemented more widely.

In the area of migrant health, however, matters have seldom proceeded in this orderly way. Inequities are not systematically monitored and investigated, and often concern only arises because of scandals that reach the press. Nevertheless, there is a great deal more empirical evidence available about health care inequities today than there was 20 years ago.

What is still seriously lacking, however, is research into the effectiveness of the innovations that are put in place. A review by Fortier and Bishop (2003) showed that out of hundreds of interventions designed to increase "cultural competence", only a handful had been evaluated. Part of the problem is the lack of priority assigned by funding agencies to research on these questions (Ingleby 2009). To achieve the goal of equitable health services for migrants, a much larger and more systematic research effort is required than has been seen up to now.

References

Berens, E., Spallek, J. and Razum, O. (2008) *Länderbericht*. MIGHEALTHNET Project (http://mighealth.net/de/images/1/19/L%C3%A4nderbericht_MIGHEALTHNET_ Deutschland.pdf, accessed 24 May 2011).

Björngren-Cuadra, C. and Cattacin, S. (2010) *Policies on Health Care for Undocumented Migrants in the EU27: Towards a Comparative Framework. Summary Report*. Malmö: Malmö University (http://www.nowhereland.info/?i_ca_id=391, accessed 24 May 2011).

Carpenter-Song, E.A., Schwallie, M.N. and Longhofer, J. (2007) Cultural competence reexamined: critique and directions for the future. *Psychiatric Services*, 58: 1362–5 (http://psychservices.psychiatryonline.org/cgi/reprint/58/10/1362, accessed 24 May 2011).

Colledge, M., van Geuns, H.A. and Svensson, P-G. (eds) (1986) *Migration and Health: Towards an understanding of the health care needs of ethnic minorities. Proceedings of a Consultative Group on Ethnic Minorities (The Hague, Netherlands, 28–30 November 1983)*. Copenhagen: WHO Regional Office for Europe.

Council of the EU (2010) *Council Conclusions on Equity and Health in All Policies: Solidarity in Health*. Brussels: Council of the European Union (http://www.consilium. europa.eu/uedocs/cms_Data/docs/pressdata/en/lsa/114994.pdf, accessed 24 May 2011).

Council of Europe (2006) *Recommendation Rec2006(18) of the Committee of Ministers to Member States on Health Services in a Multicultural Society*. Strasbourg: Council of Europe (http://tinyurl.com/39bxw2, accessed 24 May 2011).

Dittmer, J. (2009) *The Good Doctors: The Medical Committee for Human Rights and the Struggle for Social Justice in Health Care*. New York: Bloomsbury Press.

Eversley, J., Mehmedbegović, D., Sanderson, A., et al. (2010) *Language Capital: Mapping the Languages of London's Schoolchildren*. London: Central Books.

Flores, G. (2005) The impact of medical interpreter services on the quality of health care: a systematic review. *Medical Care Research and Review*, 62(3): 255–99.

Fonseca, M.L., Silva, S., Esteves, A. and McGarrigle, J. (2009) *Portuguese State of the Art Report*. MIGHEALTHNET Project (http://mighealth.net/pt/images/0/00/Mighealthnet_SOAR_eng.pdf, accessed 24 May 2011).

Fortier, J.P. and Bishop, D. (2003) *Setting the Agenda for Research on Cultural Competence in Health Care: Final Report*. Brach, C. (ed.). Rockville, MD: U.S. Department of Health and Human Services Office of Minority Health and Agency for Healthcare Research and Quality. (http://www.ahrq.gov/research/cultural.htm, accessed 30 July 2011).

García-Ramirez, M. and Hatzidimitriadou, E. (2009) User involvement and empowerment in health care practices with ethnic minority and migrant groups: a community approach. *International Journal of Migration, Health and Social Care*, 5: 2–4 (http://pierprofessional.metapress.com/index/8j5516w45t777286.pdf, accessed 24 May 2011).

Geertz, C. (1973) *The Interpretation of Cultures*. New York: Basic Books.

Guthrie, R. (1976) *Even the Rat was White*. New York: Harper and Row.

Healy, J. and McKee, M. (eds) (2004) *Accessing Health Care. Responding to Diversity*. Oxford: Oxford University Press.

HUMA (2009) *Law and practice. Access to health care for undocumented migrants and asylum seekers in 10 EU countries*. First report of the Health for Undocumented migrants and Asylum seekers network (HUMA). Paris: Médicins du Monde (http://tinyurl.com/6azbp4u, accessed 24 May 2011).

IHA (2003) *IHA cites the ten most common errors medical professionals make when communicating with patients*. Press release. La Habra, CA: Institute for Healthcare Advancement (http://mighealth.net/eu/images/7/7f/IHA_Press_release.doc accessed 24 May 2011).

Ingleby, D. (ed.) (2005) *Forced Migration and Mental Health: Rethinking the Care of Refugees and Displaced Persons*. New York: Springer.

Ingleby, D. (2006) Getting multicultural health care off the ground: Britain and the Netherlands compared. *International Journal of Migration, Health and Social Care*, 2(3/4): 4–14.

Ingleby, D. (2009) *European Research on Migration and Health*. Background paper developed within the framework of the IOM project "Assisting Migrants and Communities (AMAC): Analysis of social determinants of health and health inequalities". Geneva: International Organization for Migration.

Institute of Medicine (2005) *Complementary and Alternative Medicine in the United States*. Washington, DC: National Academies Press.

Kleinman, A., Eisenberg, L. and Good, B. (1978) Culture, illness, and care: clinical lessons from anthropologic and cross-cultural research. *Annals of Internal Medicine*, 88(2): 251–8.

Kleinman, A. and Benson, P. (2006) Anthropology in the clinic: the problem of cultural competency and how to fix it. *PLoS Medicine*, 3(10): e294 (http://artsci.wustl.edu/~anthro/research/benson/Anthropology%20in%20the%20Clinic.pdf, accessed 9 June 2011).

Kutner, M., Greenberg, E., Jin, Y. and Paulsen, C. (2006) *The Health Literacy of America's Adults. Results from the 2003 National Assessment of Adult Literacy*. Washington, DC: US Department of Education Institute of Education Sciences, National Center for Education Statistics (http://nces.ed.gov/pubsearch/pubsinfo.asp?pubid=2006483, accessed 24 May 2011).

MdM (2007) *European Survey on Undocumented Migrants' Access to Health Care*. Paris: Médicins du Monde (http://www.mdm-international.org/IMG/pdf/rapportobservatoireenglish.pdf, accessed 6 June 2011).

Mezzich, J. and Caracchi, G. (eds) (2008) *Cultural Formulation: A Reader for Psychiatric Diagnosis*. Lanham, Maryland: Jason Aronson.

Moodley, R. and Stewart, S. (2010) Integrating traditional healing practices into counselling and psychotherapy. *Counselling Psychology Quarterly*, 23(3): 239–40.

Netto, G., Bhopal, R., Lederle, N., Khatoon, J. and Jackson, A. (2010) How can health promotion interventions be adapted for minority ethnic communities? Five principles for guiding the development of behavioural interventions. *Health Promotion International*, 25(2): 248–57.

Oliver, A. and Mossialos, E. (2004) Equity of access to health care: outlining the foundations for action. *Journal of Epidemiology & Community Health*, 58(8): 655–8.

OMH (2000) *National Standards on Culturally and Linguistically Appropriate Services (CLAS) in Health Care*. Washington, DC: The Office of Minority Health, United States Department of Health and Human Services (http://minorityhealth.hhs.gov/templates/browse.aspx?lvl=2&lvlID=15, accessed 24 May 2011).

Padilla, B., Portugal, R., Ingleby, D., de Freitas, C. and Lebas, J. (2009) Health and migration in the European Union: good practices. In: Fernandes, A. and Miguel, J.P. (eds) *Health and Migration in the European Union: Better Health for All in an Inclusive Society*. Lisbon: Instituto Nacional de Saude Doutor Ricardo Jorge: 101–15 (http://www.insa.pt/sites/INSA/Portugues/Publicacoes/Outros/Paginas/HealthMigrationEU2.aspx, accessed 24 May 2011).

Peiro, M.-J. and Benedict, R. (2010) Migrant health policy: the Portuguese and Spanish EU Presidencies. *Eurohealth*, 16(1): 1–4.

PICUM (2007) *Access to Health Care for Undocumented Migrants in Europe*. Brussels: Platform for International Cooperation on Undomented Migrants (http://picum.org/picum.org/uploads/file_/Access_to_Health_Care_for_Undocumented_Migrants.pdf, accessed 6 June 2011).

Renschler, I. and Cattacin, S. (2007) Comprehensive 'difference sensitivity' in health systems. In: Björngren-Cuadra, C. and Cattacin, S. (eds) *Migration and Health: Difference Sensitivity from an Organisational Perspective*. Malmö: IMER: 37-41 (http://hdl.handle.net/2043/4289, accessed 24 May 2011).

RVZ (2000) *Allochtone Cliënten en Geestelijke Gezondheidszorg [Migrant and Ethnic Minority Clients and Mental Health Care]*. Zoetermeer: Raad vor de Volksgezondheid en Zorg [Council for Public Health and Healthcare].

Saha, S., Beach, M.C., Cooper, L.A. (2009) Patient centeredness, cultural competence, and healthcare quality. *Journal of the National Medical Association*, 100(11): 1275–85.

Simich, L. (2009) *Health Literacy and Immigrant Populations*. Policy brief prepared at the request of the Public Health Agency of Canada, Ottawa (http://canada.metropolis.net/pdfs/health_literacy_policy_brief_jun15_e.pdf, accessed 24 May 2011).

Singels, L. (2009) Ethnic health educators/care consultants in The Netherlands. In: Fernandes, A. and Pereira Miguel, J. (eds) *Health and Migration in the European Union: Better Health for All in an Inclusive Society*. Lisbon: Instituto Nacional de Saúde Doutor Ricardo Jorge: 179–81 (http://www.insa.pt/sites/INSA/Portugues/Publicacoes/Outros/Paginas/HealthMigrationEU2.aspx, accessed 24 May 2011).

UN News Centre (2010) *Secretary-General cautions against new 'politics of polarization' in Europe*. Press release, 19 October 2010. New York: UN News Centre (http://www.un.org/apps/news/story.asp?NewsID=, 36488&Cr=Europe&Cr1=, accessed 24 May 2011).

Voorham, A.J.J. (2003) *Gezondheidsbevordering voor-en-door de doelgroep. Theoretische onderbouwing en evaluatie bij migranten en ouderen. [Health promotion for and by the target group. Theoretical foundations and evaluation with migrants and elderly people]*. Rotterdam: GGD Rotterdam.

WHO Regional Office for Europe (2010) *How Health Systems can Address Health Inequities Linked to Migration and Ethnicity*. Copenhagen: WHO Regional Office for Europe.

Section VII

Conclusions

chapter sixteen

The future of migrant health in Europe

*Bernd Rechel, Philipa Mladovsky,
Walter Devillé, Barbara Rijks,
Roumyana Petrova-Benedict and
Martin McKee*

Health systems in Europe need to provide appropriate and high-quality services for increasingly diverse populations. The urgency of this need can be illustrated by projections for future migration. The European Union (EU) will continue to need migrants in the years to come, with immigration benefitting not only host societies, but also many migrants themselves. The need for continued immigration is partly due to falling birth rates and ageing populations in many European societies, resulting in a demand for foreign-born workers. This trend affects employment patterns in many sectors, including the health sector, where immigrants are needed to fill both low-skilled jobs, such as those providing basic care for elderly people, as well as high-skilled positions, with an estimated shortage of approximately 1 million health workers in the EU by 2020 (Sermeus and Bruyneel 2010).

Addressing migrant health

Migrant health needs to move higher up the political agenda in Europe. The first reason for this is that migrants, like everyone else, have a right to the highest attainable standards of physical and mental health. This right has been enshrined in numerous international and European legal instruments, such as the International Covenant on Economic, Social and Cultural Rights and the World Health Organization (WHO) constitution (WHO 1946; United Nations 1966), both of which are binding for all EU member countries. However, no EU member state has so far acceded to the International Convention on the

Protection of the Rights of All Migrant Workers and Members of Their Families (United Nations 1990). Yet, even those rights enshrined in international conventions to which EU member states have signed up all too often remain only on paper, as the commitment to implement international conventions is often weak. Although the Charter of Fundamental Rights of the European Union sets out the right of everyone to access preventive health care and to benefit from medical treatment (EU 2000), vulnerable migrants, such as asylum-seekers and undocumented migrants, still face legal obstacles in most EU countries when accessing health care. There is therefore a clear need to strengthen the legislative basis for protecting migrants' rights at both the national and European level and also to ensure implementation.

There is, furthermore, increasing recognition of the contribution of health to social well-being and economic development (Suhrcke et al. 2005; WHO 2008). Rather than being a drain on welfare systems, migrants make substantial contributions, including economic ones, to both their host societies and, by sending money to relatives at home, to their countries of origin. Remittances typically far exceed official development assistance (Fajnzylber and López 2008; World Bank 2011). Improving the health of migrants will thus bring wider benefits to the socioeconomic development of both countries of origin and destination.

A major current concern of all European health systems is equity in health service provision and health outcomes (Commission on Social Determinants of Health 2008). By addressing the health inequities faced by many migrants, health systems can become more inclusive; this is likely to benefit other vulnerable or excluded population groups, as well as society as a whole.

Recognizing the diversity of migrants today

There are a number of challenges in making health systems more responsive to the needs of migrants. One is the great diversity that exists across and within different groups of migrants, making generalizations very difficult. Migrants do not form a homogenous population, but exhibit major variations according to religion, culture, language, ethnicity and country of origin. Furthermore, there is a correlation between migration background and lower socioeconomic status, which can make it difficult to identify which of the two factors is dominant in explaining their disadvantage, although migration is also an important independent determinant of health (Davies et al. 2009). A major conclusion that can be drawn from the contributions to this book is that interventions addressing migrant health need to be tailored according to the needs of individual migrant groups, taking account of country of origin, legal and residence status, and specific economic and sociodemographic risk factors.

Migrant health and access to health services

While generalizations need to be made cautiously, the contributions to this book suggest that migrants sometimes face health issues that differ slightly from those of non-migrant populations. In terms of non-communicable disease, migrants seem to tend to have a lower risk of cancer, but a higher risk of diabetes. Migrants also have specific vulnerabilities in terms of communicable disease: they may come from high-prevalence countries where health systems are weaker and rates of communicable disease such as tuberculosis, hepatitis and HIV/AIDS generally higher. There are also persisting differences in perinatal outcomes between migrants and non-migrants in Europe, partly related to lower utilization and quality of antenatal care for migrant women: rates of stillbirth and infant mortality tend to be higher among migrants, with refugees, asylum-seekers and undocumented migrants being particularly vulnerable. Attention to migrants' mental health, in particular for refugees and asylum-seekers who have experienced traumatic events, is also warranted. Migrants are generally also at higher risk of occupational injuries and are more likely to attend work when ill.

There is also strong evidence that migrants face problems when accessing health services, exacerbated for asylum-seekers and undocumented migrants (Nørredam et al. 2006; Watson 2009; Karl-Trummer et al. 2010; Samuilova et al. 2010). The resulting health issues and challenges reflect the formal and informal barriers migrants face in accessing health care, such as legal restrictions, language barriers, cultural barriers, and lack of familiarity with how the health system of the host country operates.

The need for better evidence

The evidence base for migrant health policies, especially in relation to access to care, is still very limited (WHO 2010). Several of the chapters noted that the availability of migrant health data in Europe leaves much to be desired. Most EU countries do not collect routine data on migrant health and those that do use different definitions as a proxy for migration status (e.g. country of birth, self-reported ethnicity, nationality), so that, in addition, data are often not comparable across countries (Ingleby 2009; Rafnsson and Bhopal 2009). Furthermore, available data often refer to health status only and do not cover broader determinants of health (Gushulak 2010).

Several measures that would improve the availability and quality of data can be identified. There is a clear need for standardizing data categories and definitions across Europe, and for including questions on migration in existing data collection processes, such as censuses, national statistics and health surveys, as well as in the collection of routine health information (Juhasz et al. 2010; WHO 2010). Apart from stepping up European-wide surveys, the development and implementation of appropriate EU guidance or legislation on the collection of data on migrant health offers an option for improving the standardization of data collection and the comparability of data. Obstacles would need to be overcome since it is quite clear that this could be politically very sensitive in some countries. It will, moreover, be important to move beyond disease-based monitoring of migrant health to also collect data on age, sex and social determinants of health, as well as on health-seeking behaviours of migrants, entitlements, provider attitudes, and how health systems perform with regard to health services for migrants (Ingleby 2009; WHO 2010).

The EC has funded several projects for improving data collection on migrant health, but there is substantial scope for developing migrant health research further, in particular by means of increased collaboration at the European level. An overall European vision of the collection of migrant health data, agreed with other major stakeholders such as the International Organization for Migration (IOM) and WHO, would help to ensure a more coherent approach to improving the monitoring of migrant health in Europe.

Building on examples of "good practice"

The contributors to this book have identified a number of obstacles to improving migrant health in Europe today. These include the politically charged nature of migration in general, the right-wing backlash against immigration, and practical resource constraints in collecting data on migrants or catering for their specific needs. They have, however, also identified areas where progress is being made, outlining a number of approaches to making health services accessible and more responsive to migrants. Measures to overcome language barriers include the use of easily accessible and free professional interpreting services and the training of health workers in using them. Another approach is to address cultural differences, such as through the development of cultural competence among health workers. Ideally, this should start in undergraduate education and be part of the in-service training of practitioners. The provision of information materials on health, treatments and the overall health system to migrants and also in migrants' own language is another promising measure to ensure that they are not unduly disadvantaged compared to the rest of the population. Health managers and service providers need to invest time and organizational resources in the provision of health care to migrants.

While many of these approaches make intuitive sense and have been found useful in practice by health workers and patients, more rigorous research on the effectiveness of interventions in the area of migrant health is urgently needed, including the costs and benefits of different policies. There is also the need to implement many of the initiatives on a more sustainable and coordinated basis; without public and government involvement, structural improvements are impossible to achieve (Ingleby 2006).

A call for national and European action on migrant health

In terms of national policies on migrant health, only ten EU member states seem to have adopted specific policies on migrant health at the national level. Furthermore, there is considerable variation in these policies as to which population groups are targeted, which health issues addressed, whether providers or patients are the focus of interventions, and whether policies are actually being implemented. In England, Ireland and the Netherlands, for example, migrant policies are integrated into broader policies on ethnic minorities, while in Austria, Germany, Italy, Portugal, Spain and Sweden the focus is on first-generation migrants. There seems to be huge potential for cross-country exchanges and learning in Europe about how to develop migrant health policies (Mladovsky 2007; World Health Assembly 2008; Mladovsky 2009). It is, moreover, important, to realize that the adoption of national or sub-national migrant health policies is not simply one-way traffic. Policy aberrations and reversals are not unusual and the example of the Netherlands illustrates that progressive migrant health policies – as well as broader policies of multiculturalism – can be undermined or even reversed by political parties reliant on anti-immigration sentiments. This also serves as a reminder of the need to address the broader context of migrants living in Europe, including the social determinants of their health. European countries differ widely in their asylum, residency and citizenship policies and models of migrant incorporation. Those countries with more repressive policy regimes not only make lives harder for migrants, but are also more likely to restrict their access to health care. However, there are also positive developments, as some countries, such as Portugal and Spain, have opted for providing universal access to health care, including for undocumented migrants.

Going beyond the national level, it is clear that European policies on migrants' health and access to health care are needed. While there have been several attempts to put migrant health on the European political agenda, particularly in the context of the Portuguese and Spanish presidencies (Peiro and Benedict 2010), most of these attempts have been declarative in nature and were not followed by changes in national policies or regulations. Worryingly, in the current context of economic crisis and budgetary constraints, there is the risk that the momentum resulting from these presidencies will be lost. The EU can play a significant role in advancing migrant health in Europe, but it needs to muster the necessary political commitment and engagement for doing so sooner rather than later.

References

Commission on Social Determinants of Health (2008) *Closing the Gap in a Generation: Health equity through action on the social determinants of health.* Final Report of the Commission on Social Determinants of Health. Geneva: World Health Organization.

Davies, A.A., Basten, A. and Frattini, C. (2009) *Migration: A Social Determinant of the Health of Migrants.* Background paper developed within the framework of the IOM project "Assisting Migrants and Communities (AMAC): Analysis of social determinants of health and health inequalities". Geneva: International Organization for Migration.

EU (2000) *Charter of Fundamental Rights of the European Union.* Brussels: European Union (2000/C 364/01).

Fajnzylber, P. and Lopez, J.H. (eds) (2008) *Remittances and Development: Lessons from Latin America.* Washington, DC: The International Bank for Reconstruction and Development/The World Bank.

Gushulak, B. (2010) Monitoring migrants' health. In: *Health of Migrants – The Way Forward.* Report of a global consultation, Madrid, Spain, 3–5 March 2010. Geneva: World Health Organization: 28–42.

Ingleby, D. (2006) Getting multicultural health care off the ground: Britain and the Netherlands compared. *International Journal of Migration, Health and Social Care*, 2(3/4): 4–14.

Ingleby, D. (2009) *European Research on Migration and Health*. Background paper developed within the framework of the IOM project "Assisting Migrants and Communities (AMAC): Analysis of social determinants of health and health inequalities". Geneva: International Organization for Migration.

Juhasz, J., Makara, P. and Taller, A. (2010) *Possibilities and limitations of comparative research on international migration and health*. Promoting Comparative Quantitative Research in the Field of Migration and Integration in Europe (PROMINSTAT). Working Paper No. 09. Brussels: European Commission.

Karl-Trummer, U., Novak-Zezula, S. and Metzler, B. (2010) Access to health care for undocumented migrants in the EU: a first landscape of NowHereland. *Eurohealth*, 16(1): 13–16.

Mladovsky, P. (2007) *Research Note: Migration and Health in the EU*. Brussels: European Commission.

Mladovsky, P. (2009) A framework for analysing migrant health policies in Europe. *Health Policy*, 93(1): 55–63.

Nørredam, M., Mygind, A. and Krasnik, A. (2006) Access to health care for asylum seekers in the European Union – a comparative study of country policies. *European Journal of Public Health*, 16(3): 286–90.

Peiro, M.-J. and Benedict, R. (2010) Migrant health policy: The Portugese and Spanish EU Presidencies. *Eurohealth*, 16(1): 1–4.

Rafnsson, S. and Bhopal, R. (2009) Large-scale epidemiological data on cardiovascular diseases and diabetes in migrant and ethnic minority groups in Europe. *European Journal of Public Health*, 19(5): 484–91.

Samuilova, M., Peiro, M.-J. and Benedict, R. (2010) Access to health care for undocumented migrants in the EU: a first landscape of NowHereland. *Eurohealth*, 16(1): 26–8.

Sermeus, W. and Bruyneel, L. (2010) *Investing in Europe's Health Workforce of Tomorrow: Scope for Innovation and Collaboration*. Summary Report of the three Policy Dialogues, Leuven, Belgium, 26–30 April 2010. Brussels: European Commission.

Suhrcke, M., McKee, M., Sauto Arce, R., Tsolova, S. and Mortensen, J. (2005) *The Contribution of Health to the Economy in the European Union*. Brussels: European Commission.

UN (1966) *International Covenant on Economic, Social and Cultural Rights*. New York: United Nations.

UN (1990) *International Convention on the Protection of the Rights of All Migrant Workers and Members of Their Families*. New York: United Nations.

Watson, R. (2009) Migrants in Europe are losing out on care they are entitled to. *BMJ*, 339: b3895.

WHO (1946) *WHO Constitution*. Geneva: World Health Organization.

WHO (2008) *The Tallinn Charter: Health Systems for Health and Wealth*. Copenhagen: WHO Regional Office for Europe Ministerial Conference on Health Systems.

WHO (2010) *Health of Migrants – The Way Forward*. Report of a global consultation, Madrid, Spain, 3–5 March 2010. Geneva: World Health Organization.

World Bank (2011) *Migration and Remittances Factbook 2011*. Washington, DC: The International Bank for Reconstruction and Development/The World Bank.

World Health Assembly (2008) *Health of Migrants, Resolution 61.17*. Geneva: World Health Organization.

Index

A&E (accident and emergency) *see*
    emergency care
abbreviations xix–xx
abortions, migrants' access 69
access to health services, migrants' 67–78
   see also right to health, migrants'
   abortions 69
   barriers 71–2
   cancer screening 69
   communication 71–2, 73–4
   conceptualizing 68–9
   decision-making, health services 67
   emergency care 70, 220–1
   equity 67–8, 72–4
   formal barriers 71
   future of migrant health in Europe 246–7
   general practitioners 69–70
   good practice, health service provision
      232–3
   hospitalization 70
   human rights treaties 72–3
   indicators 70–1
   informal barriers 71–2
   integration 67
   language/language barriers 71–2, 73–4,
      204–6, 218, 233–5
   legal restrictions 71
   measuring 68–9
   mental health 175–7
   migrants' right to health 67
   migrants vs non-migrants 69–70, 71–2

   occupational health 163
   organization of health services 73
   policies 73
   preventive services 69
   reasons for concern 67–8
   reasons for differences 71–2
   reducing inequalities 72–4
   sociocultural factors 71–2, 73–4
   specialist care 70
   utilization of health services 68–9
   vaccination 69
accident and emergency (A&E) *see*
   emergency care
acculturation stress, mental health 172–3
action, call for
   future of migrant health in Europe 248–9
   occupational health 163–4
adapting health services for migrants
   see also good practice, health service
      provision
   historical background 227–9
affective disorders/depression 173–4
AMAC *see* Assisting Migrants and
   Communities
antenatal care *see* maternal and child health
apprehended aliens, trends 32–4
areas to be addressed
   policy measures 7–8
   political response 7–8
Assisting Migrants and Communities
   (AMAC) 6–7

Asylum Procedures Directive, United Nations
High Commissioner for Refugees
(UNHCR) 39–40
asylum seekers/asylum-seeking
application numbers 28–31
apprehended aliens 32–4
Asylum Procedures Directive 39–40
decisions 31, 38–40
life events 171–2
maternal and child health 143–4
mental health 169–81
policies, EU 38–40
policies, migrant health 189–90
policy differences 38–40
psychopathology 172–7
statistics 39–40
terminology 171
third-country nationals (TCNs) 38–40
trends 28–31
United Nations High Commissioner for
Refugees (UNHCR) 39–40
attitudes to data collection, monitoring
migrants' health 82–4
attitudes to migrants/immigration, political
response 7–8

Ban Ki-Moon
integration 55
right to health, migrants' 55
barriers
see also language/language barriers;
sociocultural factors
mental health 175–7
migrant population 5–6
migrants' access to health services 71–2
benefits, health, future of migrant health in
Europe 245–6
Bratislava Declaration 6
burden of disease, non-communicable
diseases (NCDs) 113–15

call for action
future of migrant health in Europe
248–9
occupational health 163–4
cancer screening, migrants' access 69
cancers
incidence 103–5, 111–12
mortality 103–5
risks 103–5, 111–12
cardiovascular disease
incidence 105–6
mortality 105–6
variations 105–6
categories of migrants, monitoring migrants'
health 82–4
central/eastern Europe
integration 17–18
international migration 17–18, 25–8
labour flows 25–8
trends 17–18, 25–8

challenges
data collection 84–6
migrant health 3–4
change, implementing
good practice, health service provision
238–9
separate vs integrated services 238–9
sustainability of changes 239
childhood diseases 128
see also maternal and child health
circular migration, trends 17–18
citizenship
policies, EU 43–6
third-country nationals (TCNs) 43–6
Committee on Economic, Social and Cultural
Rights, migrants' right to health 57–8
Committee on the Elimination of
Discrimination against Women 58–60
Common Basic Principles
policies, EU, immigration/migrant
incorporation 46–8
third-country nationals (TCNs) 46–8
communicable diseases 121–38
see also non-communicable diseases
(NCDs)
childhood diseases 128
hepatitis, viral 123–6
HIV/AIDS 126–8, 134
measles, mumps and rubella (MMR) 128
screening 128–34
tuberculosis (TB) 122–3, 129–34
viral hepatitis 123–6
communication
see also language/language barriers
migrants' access to health services 71–2,
73–4
conferences
Health and Migration in the European
Union 6–7
Migration for Employment Convention 57
countries comparison, political response 6–8
cultural factors see sociocultural factors

data collection
attitudes to 82–4
background data 86–7
conceptual challenges 84–6
methodological challenges 84–6
migration status 82–4
monitoring migrants' health 82–6
morbidity 87
mortality 87
survey data 88–94
utilization of health services 87–8
data limitations, non-communicable diseases
(NCDs) 102–3
data scarcity 4, 81–2
see also monitoring migrants' health
trends 18–19, 22–5
data sources, non-communicable diseases
(NCDs) 102–3

decision-making on health services,
  migrants' access to health services 67
decisions, asylum-seeking 31, 38–40
defining migrant population 3–4
  monitoring migrants' health 85–6
depression/affective disorders 173–4
diabetes mellitus (DM)
  incidence 106
  mortality 106–8, 113
  prevalence 106–8
discrimination
  Committee on the Elimination of
    Discrimination against Women 58–60
  workplace 163
disease burden, non-communicable diseases
  (NCDs) 113–15
disease types
  see also communicable diseases; non-
    communicable diseases (NCDs);
    occupational health
  migrant population 4–5
diversity
  EU population 101–2
  migrant population 4–5, 101–2
  migrant population, future of migrant
    health in Europe 246
DM see diabetes mellitus

eastern Europe see central/eastern Europe
emergency care 213–26
  access, migrants' 70, 220–1
  'cultural' factors 219–20, 223–4
  gender roles 219–20
  good practice 213–26
  health systems, understanding 220
  language barriers, overcoming 218
  legislation 56–7
  medical history, access 222
  migrants' access 70, 220–1
  migrants' right to health 56–7
  post-migration status 222
  practitioners' views 213–26
  staff-patient relationships 221, 224
  stressors, migration 222
  time and organizational resources 221
  treatment expectations 220
employment
  see also occupational health
  Migration for Employment Convention
    57
entitlement, health system 230–1
equity
  access to health services, migrants' 72–4
  migrants' access to health services 67–8
European Court of Human Rights, migrants'
  right to health 60–2
evidence base, future of migrant health in
  Europe 247–8

foreign labour force stocks in Europe 155–6,
  157–8

foreign population
  see also migrant population
  destinations 20–2
  flows 22–5
  increase 24–5
  origins 20–2
  stocks 19–22
  total numbers 19–20, 21
  trends 19–25
future of migrant health in Europe 245–50
  access to health services, migrants' 246–7
  benefits, health 245–6
  call for action 248–9
  diversity of migrants 246
  evidence base 247–8
  good practice, health service provision 248

gender roles, emergency care 219–20
general practitioners, migrants' access 69–70
genetic factors, maternal and child health
  146–7
good practice, emergency care 213–26
good practice, health service provision
  227–42
  access to health services, migrants' 232–3
  adapting health services for migrants
    227–42
  change, implementing 238–9
  cultural competence 237–8
  entitlement, health system 230–1
  future of migrant health in Europe 248
  health education 231–2
  'health literacy' 231–2
  health promotion 231–2
  historical background 227–9
  integrated vs separate services 239
  language/language barriers 233–5
  research policies, inclusive 229–30
  sociocultural factors 235–8
  sustainability of changes 239
  user involvement 239

Health and Migration in the European Union
  conference 6
health benefits, future of migrant health in
  Europe 245–6
health education, good practice, health
  service provision 231–2
'health literacy', good practice, health service
  provision 231–2
health promotion, good practice, health
  service provision 231–2
health services access see access to health
  services, migrants'
healthy-immigrant hypothesis, mental
  health 172–3
'healthy migrant effect' 4
help-seeking behaviour
  mental health 175–7
  sociocultural factors 175–7
hepatitis, viral 123–6

HIV/AIDS 126–8
  screening 134
hospitalization, migrants' access 70

ILO *see* International Labour Organization
incidence
  cancers 111–12
  diabetes mellitus (DM) 106
infant mortality 140–3
injuries, occupational 159–62
integrated vs separate services, good practice, health service provision 239
integration
  Ban Ki-Moon 55
  central/eastern Europe 17–18
  migrants' access to health services 67
International Labour Organization (ILO), social justice principles 57
international legal framework, migrants' right to health 56–60
international migration
  central/eastern Europe 17–18, 25–8
  trends 17–36
Ireland
  National Intercultural Health Strategy 194
  policies, migrant health 194
irregular migration, trends 32–4

labour flows
  central/eastern Europe 25–8
  trends 25–8
language/language barriers 204–6
  emergency care 218
  good practice, health service provision 233–5
  migrants' access to health services 71–2, 73–4, 233–5
legal restrictions, migrants' access to health services 71
legislation
  Committee on Economic, Social and Cultural Rights 57–8
  Council of Europe instruments 60–2
  emergency care 56–7
  employment, Migration for Employment Convention 57
  European Court of Human Rights 60–2
  European Union law 62–3
  International Covenant on Economic, Social and Cultural Rights, Article 12: 56
  international legal framework, migrants' right to health 56–60
  Migration for Employment Convention 57
  national legal framework 63–4
  refugees' status 57
  Status of Refugees 57
life-course violence model, mental health 173, 174
life events
  asylum seekers 171–2

  mental health 171–2
  refugees 171–2
Lisbon Treaty, migrants' right to health 62–3
Long-Term Residents Directive (2003), third-country nationals (TCNs) 41–3
low birth weight, maternal and child health 144–5

maltreatment/neglect 55–6
maternal and child health 139–53
  antenatal care 147–9
  asylum-seekers 143–4
  consanguineous marriage 142–3
  factors influencing perinatal outcomes 139–40
  genetic factors 146–7
  infant mortality 140–3
  low birth weight 144–5
  perinatal mortality 140–3
  preterm birth 145–6
  quality of care 148–9
  refugees 143–4
  undocumented migrants 143–4
measles, mumps and rubella (MMR) 128
mental health 169–81
  access to health services, migrants' 175–7
  acculturation stress 172–3
  affective disorders/depression 173–4
  associated factors 173–4
  asylum seekers/asylum-seeking 169–81
  barriers 175–7
  depression/affective disorders 173–4
  healthy-immigrant hypothesis 172–3
  help-seeking behaviour 175–7
  hypotheses 172–3
  life-course violence model 173, 174
  life events 171–2
  migration-morbidity hypothesis 172–3
  post-traumatic stress disorder (PTSD) 174–5
  psychopathology 172–7
  refugees 169–81
  selection hypothesis 172–3
  social health 175
  sociocultural factors 172–3, 175–7
  violence 173, 174
migrant population
  see also foreign population
  barriers 5–6
  defining 3–4, 85–6
  disease types 4–5
  diversity 4–5, 101–2
  measuring 3–4
  undocumented migrants 5
Migration for Employment Convention 57
migration-morbidity hypothesis, mental health 172–3
MMR *see* measles, mumps and rubella
monitoring migrants' health 81–98
  see also data scarcity; statistics; trends
  attitudes to data collection 82–4
  background data 86–7

categories of migrants 82–4
conceptual challenges 84–6
data collection 82–6
defining migrant population 85–6
European research projects 94–5
methodological challenges 84–6
migration status 82–4
morbidity, data collection 87
mortality, data collection 87
research 94–5
survey data 88–94
utilization of health services 87–8
morbidity, data collection 87
mortality
   cancers 103–5
   cardiovascular disease 105–6
   data collection 87
   diabetes mellitus (DM) 106–8, 113
   infant 140–3
   perinatal 140–3
multiculturalism, political response 7

National Intercultural Health Strategy,
   Ireland 194
national legal framework, migrants' right to
   health 63–4
national models of incorporation
   policies, EU 46–8
   third-country nationals (TCNs) 46–8
national policies
   see also policies, EU, immigration/migrant
      incorporation; policies, migrant health
   differences 7
   health issues addressed 186–9, 191–3
   immigration/migrant incorporation 43–6
   migrant health 186–9
   third-country nationals (TCNs) 43–6
NCDs see non-communicable diseases
neglect/maltreatment 55–6
net migration, trends 24–5
non-communicable diseases (NCDs) 101–20
   see also communicable diseases
   burden of disease 113–15
   cancers 103–5, 111–12
   cardiovascular disease 105–6
   complex patterns 108–9, 115–17
   convergence 110–11
   countries of origin yardstick 111–13
   data limitations 102–3
   data sources 102–3
   diabetes mellitus (DM) 106–8
   patterns 108–9, 115–17
   population diversity 101–2
   risks 103–5, 110–13
   smoking 104, 108, 113

occupational health 155–68
   access to health services, migrants' 163
   call for action 163–4
   discrimination 163
   employment, migrant populations 157–8

foreign labour force stocks in Europe
   155–6, 157–8
   occupational differences, Spain 157–8
   occupational diseases 159–62
   occupational injuries; 159–62
   self-reported health 159–62
   sickness presenteeism 162–3
   Spain, occupational differences 157–8
   working conditions, migrant populations
      157–8
outline, this book's 8–11

patterns, non-communicable diseases (NCDs)
   108–9, 115–17
perinatal mortality 140–3
policies, EU, immigration/migrant
   incorporation
   see also national policies; policies, migrant
      health
   asylum-seeking 38–40
   citizenship 43–6
   Common Basic Principles 46–8
   national models of incorporation 46–8
   national policies 43–6
   policy differences 38–40
   residency, long-term 41–3
   third-country nationals (TCNs) 37–51
policies, migrant health 185–201
   analysing 185–6
   asylum seekers 189–90
   health issues addressed 186–9, 191–3
   implementing 196–7
   Ireland 194
   National Intercultural Health Strategy 194
   national policies 186–9
   population groups targeted 186–91
   prioritizing 198
   research policies, inclusive 229–30
   Spain 188, 192, 195
   targeting migrants in general 186–9
   targeting patients 193–6
   targeting providers 193–6
   undocumented migrants 191
policy differences, asylum-seeking 38–40
policy measures, areas to be addressed 7–8
political response 6–8
   areas to be addressed 7–8
   Assisting Migrants and Communities
      (AMAC) 6–7
   attitudes to migrants/immigration 7–8
   Bratislava Declaration 6
   conferences 6–7
   countries comparison 6–8
   Health and Migration in the European
      Union conference 6
   multiculturalism 7
   national policies 7
   policy measures 7–8
populations see foreign population; migrant
   population; third-country nationals
   (TCNs)

post-traumatic stress disorder (PTSD) 174–5
pregnancy *see* maternal and child health
preterm birth, maternal and child health 145–6
prevalence
    diabetes mellitus (DM) 106–8
    HIV/AIDS 126–7
    smoking 104, 108, 113
    viral hepatitis 123–6
preventive services
    abortions 69
    cancer screening 69
    migrants' access to health services 69
    vaccination 69
psychopathology
    asylum seekers 172–7
    refugees 172–7
PTSD *see* post-traumatic stress disorder

refugees
    life events 171–2
    maternal and child health 143–4
    mental health 169–81
    psychopathology 172–7
    terminology 171
refugees' status
    legislation 57
    migrants' right to health 57
religious considerations 208–9
research
    European research projects 94–5
    monitoring migrants' health 94–5
residency, long-term
    Long-Term Residents Directive (2003) 41–3
    policies, EU 41–3
    third-country nationals (TCNs) 41–3
right to health, migrants' 55–66
    see also access to health services, migrants'
    Ban Ki-Moon 55
    Committee on Economic, Social and Cultural Rights 57–8
    Committee on the Elimination of Discrimination against Women 58–60
    Council of Europe instruments 60–2
    emergency care 56–7
    employment, Migration for Employment Convention 57
    European Court of Human Rights 60–2
    European Union law 62–3
    integration 55
    International Covenant on Economic, Social and Cultural Rights, Article 12: 56
    International Labour Organization (ILO), social justice principles 57
    legal framework, international 56–60
    legal framework, national 63–4
    Lisbon Treaty 62–3
    maltreatment/neglect 55–6
    migrants' access to health services 67
    Migration for Employment Convention 57

refugees' status 57
social justice principles 57
Status of Refugees 57
risks
    cancers 103–5, 111–12
    non-communicable diseases (NCDs) 103–5, 110–13

screening
    cancer 69
    communicable diseases 128–34
    HIV/AIDS 134
    tuberculosis (TB) 129–34
second-generation migrants 4
selection hypothesis, mental health 172–3
smoking, prevalence 104, 108, 113
social health, mental health 175
social justice principles, International Labour Organization (ILO) 57
sociocultural factors
    acculturation stress, mental health 172–3
    Committee on Economic, Social and Cultural Rights 57–8
    cultural competence 237–8
    culturally responsive health services 203–12
    culture, defining 204
    emergency care, 'cultural' factors 219–20, 223–4
    gender roles, emergency care 219–20
    good practice, health service provision 235–8
    help-seeking behaviour, mental health 175–7
    International Covenant on Economic, Social and Cultural Rights, Article 12: 56
    Ireland, National Intercultural Health Strategy 194
    language barriers, overcoming 204–6, 218
    mental health 172–3, 175–7
    migrants' access to health services 71–2, 73–4
    multiculturalism, political response 7
    religious considerations 208–9
    stereotypes, overcoming 206–8
Spain
    health issues addressed 188, 192
    occupational differences 157–8
    occupational injuries 159–61
    policies, migrant health 188, 192, 195
    specialist care, migrants' access 70
staff-patient relationships, emergency care 221
statistics
    see also monitoring migrants' health; trends
    asylum seekers/asylum-seeking 39–40
Status of Refugees
    legislation 57
    migrants' right to health 57
stereotypes, overcoming 206–8

survey data, monitoring migrants' health
88–94
'*syndrome méditerranéen*', overcoming
stereotypes 207

TB *see* tuberculosis
TCNs *see* third-country nationals
terminology
asylum seekers/asylum-seeking 171
refugees 171
third-country nationals (TCNs)
asylum seekers/asylum-seeking 38–40
citizenship 43–6
Common Basic Principles 46–8
EU policies, immigration/migrant
incorporation 37–51
Long-Term Residents Directive (2003)
41–3
national models of incorporation 46–8
national policies 43–6
residency, long-term 41–3
time and organizational resources,
emergency care 221
trends 17–36
see also monitoring migrants' health;
statistics
apprehended aliens 32–4
asylum-seeking 28–31
central/eastern Europe 17–18, 25–8
circular migration 17–18
data scarcity 18–19, 22–5
Europe's international migration 17–36
foreign population 19–25
international migration 17–36

irregular migration 32–4
labour flows 25–8
net migration 24–5
population, foreign 19–25
population increase 24–5
tuberculosis (TB) 122–3
screening 129–34

undocumented migrants
maternal and child health 143–4
migrant population 5
policies, migrant health 191
United Nations High Commissioner for
Refugees (UNHCR)
Asylum Procedures Directive 39–40
asylum seekers/asylum-seeking 39–40
user involvement, good practice, health
service provision 239
utilization of health services
access to health services, migrants' 68–9
data collection 87–8
monitoring migrants' health 87–8

vaccination, migrants' access 69
violence
life-course violence model 173, 174
mental health 173, 174
viral hepatitis 123–6

women migrants
see also maternal and child health
Committee on the Elimination of
Discrimination against Women 58–60
working conditions *see* occupational health